Lecture Notes in Computer Science   8896

Commenced Publication in 1973
Founding and Former Series Editors:
Gerhard Goos, Juris Hartmanis, and Jan van Leeuwen

More information about this series at http://www.springer.com/series/7412

Oscar Camara · Tommaso Mansi
Mihaela Pop · Kawal Rhode
Maxime Sermesant · Alistair Young (Eds.)

Statistical Atlases and Computational Models of the Heart

Imaging and Modelling Challenges

5th International Workshop, STACOM 2014
Held in Conjunction with MICCAI 2014
Boston, MA, USA, September 18, 2014
Revised Selected Papers

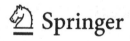 Springer

Editors

Oscar Camara
University Pompeu Fabra
Barcelona
Spain

Kawal Rhode
St. Thomas Hospital
London
United Kingdom

Tommaso Mansi
Siemens Corporate Technology
Princeton
New Jersey
USA

Maxime Sermesant
Inria
Sophia Antipolis
France

Alistair Young
University of Auckland
Auckland
New Zealand

Mihaela Pop
Sunnybrook Research Institute
Toronto
Ontario
Canada

ISSN 0302-9743
Lecture Notes in Computer Science
ISBN 978-3-319-14677-5
DOI 10.1007/978-3-319-14678-2

ISSN 1611-3349   (electronic)

ISBN 978-3-319-14678-2   (eBook)

Library of Congress Control Number: 2014959857

LNCS Sublibrary: SL 6 – Image Processing, Computer Vision, Pattern Recognition, and Graphics

Springer Cham Heidelberg New York Dordrecht London
© Springer International Publishing Switzerland 2015

Printed on acid-free paper

Springer International Publishing AG Switzerland is part of Springer Science+Business Media
(www.springer.com)

Preface

Recently, there has been considerable progress in cardiac image analysis techniques, cardiac atlases, and computational models, which can integrate data from large-scale databases of heart shape, function, and physiology. Integrative models of cardiac function are important for understanding disease, evaluating treatment, and planning intervention. However, significant clinical translation of these tools is constrained by the lack of complete and rigorous technical and clinical validation, as well as benchmarking of the developed tools. For doing so, common and available ground-truth data capturing generic knowledge on the healthy and pathological heart is required. This knowledge can be acquired through the building of statistical models of the heart. Several efforts are now established to provide web-accessible structural and functional atlases of the normal and pathological heart for clinical, research, and educational purposes. We believe all these approaches will only be effectively developed through collaboration across the full research scope of the imaging and modelling communities.

STACOM 2014 was held in conjunction with the MICCAI 2014 conference (Boston, USA), following the past four editions: STACOM 2013 (Nagoya, Japan), STACOM 2012 (Nice, France), STACOM 2011 (Toronto, Canada), and STACOM 2010 (2010, Beijing, China). STACOM 2014 provided a forum for discussion of the latest developments in the areas of statistical atlases and computational imaging and modelling of the heart. The topics of the workshop included: cardiac image processing, atlas construction, statistical modelling of cardiac function across different patient populations, cardiac mapping, cardiac computational physiology, model customization, atlas-based functional analysis, ontological schemata for data and results, integrated functional and structural analyses, as well as the pre-clinical and clinical applicability of these methods. STACOM 2014 drew submissions from around the World and 30 selected papers were invited to be published by Springer in this *Lecture Notes in Computer Science* volume. Besides regular contributions concerning the state-of-the-art cardiac image analysis techniques, computational models that integrate data from large-scale databases of heart shape, as well as function and physiology, additional efforts of this year's STACOM 2014 workshop were focused on two imaging and modelling challenges described below.

Motion Correction challenge. Dynamic contrast MR myocardial perfusion imaging has evolved into an accurate technique for diagnosis of coronary artery disease. To quantify the time-series data, motion-free data is desired. The problem is then to handle the inter-frame motion artifact caused by respiration, which makes quantitative analyses difficult. Several methods have been proposed in the last decade, which can be categorized into two groups: rigid and non-rigid registration techniques. Rigid registration is computationally more efficient, robust to noise, and provides better consistency. Non-rigid registration however provides better alignment if there is cardiac motion due to for example through-plane motion, but it is more susceptible to noise and requires more computation. It is also not clear if images with tissue from out of plane should be used, or if instead the time frame should be discarded. However, all of these methods are still limited in clinical acceptance, and this is due in part to the absence of unbiased algorithmic validation framework using a common multi-centre dataset. The STACOM 2014 *Motion Correction challenge* was designed to test the hypothesis that there is no significant differences in terms of perfusion values from MR images that have been corrected either by non-rigid or rigid methods. Data and results from this challenge have highlighted the range of methods available and objectively characterized them in terms of the resulting blood flow.

LV mechanics challenge. Understanding the mechanical behaviour of the heart is important in the evaluation of cardiac disease. In particular, patients with heart failure can present with a spectrum of symptoms from preserved to reduced ejection fraction. Currently it is difficult to determine the passive stiffness properties as well as the active tension development during systole. Recently, a number of methods were proposed for utilizing image information to reverse engineer the mechanical properties of the heart. These take the form of mathematical simulations of the cardiac cycle. However, there was no objective comparison of the characteristics of these approaches. The STACOM 2014 *LV mechanics challenge* was designed to compare the behaviour of different methods used to simulate the systolic and diastolic mechanics of the left ventricle. The data include mesh point clouds and binary masks defining the LV geometry, and muscle fibre orientations derived from ex-vivo diffusion tensor MRI. Geometries at three states in the cardiac cycle were given: unloaded (diastasis), end of inflation (end-diastole), and end of contraction (end-systole). In-vivo left ventricular pressures and volumes were also provided throughout the cardiac cycle. This challenge enables discussion of which boundary conditions and what assumptions should be made for clinical evaluation of heart stiffness and contractility.

We hope that the results obtained by these two challenges, along with all regular paper contributions, will act to accelerate progress in the important areas of heart function and structure analysis.

September 2014

Oscar Camara
Tommaso Mansi
Mihaela Pop
Kawal Rhode
Maxime Sermesant
Alistair Young

Organization

We would like to thank all organizers, additional reviewers, contributing authors, and sponsors for their time, effort, and financial support in making STACOM 2014 a successful event.

Chairs

Oscar Camara	Universitat Pompeu Fabra, Barcelona, Spain
Tommaso Mansi	Siemens Corporation, Corporate Technology, Imaging and Computer Vision, Princeton, USA
Mihaela Pop	Sunnybrook Research Institute, University of Toronto, Canada
Kawal Rhode	King's College London, UK
Maxime Sermesant	Inria, Asclepios Project, Sophia Antipolis, France
Alistair Young	University of Auckland, New Zealand

Challenges – Organizing Teams

MoCo challenge: Edward DiBella, Avan Suinesiaputra, Alistair Young

LV mechanics challenge: Vicky Wang, Martyn Nash, Alistair Young

Additional Referees and Scientific Advisors

We would like to acknowledge the following reviewers who, in addition to the chairs and challenge organizers of the workshop provided scientific feedback to the participants on their papers:

Julien Bardonnet
Constantine Butakoff
Nicholas Duchateau
Mathieu De Craene
Rocio Cabrera Lozoya
Loic le Folgoc
Marco Lorenzi
Stephanie Marchesseau

Dominik Neumann
Tiziano Passerini
Mihai Scutaru
Ingmar Voigt
Graham Wright
Robert Xu
Huanhuan Yang

Sponsor Relations

Mihaela Pop	Sunnybrook Research Institute, University of Toronto, Canada

Webmaster

Avan Suinesiputra   University of Auckland, New Zealand

OCS – Springer Conference Submission System

Mihaela Pop   Sunnybrook Research Institute, University of
                                     Toronto, Canada
Maxime Sermesant   Inria, Asclepios Project, Sophia Antipolis, France

Sponsors

We are extremely grateful for the industrial funding support. STACOM 2014 workshop received financial support from the following sponsors:

SciMedia Ltd (http://www.scimedia.com/)

VisualSonics (http://visualsonics.com)

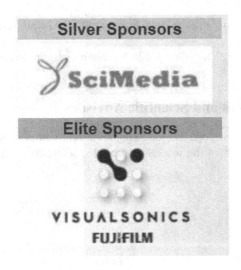

Contents

Regular Papers

MoCo (Motion Correction) Challenge

Advanced Normalization Tools for Cardiac Motion Correction

Nicholas J. Tustison$^{(\boxtimes)}$, Yang Yang, and Michael Salerno

University of Virginia, Charlottesville, VA 22903, USA
ntustison@virginia.edu

Abstract. We present our submission to the STACOM 2014 MoCo challenge for motion correction of dynamic contrast myocardial perfusion MRI. Our submission is based on the publicly available Advanced Normalization Tools (ANTs) specifically tailored for this problem domain. We provide a brief description with actual code calls to facilitate reproducibility. Time plots and K^{trans} values, based on the validation methodology of [11], are also provided to determine clinically relevant performance levels.

Keywords: ANTs · Image registration · Motion estimation · Myocardial perfusion

1 Introduction

Motion correction for dynamic contrast MR myocardial perfusion is of significant research interest and has resulted in several techniques generally characterized as rigid or non-rigid image registration-based. To bring together interested researchers for discussion and comparison of methods for correction of motion artefacts and the development of performance benchmarks of such techniques, the STACOM 2014 workshop committee organized a motion correction challenge to be held in conjunction with MICCAI 2014.

We describe the submission of our non-rigid motion correction approach below which is both publicly available and open source.[1] This facilitates reproducibility for other researchers who wish to investigate the methods proposed and perhaps formulate configurations which improve existing performance levels.

2 Materials and Methods

2.1 Evaluation Data

As described by the challenge organizers:

> *The evaluation dataset consists of 10 cases from two centres: the University of Utah and University of Auckland. For each case, a single short axis slice time series at rest and at stress is provided. The Utah datasets*

---

[1] https://github.com/stnava/ANTs

© Springer International Publishing Switzerland 2015
O. Camara et al. (Eds.): STACOM 2014, LNCS 8896, pp. 3–12, 2015.
DOI: 10.1007/978-3-319-14678-2_1

were acquired using a saturation-recovery radial turboFLASH sequence at rest and during adenosine infusion (140 ?g/kg/min), as described in [5]. Contrast was 5 cc/s injection of Multihance (Gd-BOPTA) at 0.02 mmol/kg for the rest and 0.03 mmol/kg for the stress. Four of these subjects have known coronary artery disease. The Auckland cases were acquired using a saturation-recovery Cartesian turboFLASH sequence at rest and during adenosine infusion (140 µg/kg/min). Contrast was 0.04 mmol/kg Omniscan (gadodiamide). None of the Auckland cases have overt coronary disease. Expert-drawn contours only at a reference frame, chosen when contrast is present in both ventricles, were provided to the participants.

2.2   Preprocessing and Image Registration

We used the Advanced Normalization Tools (ANTs) package as the basis of our motion correction estimation framework as it provides a suite of utilities for image preprocessing and registration which have exhibited excellent performance in a variety of applications and challenges. For example, the popular Symmetric Normalization (SyN) algorithm [1,2] performed well in a recent evaluation of popular deformable registration algorithms on human brain images [7]. Similarly, ANTs image registration and other capabilities were instrumental in recent MICCAI challenge performances including the lung-based EMPIRE10 (pulmonary CT) [9] and BRATS2013 (multimodal MRI, brain tumor) [8].

Normalization to the reference frame employs a pairwise registration strategy whereby each image is registered to its successive temporal neighbor using a recently developed SyN variation where the smoothing kernel is based on B-splines [14]. As originally formulated, the SyN transform is an explicit symmetrization of the well-known Large Deformation Diffeomorphic Metric Mapping (LDDMM) framework [4] which computes the geodesic solution between image pairs in the space of diffeomorphisms, i.e. differentiable mappings which have differentiable inverses [6]. One of the benefits of LDDMM (and SyN) is that it yields both the forward and inverse transforms between images I and J, which we denote as $I \underset{b}{\rightsquigarrow} J$ (where 'b' denotes "B-spline SyN"). Note that the image of the last time frame is registered to the image at the first time frame. Thus, to transform any image, I_t, at time point, t, to the reference image, I_R, temporally located at time, $t = r$, we simply concatenate the transforms either forwards

$$I_R \underset{b_r}{\rightsquigarrow} \underset{b_{r+1}}{\rightsquigarrow} \cdots \underset{b_{t-2}}{\rightsquigarrow} \underset{b_{t-1}}{\rightsquigarrow} I_t \qquad (1)$$

or backwards

$$I_R \underset{b_{r-1}}{\rightsquigarrow} \underset{b_{r-2}}{\rightsquigarrow} \cdots \underset{b_{t+1}}{\rightsquigarrow} \underset{b_t}{\rightsquigarrow} I_t. \qquad (2)$$

By concatenating transforms, only a single interpolation is performed for each normalization to the reference frame.

Given the temporal image variability and other confounds (e.g., noise), a multivariate image registration strategy was employed. Conventional image registration approaches are often limited to a single metric choice with a single "fixed" and "moving" image pair. In contrast, we use multiple image pairs and corresponding metrics which is made possible by recent developmental work to the Insight Toolkit [3]. These additional image pairs were created using several processing steps. Preprocessing for each image included N4 bias correction to minimize low frequency intensity variation artifacts commonly associated with MRI [15]. From each bias corrected image we created the following two images: (1) an image derived from a noise reduction filtering procedure meant to preserve structure [12] known as "SUSAN" from the FMRIB Software Library (FSL)[2] and (2) a Laplacian-based edge-detection image derived from the SUSAN image. A sample set of these images for one of the MoCo data is found in Figure 1.

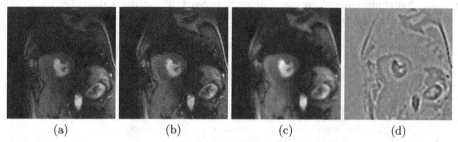

(a)   (b)   (c)   (d)

Fig. 1. Sample auxiliary images from the MoCo data set (Subject 9 (Rest): Frame 23). Shown are the (a) original, (b) N4 bias corrected, (c) SUSAN, and (d) Laplacian images

Each of these three sets of derived images are used to drive a deformable B-spline SyN pairwise registration for each temporal neighboring image pair where a weighted minimization of the three similarity metrics produced the resulting correspondence. For these data, we used equal weighting for each image pair/similarity metric which was based on a very limited heuristical assessment of the data. Investigation into relative weighting schemes might increase performance levels particularly for varying data qualities. For example, given less noisy data, decreasing the weighting of the contribution of the SUSAN-based image pairing might be helpful as noise would be less of a factor.

This process is most clearly described by the `antsRegistration` program call given in Listing 1.1.[3] Each fixed and moving image pair was histogram matched [10] and intensity-truncated to b extreme values. The choice of similarity metric for each image pair was motivated by the characteristics of each individual set

---

[2] http://fsl.fmrib.ox.ac.uk/fsl/fslwiki/

[3] In many situations, the deformable registration portion of the total alignment strategy is preceded by one or more linear registrations (e.g., center of mass alignment, affine registration). This is easily accommodated into the `antsRegistration` command line syntax. However, for this specific problem domain, it was found that such pre-deformable alignment steps were unnecessary.

and the need to balance an aggressive alignment of strong image features while minimizing displacements caused by incorrect correspondences. The N4 bias corrected images were incorporated into the motion correction strategy since they were closest to the original imaging data. Given the relative amount of noise, we used a neighborhood cross correlation (CC) metric (window radius = 6 voxels) which evaluates the linear intensity relationship between neighborhood regions at corresponding points in the image pair. This metric is the default similarity metric choice used in ANTs-based image registration [1] and helps mitigate the effects of noise. In contrast, because of the smoothing effects of SUSAN and the Laplacian filtering, we used the more aggressive Demons metric [13] which can be viewed as a second order minimization of the sum-of-squared differences (SSD) objective function.

A multi-resolution approach consisting of three levels with each successive level corresponding to double the resolution of the previous level was used with varying isotropic smoothing used at each level. For specific parameter choices, we refer the reader to Listing 1.1.

```
// Input image pairs include:
//   * N4 bias corrected
//   * Structure-preserving noise reduction (SUSAN) of N4 images
//   * Laplacian filtering of N4 images.

antsRegistration  --dimensionality 2
                  --output ${registrationPrefix} \
                  --winsorize-image-intensities [0.01,0.99] \
                  --use-histogram-matching 1 \
                  --transform BSplineSyN[0.1,2x2,0] \
                  --metric CC[${n4Fixed},${n4Moving},1,6] \
                  --metric Demons[${susanFixed},${susanMoving},1,1] \
                  --metric Demons[${laplacianFixed},${laplacianMoving},1,1] \
                  --convergence [100x70x50,1e-8,10] \
                  --shrink-factors 4x2x1 \
                  --smoothing-sigmas 1x0.5x0vox
```

Listing 1.1. `antsRegistration` call used for the pairwise registration.

Once all the pairwise transforms are generated between each set of temporal neighbors, we normalize all the original images to the reference frame by concatenating all the transforms using the program `antsApplyTransforms` which performs only a single interpolation per normalization regardless of the number of transforms specified.

3 Evaluation

As described by the challenge organizers:

> We will validate the motion correction algorithms based on flow indices. That is, the registered datasets will be processed to
> - create time curves for each of 6 tissue regions,
> - create an arterial input function (AIF) from the automatically determined blood pool curves within the endocardial border,

- *subtract off the average of the initial pre-contrast frames and normalize by estimated coil sensitivity differences so that the time curves are proportional to gadolinium concentration, and*
- *fit the data to a compartment model to obtain myocardial blood flow MBF in ml/g/min [11].*

The score will be the sum of squared differences of the Myocardial Blood Flow (MBF) index with the registration method, compared to MBF of a pseudo-gold standard obtained from manually drawn contours from experienced analysts.[4]

Implementation of the validation methodology was provided by the workshop organizers which were applied to all motion-corrected 10 gated image sets and the single ungated data set. The resulting time curves and model fits are given in Figures 2, 3, and 4 with the K^{trans} values given in Tables 1.

Table 1. K^{trans} values for all data for all 6 ROIs

	ROI_1	ROI_2	ROI_3	ROI_4	ROI_5	ROI_6
MoCo_01 (rest)	0.7646	0.793	0.6472	0.6223	1.1396	0.6169
MoCo_01 (stress)	2.991	3.3591	3.3946	3.8864	3.6427	2.9233
MoCo_02 (rest)	1.26	0.8393	0.8038	0.8026	0.621	0.9659
MoCo_02 (stress)	3.6184	4.7307	2.4689	2.1684	2.0884	4.6189
MoCo_03 (rest)	1.3238	1.0138	1.9537	1.4278	0.6698	1.2323
MoCo_03 (stress)	4.6317	4.482	2.5719	2.2236	1.2169	3.3639
MoCo_04 (rest)	2.4826	1.958	1.7667	2.0848	3.0735	2.516
MoCo_04 (stress)	6.6083	10.1963	9.2774	10.0296	10.7357	8.875
MoCo_05 (rest)	1.6678	1.4952	0.8095	0.8683	1.1663	1.318
MoCo_05 (stress)	2.4283	2.6987	2.0908	1.9775	2.3872	3.0467
MoCo_06 (rest)	0.9946	1.2878	1.1367	0.7262	0.8156	0.865
MoCo_06 (stress)	2.1543	2.6292	2.1322	2.59	1.4002	1.4648
MoCo_07 (rest)	0.6009	0.5397	0.4214	0.2904	0.8107	1.234
MoCo_07 (stress)	2.8381	2.2815	1.8141	1.7029	2.7065	2.8503
MoCo_08 (rest)	1.0315	0.8754	0.7959	0.7106	0.9726	1.0769
MoCo_08 (stress)	3.1103	2.9066	2.2222	2.369	2.4781	1.796
MoCo_09 (rest)	1.0073	0.8589	0.7194	0.8689	1.1375	1.1258
MoCo_09 (stress)	1.939	0.9883	1.0515	1.6527	1.9416	2.2943
MoCo_10 (rest)	2.734	2.3579	2.2832	2.3316	2.822	2.743
MoCo_10 (stress)	2.2161	3.8051	2.9618	2.234	5.6507	2.9052
Ungated	2.3471	3.0672	2.6664	3.7773	3.5338	2.7093

---

[4] http://www.cardiacatlas.org/web/stacom2014/moco-validation

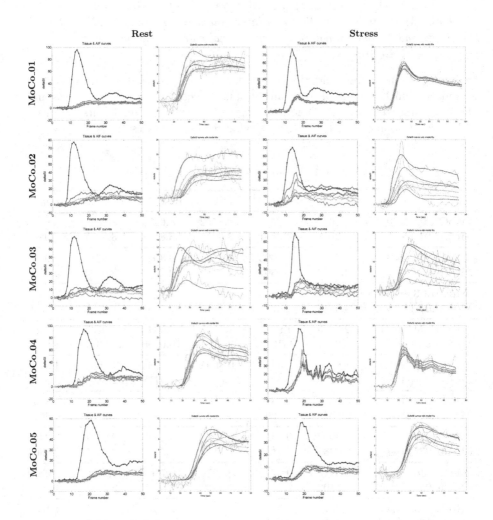

Fig. 2. Validation time curves consisting of tissue and arterial input function time plots for the first five gated data sets

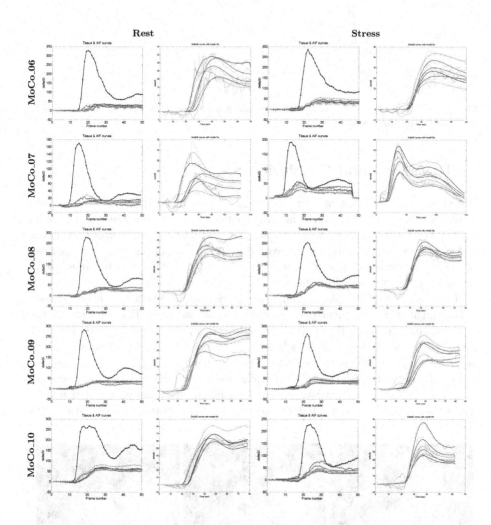

Fig. 3. Validation time curves consisting of tissue and arterial input function time plots for the gated data sets 6–10

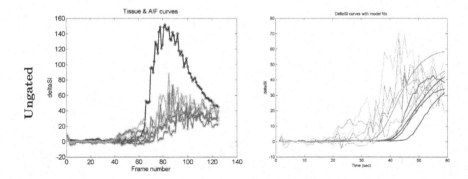

Fig. 4. Validation time curves consisting of tissue and arterial input function time plots for the ungated data set

4   Discussion and Conclusions

Based on visual assessment, our correction motion method seems to work well. However, such qualitative verification is far from ideal as the true measure of its utility is tied directly to its ability to produce useful clinical measures (hence, the motivation for the validation framework provided by the organizers). Comparison of our results with results produced by other teams will certainly prove useful in assessing the proposed methods.

Confounds such as noise, through-plane motion, and lack of contrast caused errors during the alignment optimization over all subjects. For example, in the ungated case shown in Figure 5 there is definite motion between frames $t = 77$ and $t = 78$ (wall thinning) which is not captured by our methodology. This is to be expected given the conservative approach to minimize the effects of noise. However, considering the different motion characteristics between the two types of data, the heuristically-chosen optimal parameters selected for the gated data might be suboptimal for the ungated data. Further investigation with

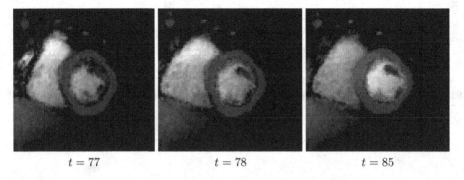

$t = 77$ $t = 78$ $t = 85$

Fig. 5. Wall thinning between $t = 77$ and $t = 78$ not captured by the proposed ANTs registration configuration. For completeness, we show the reference image ($t = 85$)

additional ungated data would be necessary for tuning a different, targeted set of parameters.

One other major potential issue with our method is the dependency on good pairwise normalizations to be able to infer correct correspondences back to the reference frame. Any error in the chain of transforms will be propagated in normalizing a particular image back to the reference frame. The general principle of incorporating prior knowledge to improve solution strategies is definitely an avenue we are pursuing for future work. One extension we are currently investigating is the use of optimal shape and intensity templates derived from the subject image data. By coalescing similar images into subgroups of optimal templates and calculating the transforms between them, optimal transformation paths between images can be found using graph-theoretic methods.

References

1. Avants, B.B., Epstein, C.L., Grossman, M., Gee, J.C.: Symmetric diffeomorphic image registration with cross-correlation: evaluating automated labeling of elderly and neurodegenerative brain. Med. Image Anal. **12**(1), 26–41 (2008)
2. Avants, B.B., Tustison, N.J., Song, G., Cook, P.A., Klein, A., Gee, J.C.: A reproducible evaluation of ANTs similarity metric performance in brain image registration. Neuroimage **54**(3), 2033–2044 (2011)
3. Avants, B.B., Tustison, N.J., Stauffer, M., Song, G., Wu, B., Gee, J.C.: The insight toolkit image registration framework. Front Neuroinform. **8**, 44 (2014)
4. Beg, M.F., Miller, M.I., Trouve, A., Younes, L.: Computing large deformation metric mappings via geodesic flows of diffeomorphisms. International Journal of Computer Vision **61**(2), 139–157 (2005)
5. DiBella, E.V.R., Fluckiger, J.U., Chen, L., Kim, T.H., Pack, N.A., Matthews, B., Adluru, G., Priester, T., Kuppahally, S., Jiji, R., McGann, C., Litwin, S.E.: The effect of obesity on regadenoson-induced myocardial hyperemia: a quantitative magnetic resonance imaging study. Int. J. Cardiovasc. Imaging **28**(6), 1435–1444 (2012)
6. Dupuis, P., Grenander, U.: Variational problems on flows of diffeomorphisms for image matching. Q. Appl. Math. **LVI**, 587–600 (1998)
7. Klein, A., Andersson, J., Ardekani, B.A., Ashburner, J., Avants, B., Chiang, M.C., Christensen, G.E., Collins, D.L., Gee, J., Hellier, P., Song, J.H., Jenkinson, M., Lepage, C., Rueckert, D., Thompson, P., Vercauteren, T., Woods, R.P., Mann, J.J., Parsey, R.V.: Evaluation of 14 nonlinear deformation algorithms applied to human brain MRI registration. Neuroimage **46**(3), 786–802 (2009)
8. Menze, B., Jakab, A., Bauer, S., Kalpathy-Cramer, J., Farahani, K., Kirby, J., Burren, Y., Porz, N., Slotboom, J., Wiest, R., Lanczi, L., Gerstner, E., Weber, M.A., Arbel, T., Avants, B., Ayache, N., Buendia, P., Collins, L., Cordier, N., Corso, J., Criminisi, A., Das, T., Delingette, H., Demiralp, C., Durst, C., Dojat, M., Doyle, S., Festa, J., Forbes, F., Geremia, E., Glocker, B., Golland, P., Guo, X., Hamamci, A., Iftekharuddin, K., Jena, R., John, N., Konukoglu, E., Lashkari, D., Antonio Mariz, J., Meier, R., Pereira, S., Precup, D., Price, S., Riklin-Raviv, T., Reza, S., Ryan, M., Schwartz, L., Shin, H.C., Shotton, J., Silva, C., Sousa, N., Subbanna, N., Szekely, G., Taylor, T., Thomas, O., Tustison, N., Unal, G., Vasseur, F., Wintermark, M., Hye Ye, D., Zhao, L., Zhao, B., Zikic, D., Prastawa, M., Reyes, M., Van Leemput, K.: The multimodal brain tumor image segmentation benchmark (BRATS) (2014). http://hal.inria.fr/hal-00935640

 9. Murphy, K., van Ginneken, B., Reinhardt, J.M., Kabus, S., Ding, K., Deng, X., Cao, K., Du, K., Christensen, G.E., Garcia, V., Vercauteren, T., Ayache, N., Commowick, O., Malandain, G., Glocker, B., Paragios, N., Navab, N., Gorbunova, V., Sporring, J., de Bruijne, M., Han, X., Heinrich, M.P., Schnabel, J.A., Jenkinson, M., Lorenz, C., Modat, M., McClelland, J.R., Ourselin, S., Muenzing, S.E.A., Viergever, M.A., De Nigris, D., Collins, D.L., Arbel, T., Peroni, M., Li, R., Sharp, G.C., Schmidt-Richberg, A., Ehrhardt, J., Werner, R., Smeets, D., Loeckx, D., Song, G., Tustison, N., Avants, B., Gee, J.C., Staring, M., Klein, S., Stoel, B.C., Urschler, M., Werlberger, M., Vandemeulebroucke, J., Rit, S., Sarrut, D., Pluim, J.P.W.: Evaluation of registration methods on thoracic CT: the EMPIRE10 challenge. IEEE Trans. Med. Imaging **30**(11), 1901–1920 (2011)
10. Nyúl, L.G., Udupa, J.K., Zhang, X.: New variants of a method of MRI scale standardization. IEEE Trans. Med. Imaging **19**(2), 143–150 (2000)
11. Pack, N.A., DiBella, E.V.R.: Comparison of myocardial perfusion estimates from dynamic contrast-enhanced magnetic resonance imaging with four quantitative analysis methods. Magn. Reson. Med. **64**(1), 125–137 (2010)
12. Smith, S.M., Brady, J.M.: SUSAN - a new approach to low level image processing. International Journal of Computer Vision **23**(1), 45–78 (1997)
13. Thirion, J.P.: Image matching as a diffusion process: an analogy with Maxwell's demons. Med. Image Anal. **2**(3), 243–260 (1998)
14. Tustison, N.J., Avants, B.B.: Explicit B-spline regularization in diffeomorphic image registration. Front Neuroinform. **7**, 39 (2013)
15. Tustison, N.J., Avants, B.B., Cook, P.A., Zheng, Y., Egan, A., Yushkevich, P.A., Gee, J.C.: N4ITK: improved N3 bias correction. IEEE Trans. Med. Imaging **29**(6), 1310–1320 (2010)

Deformable Image Registration and Intensity Correction of Cardiac Perfusion MRI

Mehran Ebrahimi$^{(\boxtimes)}$ and Sancgeetha Kulaseharan

Faculty of Science, University of Ontario Institute of Technology,
2000 Simcoe Street North, Oshawa, ON L1H 7K4, Canada
mehran.ebrahimi@uoit.ca, sancgeetha.kulaseharan@uoit.net

Abstract. Dynamic contrast Magnetic Resonance myocardial perfusion imaging has evolved into an accurate technique for the diagnosis of coronary artery disease. In this manuscript, we introduce and evaluate the performance of a non-rigid joint multi-level image registration and intensity correction algorithm on a common dataset. An objective functional is formed for which the corresponding Hessian and Jacobian is computed and employed in a multi-level Gauss-Newton minimization approach. In this paper, our experiments are based on elastic regularization on the transformation and total variation on the intensity correction. Our preliminary validations suggest that the registration scheme provides suitable motion correction if the parameters in the algorithm are properly tuned.

Keywords: Image registration · Inverse problems · Intensity correction · Optimization · Multi-level

1 Introduction

Dynamic contrast MR myocardial perfusion imaging has evolved into an accurate technique for the diagnosis of coronary artery disease. T1-weighted images are rapidly acquired every heartbeat to track the uptake and washout of a contrast agent. The diagnosis is based on time-series signal intensity data typically from rest and pharmacological stress images. Quantification of myocardial perfusion can be a useful adjunct to visual analysis, and can be valuable in other contexts. To quantify the time-series data, motion-free data is desired. However, at least 40 seconds of data are typically used to obtain regional perfusion values in the myocardium. Breath-holding becomes a major issue, particularly for patients and during pharmacological stress imaging. The problem is then to handle the inter-frame motion artefact caused by respiration, which makes quantitative analyses difficult.

In this manuscript, we present preliminary validations of a non-rigid joint motion and intensity correction algorithm that has been recently introduced in [4] and evaluate it on a common dataset. A key ingredient of the approach is the integration of intensity change compensation and motion correction into a unified

© Springer International Publishing Switzerland 2015
O. Camara et al. (Eds.): STACOM 2014, LNCS 8896, pp. 13–20, 2015.
DOI: 10.1007/978-3-319-14678-2_2

model. Rather than dividing the task into two sub-problems and treating these sub-problems sequentially and independently, the new approach assumes that these sub-problems are in fact related and mutually dependent. The algorithm is therefore based on a generalized variational framework, which integrates changes of positions and changes of intensities into a combined optimization framework. Recently in [5], a general PDE-framework for registration of contrast enhanced images was introduced. A PDE with a steady-state solution that corresponds to the solution of the described problem is derived and solved numerically. Furthermore, [14] model the intensity correction as a multiplicative term. However, this is not sufficient because loosely speaking if the intensity of a pixel is zero in one image and non-zero in another one, a multiplicative intensity correction factor cannot fix this. The scheme used in this manuscript is similar to [5], except that a more generalized regularization expression is employed. Furthermore, the more efficient Gauss-Newton approach in a multi-level implementation [13,15] is used as opposed to the steepest descent method in [5].

2   Data

The dataset consists of 10 cases from two centres: the University of Utah and University of Auckland. For each case, a single short axis slice time series at rest and at stress is provided. The Utah datasets were acquired using a saturation-recovery radial turboFLASH sequence at rest and during adenosine infusion ($140\,\mu g/kg/min$), as described in [3]. Contrast was 5 cc/s injection of Multihance (Gd-BOPTA) at $0.02\,mmol/kg$ for the rest and $0.03\,mmol/kg$ for the stress. Four of these subjects have known coronary artery disease. The Auckland cases were acquired using a saturation-recovery Cartesian turboFLASH sequence at rest and during adenosine infusion ($140\,\mu g/kg/min$). Contrast was $0.04\,mmol/kg$ Omniscan (gadodiamide). Expert-drawn contours were also provided at a chosen reference frame for each rest and stress case study.

3   Multi-level Joint Image Registration and Intensity Correction

Consider the registration problem of a template image T to a reference image R, where T is a realization of R deformed via a transformation y and the intensity of this realization is changed via an extra additive [image] term w.

The d-dimensional reference and template images are represented by mappings $R, T : \Omega \subset \mathbb{R}^d \to \mathbb{R}$ of compact support. The goal is to find the transformation $y : \mathbb{R}^d \to \mathbb{R}^d$ and a compactly supported intensity correction image $w : \Omega \subset \mathbb{R}^d \to \mathbb{R}$ such that $T[y] + w$ is similar to R, in which $T[y]$ is the transformed template image and $T[y] + w$ is the intensity-corrected deformed image. A formulation of the joint image registration and intensity correction of a template image T to a reference image R can be written as the following problem.
Problem. Given two images $R, T : \Omega \subset \mathbb{R}^d \to \mathbb{R}$, find a transformation

$y : \mathbb{R}^d \to \mathbb{R}^d$ and an intensity correction image $w : \Omega \subset \mathbb{R}^d \to \mathbb{R}$ that minimize the joint objective functional

$$\mathcal{J}[y; w] := \mathcal{D}[\mathcal{T}[y] + w, \mathcal{R}] + \alpha \mathcal{S}[y - y^{\text{ref}}] + \beta \mathcal{Q}[w].$$

Here, $\mathcal{D}$ measures the dissimilarity of $\mathcal{T}[y] + w$ and $\mathcal{R}$, and $\alpha \mathcal{S} + \beta \mathcal{Q}$ is a regularization expression on $[y; w]$. It is assumed that $y^{\text{ref}}(x) = x$. Furthermore, sum of squared distances (SSD) is used as the dissimilarity measure, the elastic regularization is applied to the transformation [12,13], and the total variation (TV) [17,18] penalty is used on the additive intensity correction image. All of this can be summarized as

$$\mathcal{D}[\mathcal{T} + w, \mathcal{R}] = \mathcal{D}^{\text{SSD}}[\mathcal{T} + w, \mathcal{R}]$$
$$= \frac{1}{2} \int_\Omega (\mathcal{T}(x) + w(x) - \mathcal{R}(x))^2 \, dx,$$

$$(1)$$

$$\mathcal{S}[y] = \frac{1}{2} \int_\Omega \mu \langle \nabla y, \nabla y \rangle + (\lambda + \mu)(\nabla \cdot y)^2 \, dx,$$

$$(2)$$

$$\mathcal{Q}[w] = TV_\epsilon[w] = \int_\Omega \sqrt{\|\nabla w(x)\|^2 + \epsilon} \, dx$$

$$\approx \int_\Omega \|\nabla w(x)\| \, dx. \qquad (3)$$

Here we employ a discretize-then-optimize paradigm using a Gauss-Newton approach (see [13,15] and the FAIR software [13] for details) to minimize the functional in Equation (1). For practical implementations of the Hessian and Jacobian of the regularizer and the TV operators see [13,18]. We also consider different discrete representations of the joint image registration/intensity correction problem, and address the discrete problems sequentially in the so-called multi-level approach. Starting with the coarsest and thus inexpensive problem, a solution is computed, which then serves as a starting guess for the next finer discretization, see [13]. This procedure has several advantages. It adds additional regularization to the registration problem (more weight is given to more important structure), it is very efficient (typically, most of the work is done on the computationally inexpensive coarse representations, and only a refinement is required on the costly finest representation), it preserves the optimization character of the problem and thus allows the use of established schemes for line searches and stopping. The use of this technique leads to optimal schemes in the sense that only a fixed number of arithmetic operations is expected for every data point.

4   Results and Validation

We performed a series of pair-wise intensity-based registration experiments using the described method taking the reference image $R(\mathbf{x})$ as the frame for which the expert-drawn contour is available. Here we present an example of these experiments for a pair of images in the stress case of 8-th dataset. The reference image in Figure 1(b) corresponds to the reference in stress case of study #8 (frame #21), and the template image Figure 1(a) is the last image in that sequence (frame #50). Using the multi-level Gauss-Newton approach, we are not only able to compute a reasonable displacement field Figure 1(d) but also an intensity correction term displayed in Figure 1(g). Due to this intensity correction term, we are now enabled to display the final registered and intensity corrected image $T(yc) + w(xc)$. In this experiment, we used the main parameters $\alpha = 50$, $\beta = 1$, $\epsilon = 1$, $\mu = 1$, and $\lambda = 0$, along with an Armijo line search [15] and a 2D linear interpolation [13]. The experimental result of our implementation is presented in Figure 1 for level 7, and the result of the previous levels 3 to 6 are displayed in Figure 2 (a) to (d). As it can be observed, the method has effectively separated the intensity changes of the two images being registered.

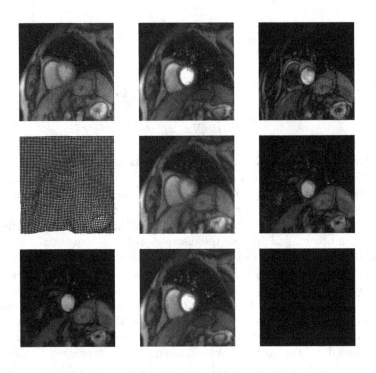

Fig. 1. Multi-level Gauss-Newton approach to joint image registration and intensity correction of stress dataset #8 for level 7:
(a) Template $T(\mathbf{x})$ (frame #50). (b) Reference $R(\mathbf{x})$ (frame #21). (c) $|T(\mathbf{x}) - R(\mathbf{x})|$.
(d) Grid $\mathbf{y}$. (e) Transformed template $T(\mathbf{y})$. (f) $|T(\mathbf{y}) - R(\mathbf{x})|$.
(g) Intensity correction $|\mathbf{w}(\mathbf{x})|$. (h) $T(\mathbf{y}) + \mathbf{w}(\mathbf{x})$. (i) $|T(\mathbf{y}) + \mathbf{w}(\mathbf{x}) - R(\mathbf{x})|$.

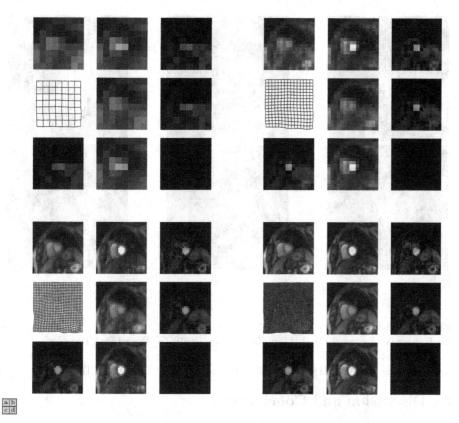

Fig. 2. Multi-level Gauss-Newton approach to joint image registration and intensity correction of stress dataset #8 for levels (a) 3. (b) 4. (c) 5. (d) 6. The order of displayed images are consistent with images displayed for the level 7 in Figure 1.

Figure 3 displays the final result for dataset #8, where the top row is relating to the rest and the bottom row is relating to to stress cases both taking frame #50 as the template and the corresponding references are frames #22 for rest and #21 for the stress case. The corresponding fixed location of contours for each case is also presented for comparison. It can be visually observed that the contours are correctly placed on the registered template images (c) and (f) compared to to their corresponding unregistered template images (b) and (e), while the motion is relatively smaller in the rest image (top row) compared to the stress image (bottom row).

Finally, Figure 4 shows results relating to dataset #8, top two rows are related to rest, and bottom 2 rows are related to stress. The graphs on the left and right respectively correspond to pre-registration and post-registration. Graphs on odd rows relate to tissue and AIF curves, and graphs on even rows represent Delta Si curves with model fits. Detailed information about obtaining these graphs is available in [16].

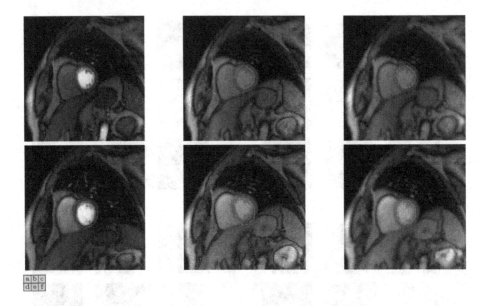

Fig. 3. Rest dataset #8:
(a) Reference (frame #22) (b) Template (frame #50) (c) Registered Template
Stress dataset #8:
(d) Reference (frame #21) (e) Template (frame #50) (f) Registered Template.

5   Discussion and Conclusion

It can be visually observed that the introduced algorithm has reasonably registered the pair of images. In addition, by comparing the tissue and AIF and
Delta Si curves in Figure 4 before (left) and after (right) registration we realize
smoother curves are obtained as a result of motion correction.

In our scheme, no prior rigid registration was performed on the acquired
datasets. Choosing the main parameters of the algorithm, i.e. α and β, can
significantly affect the result of the registration algorithm. These parameters
are required to be tuned to yield superior registration results. A larger value
of α allows less motion and attributes image intensity changes to the contrast
enhancement. Inversely, a larger value of β tends to associate any variation of
the image intensity to the motion, and allows the template image to move more
freely which may lead to physically implausible motion in its extreme. In general,
any registration algorithm requires setting a number of parameters and may fail
if the parameters are not tuned properly. Finding a right balance among the
parameters in our described algorithm proved to be challenging. Overall, the
registration of the first five cases (1-5) was found to be more challenging than
the last five cases (6-10) using our described method and we tried to further tune
the parameters for the first five cases. As expected, registration of rest cases was
found to be less challenging than the stress cases due to the fact that less motion
was present in the rest image series.

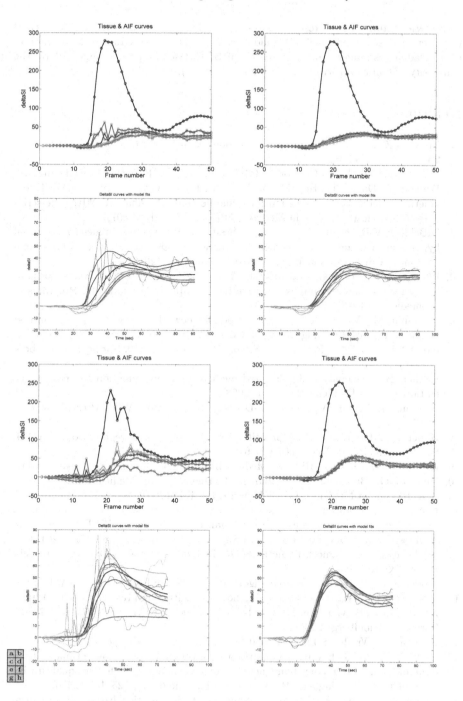

Fig. 4. Results relating to dataset #8, Top 2 rows: Rest, Bottom 2 rows: Stress, Left: Pre-registration, Right: Post-registration, Odd rows: Tissue and AIF curves, Even rows: Delta Si curves with model fits

Acknowledgments. This research was supported in part by the Natural Sciences and Engineering Research Council of Canada (NSERC) Discovery Grant of M. Ebrahimi. Undergraduate summer student research of S. Kulaseharan was supported by the University of Ontario Institute of Technology (UOIT).

References

1. Brown, L.G.: A survey of image registration techniques. ACM Computing Surveys **24**(4), 325–376 (1992)
2. Buonaccorsi, G.A., O'Connor, J.P.B., Caunce, A., Roberts, C., Cheung, S., Watson, Y., Davies, K., Hope, L., Jackson, A., Jayson, G.C., Parker, G.J.M.: Tracer kinetic model-driven registration for dynamic contrast-enhanced MRI time-series data. Magnetic Resonance in Medicine **58**(5), 1010–1019 (2007)
3. DiBella, E.V.R., et al.: The effect of obesity on regadenoson-induced myocardial hyperemia: a quantitative magnetic resonance imaging study. The International Journal of Cardiovascular Imaging **28**(6), 1435–1444 (2012)
4. Ebrahimi, M., Lausch, A., Martel, A.L.: A gauss-newton approach to joint image registration and intensity correction. Computer Methods and Programs in Biomedicine **112**(3), 398–406 (2013)
5. Ebrahimi, M., Martel, A.L.: A general pde-framework for registration of contrast enhanced images. In: Yang, G.-Z., Hawkes, D., Rueckert, D., Noble, A., Taylor, C. (eds.) MICCAI 2009, Part I. LNCS, vol. 5761, pp. 811–819. Springer, Heidelberg (2009)
6. Fischer, B., Modersitzki, J.: Ill-posed medicine - an introduction to image registration. Inverse Problems **24**, 1–19 (2008)
7. Ardeshir Goshtasby, A.: 2-D and 3-D Image Registration. Wiley Press, New York (2005)
8. Haber, E., Modersitzki, J.: A multilevel method for image registration. SIAM J. Sci. Comput. **27**(5), 1594–1607 (2006)
9. Hajnal, J., Hawkes, D., Hill, D.: Medical Image Registration. CRC Press (2001)
10. Hill, D.L.G., Batchelor, P.G., Holden, M., Hawkes, D.J.: Medical image registration. Physics in Medicine and Biology **46**, R1–R45 (2001)
11. Lausch, A., Ebrahimi, M., Martel, A.: Image registration for abdominal dynamic contrast-enhance magnetic resonance images. In: 8th IEEE International Symposium on Biomedical Imaging: From Nano to Macro, pp. 561–565 (2011)
12. Modersitzki, J.: Numerical methods for image registration. Oxford University Press, Oxford (2004)
13. Modersitzki, J.: (FAIR) Flexible Algorithms for Image Registration. SIAM (2009)
14. Modersitzki, J., Wirtz, S.: Combining homogenization and registration. In: Pluim, J.P.W., Likar, B., Gerritsen, F.A. (eds.) WBIR 2006. LNCS, vol. 4057, pp. 257–263. Springer, Heidelberg (2006)
15. Nocedal, J., Wright, S.J.: Numerical Optimization, 2nd edn. Springer (2006)
16. Pack, N., DiBella, E.V.R.: Comparison of myocardial perfusion estimates from dynamic contrast-enhanced magnetic resonance imaging with four quantitative analysis methods. Magnetic Resonance in Medicine **64**(1), 125–137 (2010)
17. Rudin, L.I., Osher, S., Fatemi, E.: Nonlinear total variation based noise removal algorithms. Physica D: Nonlinear Phenomena **60**(1–4), 259–268 (1992)
18. Vogel, C.R.: Computational Methods for Inverse Problems. SIAM (2002)

Comparison of Linear and Non-linear 2D+T Registration Methods for DE-MRI Cardiac Perfusion Studies

Gert Wollny[1]([✉]) and María-Jesus Ledesma-Carbayo[2]

[1] BIT ETSI Telecomunicación, Universidad Politécnica de Madrid, Madrid, Spain
gw.fossdev@gmail.com
[2] Ciber BBN, Zaragoza, Spain

Abstract. A series of motion compensation algorithms is run on the challenge data including methods that optimize only a linear transformation, or a non-linear transformation, or both – first a linear and then a non-linear transformation. Methods that optimize a linear transformation run an initial segmentation of the area of interest around the left myocardium by means of an *independent component analysis* (ICA) (*ICA-**). Methods that optimize non-linear transformations may run directly on the full images, or after linear registration. Non-linear motion compensation approaches applied include one method that only registers pairs of images in temporal succession (*SERIAL*), one method that registers all image to one common reference (*AllToOne*), one method that was designed to exploit quasi-periodicity in free breathing acquired image data and was adapted to also be usable to image data acquired with initial breath-hold (*QUASI-P*), a method that uses ICA to identify the motion and eliminate it (*ICA-SP*), and a method that relies on the estimation of a *pseudo ground truth* (*PG*) to guide the motion compensation.

1 Introduction

Various motion compensation methods are presented that are applied to the first-pass gadolinium-enhanced myocardial perfusion data provided in the motion compensation challenge. All these methods were implemented by using a freely available toolkit for gray scale image processing MIA [1].

The motion compensation schemes include methods that (1) use an *independent component analysis* (ICA) to segment the area of interest around the left myocardium, and to identify motion and eliminate it [2], (2) a method, *QUASI-P*, initially designed for the application to free breathing data [3], but here adapted to be applicable to data acquired with initial breath hold, (3) two generic methods, *SERIAL* and *AllToOne*, that only require that the data to comprise intra-subject tracking of movement, and (4) a method that uses *pseudo ground truth* (*PG*) to guide the motion compensation [4].

The ICA-based methods can be run with both – linear and non-linear registration, all other methods rely on non-linear registration to achieve motion

© Springer International Publishing Switzerland 2015
O. Camara et al. (Eds.): STACOM 2014, LNCS 8896, pp. 21–31, 2015.
DOI: 10.1007/978-3-319-14678-2_3

compensation. In the following the image registration back-end and methods are described in more detail.

2   Methods

2.1   Image Registration

Given a d-dimensional domain $\Omega \subset \mathbb{R}^d$ and a space of images $\mathbb{I} = \{I | I : \Omega \to \mathbb{R}\}$, and given a study image $S \in \mathbb{I}$ and a reference image $R \in \mathbb{I}$, registration aims at transforming the study image S with respect to the reference image R, so that structures at the same coordinates in both images represent the same object. In practice, given a space of allowed transformation $\mathbb{T}$ this is achieved by finding a transformation $T_{\mathrm{reg}} \in \mathbb{T}$ that minimizes a given cost function $F_{\mathrm{cost}} : \mathbb{I} \times \mathbb{I} \to \mathbb{R}$, while constraining the transformation through the joint minimization of an energy term $E : \mathbb{T} \to \mathbb{R}$:

$$T_{\mathrm{reg}} := \arg \min_{T \in \mathbb{T}} \left(F_{\mathrm{cost}}(S_T, R) + \kappa E(T) \right). \tag{1}$$

The cost function F_{cost} accounts for the mapping of similar structures. $E(T)$ ensures topology preservation, which is necessary to maintain structural integrity in the study image, and it thus introduces a smoothness constraint on the transformation T. The parameter κ is a weighting factor that balances registration accuracy and transformation smoothness.

Based on the allowed transformation space $\mathbb{T}$ one can distinguish between linear and non-linear registration. With linear registration, $\mathbb{T}$ the topology is always preserved, hence the additional energy term $E(T)$ is not required; consequently κ is set to zero in this case. In non-linear registration, this preservation of topology is not guaranteed and it is advisable to add an energy term $E(T)$ with a positive weight κ.

Cost Functions. In our application, the cost function F is derived from a so-called voxel-similarity measure that takes into account the intensities of the whole image domain. As a consequence, the driving force of the registration is calculated directly from the given image data.

Specifically, we employ three image similarity measures:

1. The *sum of squared differences* (SSD)

$$F_{\mathrm{SSD}}(S, R) := \frac{1}{2} \int_{\Omega} (S(\mathbf{x}) - R(\mathbf{x}))^2 \, d\mathbf{x}, \tag{2}$$

2. *normalized gradient fields* (NGF) as given in [3]; i.e. with the image noise level η and ϵ a measure for boundary "jumps" (locations with a high gradient) that is defined as

$$\epsilon := \eta \frac{\int_{\Omega} |\nabla I(\mathbf{x})| d\mathbf{x}}{\int_{\Omega} d\mathbf{x}}, \tag{3}$$

and the normalized gradient

$$\mathbf{n}_\epsilon(I, \mathbf{x}) := \frac{\nabla I(\mathbf{x})}{\sqrt{\sum_{i=1}^{d} (\nabla I(\mathbf{x}))_i^2 + \epsilon^2}}, \tag{4}$$

the NGF cost function for images of dimension d is defined by

$$F_{\mathrm{NGF}}(S, R) := \frac{1}{2} \int_\Omega \left(\|\mathbf{n}_\epsilon(R, x)\|^2 - \frac{\langle \mathbf{n}_\epsilon(R, x), \mathbf{n}_\epsilon(S, x) \rangle^2}{\|\mathbf{n}_\epsilon(R, x)\| \|\mathbf{n}_\epsilon(S, x)\|} \right)^2 dx, \tag{5}$$

3. *localized normalized cross correlation* (LNCC)

$$F_{\mathrm{NGF}}(S, R, W) := \frac{1}{\#\Omega} \sum_{\mathbf{x} \in \Omega} ncc(S, R, \mathbf{x}, W) \tag{6}$$

with k defining the neighborhood window $W := \{-k, k\}^2$ on which the cross correlation is evaluated according to

$$ncc(S, R, \mathbf{x}, W) := \frac{\left(\sum_{\mathbf{d} \in W} R(\mathbf{x} + \mathbf{d}) S(\mathbf{x} + \mathbf{d}) \right)^2}{\sum_{\mathbf{d} \in W} R^2(\mathbf{x} + \mathbf{d}) \sum_{\mathbf{d} \in W} S^2(\mathbf{x} + \mathbf{d})} \tag{7}$$

SSD can be used when study and reference image exhibit similar intensity distributions – e.g. when synthetic references are used for registration, and NGF and LNCC are used otherwise. Here, NGF and LNCC have an advantage over statistical measures like *mutual information*, since they are truly local similarity measure that can accommodate the local intensity change induced by the contrast agent passing through the heart ventricles and the myocardium. In addition, NGF has the advantage that it is fairly easy to implement and as a low computational cost.

Transformation Spaces. For linear registration we restrict the transformation space to either *translations* only, or to *rigid* transformations (i.e. translations and rotations), or *affine* transformations.

For non-linear registration methods the transformation space $\mathbb{T}$ is restricted to transformations that can be described by a B-splines based model [5], and the regularization E is based on the separate norms of the second derivative of each of the deformation components [6]. The balance between smoothness of the resulting transformation and the amount of non-rigidity that allows for the registration of smaller features can be fine tuned by setting the B-spline coefficient rate c_{rate} and the weighting factor κ accordingly. For both parameters, higher values result in smoother transformations that preserve the per-voxel volume better but come at the cost of a reduced ability to register small features.

2.2 Motion Compensation Schemes

Independent Component Analysis Based Schemes. Various of the applied motion compensation schemes make use of *independent component analysis* to create synthetic, motion-free references to guide the registration. Here a multi-pass approach is taken: In the first step, an ICA is run. Then the resulting components are classified based on a wavelet analysis of the mixing matrix, and the component representing motion is discarded. In addition, in the first pass the left and right ventricle cavity is identified and segmented, and the region of interest containing the left ventricle myocardium is extracted to restrict the following registration to this area. Synthetic reference images are then created by mixing the motion-free components, and the original images are registered to these references by optimizing SSD. Since initially the synthetic references are rather blurry, the method is run various times to achieve full motion compensation. The details of this method are described in [2], and a minor adjustment to identify a failed segmentation based on the size of the heart was added [7].

In its original implementation all images would be registered to a mean of the breathing motion that does normally not correspond to a specific image of the original series. Therefore, in order to accommodate the requirement of the challenge that all images need to be aligned to a predefined reference image, the algorithm was changed so that in each pass the registration of the reference image was inverted, i.e. the synthetic reference was registered to its corresponding original image, and the resulting transformation is applied to all other registered images.

This method was applied correcting for translations only (ICA-T), thereby mimicking [8], correcting a rigid transformation (ICA-R), an affine transformation (ICA-A), and a B-Spline based transformation (ICA-SP). In addition, we run combinations of these ICA-based linear and non-linear motion compensation schemes, i.e. ICA-T+SP and ICA-A+SP.

Note, that this method was originally designed to be applied to data acquired free breathing, but synthetic experiments indicated that the method can also be applied to data that was acquired with initial breath hold [2].

QUASI-P. The algorithm implements the method proposed in [3] that was initially designed to be run on free breathing aquired data. Here, the quasi-periodicity of free breathing was used to identify key frames that are already closely aligned, and registered using NGF to an automatically chosen reference frame. Then, by linearly combining these pre-aligned images synthetic references are created and the remaining images are registered to their synthetic counterparts by optimizing SSD.

Since five series the data provided for the challenge was acquired with initial breath hold, and the challenge rules require that all images are aligned to a predefined reference the algorithm was changed in two aspects: Firstly, instead of estimating the global reference image automatically, it was set, and secondly, when creating the initial subset it was made sure that the temporal distance between two consecutive images was not larger than seven acquisition frames. Without such a limitation it may happen that the algorithm does not add enough time points to the initial set, resulting in a failure of the second registration step that results from badly created synthetic references.

Generalized Non-linear Motion Compensation Schemes. We also run registration schemes that make no assumptions about the data other than that it comprises an intra-subject tracking of movement. Specifically, two approaches were run:

SERIAL: Here, only images in temporal succession are registered and then the transformations are applied accumulated. As registration criterion we used a weighted combination of NGF and SSD as proposed in [9].

AllToOne: With this method we register all images to one global reference by using LNCC as registration criterion.

In both cases, a B-spline transformation was optimized.

Pseudo Ground Truth. This method considers the estimation of a *pseudo ground truth (PG)* [4] in order to create synthetic reference images that are then used to compensation for the motion. This algorithm requires the images to be already linearly registered, otherwise the estimation of the pseudo ground truth will fail [2]. Hence we first run an ICA-based linear motion compensation scheme then followed by the *PG*. The implementation of the estimation of *PG* we used differs somewhat from the algorithm described in [4]. Specifically, instead of using a demons based registration scheme we use the same B-Spline based method for image registration as given above, and instead of using Gaussian elimination to solve the PG estimation problem, we used the L-BFGS algorithm ([10]). Like the ICA-based methods, this algorithm is also run in a multi-pass scheme.

In summary, the combined motion compensation algorithm we run here are *ICA-T+PG* and *ICA-A+PG*.

3   Experiments

Above registration schemes were applied to the provided challenge data. For the various methods the registration parameters were set as follows:

For optimization of linear transformations we used the simplex algorithm [11] (breaking condition for the simplex algorithm was set to 0.01, and its start step size to 0.001). For non-linear registrations run with the ICA-based schemes and PG we used *rank-1 method of the shifted limited-memory variable metric algorithm* (VAR1) [12] as optimizer. In all other cases a gradient descent optimizer was applied. For non-linear registrations with multi-pass schemes we used an initial B-spline knot spacing of 16 and a regularization weight κ of 10. With each new pass, these quantities were divided by 2. For all multi-pass schemes at most three registration passes were run. With *AllToOne*, *QUASI-P*, and *SERIAL*, we set the B-spline knot spacing to 5 and the regularization weight κ to 0.1.

For best reproducibility the experiments were obtained by running the motion compensation within a virtualized Ubuntu Linux 14.04 (i386) environment that can be downloaded as virtual hard disk [13], but with MIA [1] updated to version 2.2.2. The scripts used to run the experiments are made available at https://sourceforge.net/projects/mia/files/Scripts/

4   Results

Visual inspection of the results show a mixed picture. No method provides a visually pleasing motion compensation for all cases.

Specifically, in many cases QUASI-P fails to provide motion compensation at the beginning of the series and even deforms the image area containing the LV myocardium beyond recognition (Fig. 1 (a)), a problem with QUASI-P that that can be attributed to the generation of synthetic references by using linear interpolation between time steps [3]. Similar registration errors can be observed to a lesser extend by using the *AllToOne* approach (Fig. 1 (b)).

The identification of the LV and RV cavities, and consequently, the segmentation of a ROI around the LV myocardium failed for the data sets 1,3,5, and 9 aquired under stress, as well as for the un-gated data. Here, linear registration

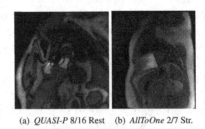

(a) *QUASI-P* 8/16 Rest   (b) *AllToOne* 2/7 Str.

Fig. 1. *QUASI-P* sometimes not only fails to achieve motion compensation, but also results in a deformation of key images of the series (a). Likewise, *AllToOne* also may result in such deformations when registering images at the beginning of the series (b), but the frequency of such occurrences is lower than with *QUASI-P*.

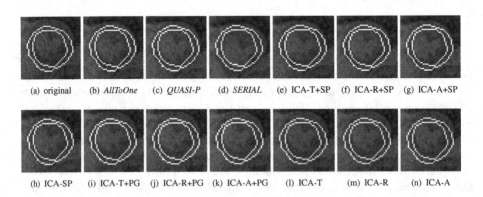

(a) original   (b) *AllToOne*   (c) *QUASI-P*   (d) *SERIAL*   (e) ICA-T+SP   (f) ICA-R+SP   (g) ICA-A+SP

(h) ICA-SP   (i) ICA-T+PG   (j) ICA-R+PG   (k) ICA-A+PG   (l) ICA-T   (m) ICA-R   (n) ICA-A

Fig. 2. Data set 5 (stress): Results for slice 50 (cropped) and all applied methods. The linear registration based methods (l-m) because the ROI around the myocardium could not be segmented for this data set. Running PG as additional non-linear registration (i-k) after a failed linear registration does also not result in an alignment as good as with all the other methods.

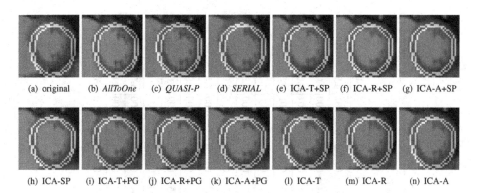

(a) original   (b) *AllToOne*   (c) *QUASI-P*   (d) *SERIAL*   (e) ICA-T+SP   (f) ICA-R+SP   (g) ICA-A+SP

(h) ICA-SP   (i) ICA-T+PG   (j) ICA-R+PG   (k) ICA-A+PG   (l) ICA-T   (m) ICA-R   (n) ICA-A

Fig. 3. Data set 8 (stress): Results for slice 45 (cropped) and all applied methods. Here, *AllToOne* (b) and *QUASI-P* (c) and all ICA*SP methods (e-h) show a good alignment for this slice, whereas the other methods that include non-linear registration (d, i-k) this alignment is not as good, but still better than without correction (a). Applying only linear registration (l-n) shows a still notable but small improvement over the uncorrected data (a) for this slice.

methods ICA-T, ICA-R, and ICA-A could not provide any notable motion compensation which is illustrated in the example images in Fig. 2 (l-m). Since the ICA-*-PG methods require initial linear registration, the also failed to provide notable motion compensation for these data sets.

As another example we present slice 45 from data set 8, stress (Fig. 3). Here the picture is a bit different: *AllToOne*, *QUASI-P* and all the combinations utilizing ICA-SP (either solely, or with initial linear registration) provide visually good results, While the other methods provide still provide a better alignment than without motion compensation, judging only from visual inspection the improvement achieved by only running linear registration is quite small.

The obtained avarage MBF values corrected for the AIF are reported below, in Table 1 for the rest studies, and in Table 2 for the stress studies. The values were obtained by running the according Matlab scripts provided by the challenge organizers and evaluating the average of the per section MBF values.

We also applied all methods to the ungated data. The segmentation of the LV region with the ICA based methods failed, and consequently no motion compensation was achieved by applying linear registration methods only. ICA-SP provided visually pleasing results, *AllToOne*, *QUASI-P*, and *SERIAL* provide a mixed picture over the time series, introducing rather erratic deformations in the images in parts of the series. Running GT (after the failed linear registration) also provided motion compensation.

Table 1. Average MBF values for the rest studies, and the ungated study

Method	1	2	3	4	5	6	7	8	9	10	Ungated
unregistered	0.53 ± 0.05	0.67 ± 0.13	1.06 ± 0.61	1.30 ± 0.14	1.18 ± 0.02	1.71 ± 0.16	0.44 ± 0.02	0.60 ± 0.00	0.54 ± 0.01	0.79 ± 0.01	4.25 ± 4.83
AllToOne	0.52 ± 0.00	0.38 ± 0.07	0.71 ± 0.20	1.44 ± 0.07	0.80 ± 0.04	1.70 ± 1.44	0.29 ± 0.01	0.53 ± 0.02	0.54 ± 0.01	0.78 ± 0.00	8.03 ± 5.68
ICA-A+PG	0.58 ± 0.00	0.70 ± 0.10	1.26 ± 0.23	1.66 ± 0.02	0.95 ± 0.10	2.79 ± 3.51	0.39 ± 0.00	0.72 ± 0.01	0.58 ± 0.00	0.84 ± 0.01	3.59 ± 2.96
ICA-A+SP	0.56 ± 0.01	0.66 ± 0.11	1.16 ± 0.14	1.58 ± 0.01	0.97 ± 0.07	2.04 ± 0.89	0.32 ± 0.00	0.57 ± 0.00	0.55 ± 0.00	0.81 ± 0.01	3.58 ± 2.64
ICA-A	0.58 ± 0.00	0.69 ± 0.10	1.21 ± 0.23	1.60 ± 0.04	1.05 ± 0.09	1.87 ± 0.42	0.37 ± 0.00	0.66 ± 0.00	0.57 ± 0.00	0.82 ± 0.00	4.35 ± 5.68
ICA-R+PG	0.61 ± 0.00	0.67 ± 0.09	1.39 ± 0.17	1.61 ± 0.04	0.98 ± 0.03	2.83 ± 3.13	0.40 ± 0.00	0.71 ± 0.01	0.55 ± 0.01	0.82 ± 0.00	3.94 ± 2.32
ICA-R+SP	0.57 ± 0.01	0.68 ± 0.10	1.14 ± 0.17	1.57 ± 0.01	0.99 ± 0.07	1.95 ± 0.59	0.32 ± 0.00	0.52 ± 0.00	0.55 ± 0.00	0.88 ± 0.15	3.66 ± 3.07
ICA-R	0.61 ± 0.00	0.65 ± 0.10	1.27 ± 0.31	1.50 ± 0.06	1.22 ± 0.02	1.96 ± 0.56	0.38 ± 0.00	0.66 ± 0.00	0.53 ± 0.01	0.82 ± 0.00	3.58 ± 5.22
ICA-T+PG	0.61 ± 0.00	0.67 ± 0.09	1.39 ± 0.17	1.61 ± 0.04	0.98 ± 0.03	2.83 ± 3.13	0.40 ± 0.00	0.71 ± 0.01	0.55 ± 0.01	0.82 ± 0.00	3.94 ± 2.32
ICA-T+SP	0.57 ± 0.00	0.67 ± 0.10	1.08 ± 0.16	1.56 ± 0.01	0.99 ± 0.09	2.01 ± 0.61	0.30 ± 0.01	0.56 ± 0.00	0.55 ± 0.00	0.85 ± 0.09	3.60 ± 2.96
ICA-T	0.62 ± 0.00	0.67 ± 0.10	1.21 ± 0.42	1.49 ± 0.07	1.18 ± 0.01	1.99 ± 0.59	0.39 ± 0.00	0.65 ± 0.00	0.53 ± 0.01	0.82 ± 0.00	3.02 ± 2.34
ICA-SP	0.52 ± 0.01	0.68 ± 0.09	1.15 ± 0.08	1.60 ± 0.01	0.98 ± 0.09	1.78 ± 0.58	0.27 ± 0.01	0.56 ± 0.00	0.54 ± 0.01	0.81 ± 0.00	3.54 ± 1.60
QUASI-P	0.51 ± 0.01	0.68 ± 0.16	1.11 ± 0.10	1.39 ± 0.06	0.92 ± 0.03	1.73 ± 0.71	0.30 ± 0.01	0.72 ± 0.02	0.67 ± 0.02	0.73 ± 0.00	3.10 ± 0.07
SERIAL	0.65 ± 0.05	0.69 ± 0.07	1.29 ± 0.57	1.74 ± 0.08	0.81 ± 0.04	1.42 ± 0.06	0.41 ± 0.01	0.60 ± 0.01	0.53 ± 0.01	0.77 ± 0.00	5.57 ± 12.59

Table 2. Average MBF values for the stress studies

Method	1	2	3	4	5	6	7	8	9	10
unregistered	2.17 ± 1.04	3.46 ± 2.31	2.87 ± 2.49	5.96 ± 1.68	2.87 ± 2.45	1.57 ± 0.25	0.90 ± 0.00	1.60 ± 0.45	0.88 ± 0.16	0.87 ± 0.06
AllToOne	2.68 ± 0.06	1.91 ± 0.29	1.72 ± 2.68	5.43 ± 0.61	2.09 ± 0.08	1.29 ± 0.04	0.68 ± 0.03	1.31 ± 0.16	0.98 ± 0.19	0.80 ± 0.05
ICA-A+PG	2.35 ± 1.20	3.92 ± 3.12	3.79 ± 5.34	4.86 ± 0.78	2.10 ± 0.34	1.35 ± 0.03	0.95 ± 0.00	1.59 ± 0.09	0.87 ± 0.10	0.89 ± 0.09
ICA-A+SP	2.30 ± 1.23	3.42 ± 2.53	3.36 ± 4.96	1.42 ± 0.38	2.23 ± 0.72	1.33 ± 0.02	0.53 ± 0.21	1.53 ± 0.06	0.94 ± 0.09	0.85 ± 0.08
ICA-A	2.29 ± 1.19	3.59 ± 2.27	2.77 ± 2.78	5.91 ± 1.98	2.85 ± 2.23	1.32 ± 0.07	0.88 ± 0.01	1.52 ± 0.08	0.86 ± 0.16	0.86 ± 0.09
ICA-R+PG	2.29 ± 1.14	4.28 ± 3.77	3.83 ± 5.48	5.03 ± 1.32	2.09 ± 0.32	1.40 ± 0.07	1.02 ± 0.00	1.63 ± 0.14	0.87 ± 0.10	0.90 ± 0.09
ICA-R+SP	2.20 ± 1.03	3.32 ± 2.16	3.18 ± 4.91	3.91 ± 2.44	2.25 ± 0.54	1.32 ± 0.02	0.90 ± 0.00	1.50 ± 0.07	0.95 ± 0.10	0.85 ± 0.07
ICA-R	2.20 ± 1.18	3.52 ± 2.36	3.01 ± 2.83	5.84 ± 1.04	2.85 ± 2.28	1.35 ± 0.04	0.91 ± 0.00	1.57 ± 0.17	0.89 ± 0.16	0.86 ± 0.10
ICA-T+PG	2.29 ± 1.14	4.28 ± 3.77	3.83 ± 5.48	5.03 ± 1.32	2.09 ± 0.32	1.40 ± 0.07	1.02 ± 0.00	1.63 ± 0.14	0.87 ± 0.10	0.90 ± 0.09
ICA-T+SP	2.17 ± 0.97	3.42 ± 2.41	3.26 ± 4.66	3.51 ± 0.72	2.20 ± 0.59	1.33 ± 0.03	0.85 ± 0.00	1.50 ± 0.06	0.95 ± 0.09	0.85 ± 0.08
ICA-T	2.23 ± 1.16	3.24 ± 2.52	3.06 ± 2.69	5.89 ± 1.06	2.85 ± 2.30	1.38 ± 0.04	0.92 ± 0.00	1.57 ± 0.19	0.89 ± 0.16	0.85 ± 0.10
ICA-SP	2.16 ± 0.69	4.02 ± 4.68	3.29 ± 4.78	5.28 ± 1.22	2.19 ± 0.74	1.27 ± 0.07	0.87 ± 0.01	1.40 ± 0.22	0.94 ± 0.11	0.88 ± 0.16
QUASI-P	1.80 ± 0.54	3.79 ± 3.62	3.28 ± 6.03	2.76 ± 0.63	2.20 ± 0.11	1.07 ± 0.03	0.96 ± 0.00	1.37 ± 0.02	0.93 ± 0.08	0.80 ± 0.04
SERIAL	2.76 ± 0.44	3.77 ± 3.33	3.26 ± 3.09	4.87 ± 0.76	1.98 ± 0.17	1.26 ± 0.05	0.99 ± 0.03	1.55 ± 0.07	0.66 ± 0.17	0.84 ± 0.08

5   Conclusion

We applied a series of 13 motion compensation methods based on image registration to the challenge data, out of these two (*AllToOne* and *SERIAL*) a generalized registration methods, and QUASI-P and all ICA based methods were specifically designed for free breathing data. The ICA based methods provide a method to identify and segment the heart ventricular cavities, and therefore they provide the possibility to restrict the registration to this area making the application of linear registration methods possible. If this segmentation failed, however, linear registration could no provide motion compensation, since the non-moving body parts in the image dominate. The linear methods were also combined with a ICA based and a PG based non-linear registration method. Both provided additional motion compensation but in the cases when linear registration failed the ICA based method usually provided visually better motion compensation than the PG method.

The main advantage of non-linear registration is that registrations is independent of an initial segmentation of the ROI. Also with ungated data, the additional deformation of the beating heart can only be captured by non-linear registration. Linear registration, on the other hand, is faster and is not not prone to registration errors like can be seen in fig. 1.

References

1. Wollny, G., Hublin, J., Ledesma-Carbayo, M.J., Skinner, M., Kellman, P., Hierl, T.: MIA - A Free and Open Source Software for Gray Scale Medical Image Analysis. Source Code for Biology and Medicine **8:20** (2013)
2. Wollny, G., Kellman, P., Santos, A., Ledesma-Carbayo, M.J.: Automatic Motion Compensation of Free Breathing acquired Myocardial Perfusion Data by Using Independent Component Analysis. Medical Image Analysis **16**(5), 1015–1028 (2012)
3. Wollny, G., Ledesma-Carbayo, M.J., Kellman, P., Santos, A.: Exploiting Quasiperiodicity in Motion Correction of Free-Breathing Myocardial Perfusion MRI. IEEE Trans. Med. Imag. **29**(8), 1516–1527 (2010)
4. Li, C., Sun, Y.: Nonrigid registration of myocardial perfusion MRI using pseudo ground truth. In: Yang, G.-Z., Hawkes, D., Rueckert, D., Noble, A., Taylor, C. (eds.) MICCAI 2009, Part I. LNCS, vol. 5761, pp. 165–172. Springer, Heidelberg (2009)
5. Kybic, J., Unser, M.: Fast Parametric Elastic Image Registration. IEEE Trans. Image Process. **12**(11), 1427–1442 (2003)
6. Rohlfing, T., Maurer Jr., C.R., Bluemke, D.A., Jacobs, M.A.: Volume-Preserving Nonrigid Registration of MR Breast Images Using Free-form Deformation with an Incompressibility Constraint. IEEE Trans. Med. Imag. **22**, 730–741 (2003)
7. Wollny, G., Kellman, P.: Free breathing myocardial perfusion data sets for performance analysis of motion compensation algorithms. GigaScience **3:23** (2014)
8. Gupta, V., Hendriks, E., Milles, J., Van Der Geest, R., Jerosch-Herold, M., Reiber, J., Lelieveldt, B.: Fully Automatic Registration and Segmentation of First-pass Myocardial Perfusion MR Image Sequences. Academic Radiology **17**(11), 1375–1385 (2010)

9. Wollny, G., Ledesma-Carbayo, M.J., Kellman, P., Santos, A.: A new similarity measure for non-rigid breathing motion compensation of myocardial perfusion MRI. In: Proc. of the 30th Int. Conf. of the IEEE-EMBS, Vancouver, BC, Canada, pp. 3389–3392 (2008)
10. Fletcher, R.: Practical Methods of Optimization, 2nd edn. Wiley (2000)
11. Nelder, J., Mead, R.: A Simplex Method for Function Minimization. Computer Journal **7**, 308–313 (1965)
12. Vlcek, J., Luksan, L.: Shifted limited-memory variable metric methods for large-scale unconstrained minimization. J. Computational Appl. Math. **186**, 365–390 (2006)
13. Wollny, G., Kellman, P.: Supporting material for: Free breathing myocardial perfusion data sets for performance analysis of motion compensation algorithms. Giga-Science, Database (2014). http://dx.doi.org/10.5524/100106

Motion Correction for Dynamic Contrast-Enhanced CMR Perfusion Images Using a Consecutive Finite Element Model Warping

Nils Noorman[1,2], James Small[1], Avan Suinesiaputra[1(✉)],
Brett Cowan[1], and Alistair A. Young[1]

[1] Department of Anatomy with Radiology, University of Auckland,
Auckland, New Zealand
a.suinesiaputra@auckland.ac.nz
[2] Biomedical NMR, Department of Biomedical Engineering,
Eindhoven University of Technology, Eindhoven, The Netherlands

Abstract. We present results of a non-rigid registration algorithm to correct breathing motion in cardiac MR perfusion sequences applied to the STACOM 2014 Motion Correction Challenge dataset. The algorithm is based on the finite element method whereby a 2D free form deformation model is deformed to match image features. Image warping is performed through global-to-local mapping of motion parameters. To overcome the contrast intensity problem in the perfusion images, the registration was applied consecutively between adjacent frames. Eleven cases were provided by the challenge: Ten cases were ECG-gated MR perfusion images with rest and adenosine-induced stress series, while the last case was an ungated MR perfusion stress acquisition. The algorithm achieved good results in terms of modified Hausdorff distance: 1.31 ± 0.93 pixels (max: 6.5 pixel), horizontal shifting < 4.5 pixels, and vertical shifting: < 4 pixels. Moderate Jaccard index: 0.57 ± 0.14 was achieved.

1 Introduction

Cardiac Magnetic Resonance (CMR) perfusion imaging has developed rapidly over the past few years, and has evolved into an accurate diagnostic tool for coronary artery disease with excellent prognostic value [2]. The protocol usually involves an administration of contrast agent followed by rapid acquisitions when the contrast uptake occurs in the myocardium. Typically, several short axis slices are acquired every heartbeat to analyse the contrast intensity profile.

The main problem for post-processing analysis of MR perfusion study is the imaging artefacts caused by breathing motion. During the contrast kinetics, data are acquired over at least 40 seconds after bolus administration. A patient must therefore perform a breath-hold for at least 40 seconds, which is problematic for elderly and patients with chronic heart disease, particularly under stress conditions. The result is a large shifting of the heart relative to the image plane,

O. Camara et al. (Eds.): STACOM 2014, LNCS 8896, pp. 32–40, 2015.
DOI: 10.1007/978-3-319-14678-2_4

which substantially affects the calculated perfusion value. A number of image processing techniques has been proposed to correct this motion artifact. An extensive survey of different motion correction algorithms is presented in [4].

We have previously developed a method to register two cardiac MR images [6], which can track motion in a cine-MRI study [5]. Our method uses free form deformations using a finite element (FE) model formulation where a 2D rectangular lattice is deformed following the movement of wall motion. This method has previously demonstrated good tracking results of endocardial and epicardial borders to quantify cardiac function. In this work, we applied this method to compensate motion caused by breathing in a MR perfusion sequence. The difficulty of tracking breathing motion in the perfusion MRI is that contrast strongly changes the intensity during the uptake and washout of the contrast agent. As such, tracking image features by the FE model becomes unreliable, particularly in the early pre-contrast uptake and late washed-out contrast frames. We modified the algorithm not to track directly breathing motion from a pre-defined reference frame, but consecutively creating reference images from adjacent frames. We also added an initial rigid registration algorithm, which coarsely tracks the location of the myocardium, resulting in a more effective registration by the non-rigid transformation.

2 Methodology

2.1 Initial Rigid Registration

A coarse rigid registration is performed to remove the most severe breathing artefacts. The original reference image is cropped using the reference mask. The Canny edge detection algorithm is applied to two consecutive images, followed by a Gaussian blurring of the resulting images [1]. Since the edge between myocardium and the lungs are strong edges, the threshold for the Canny edge detection is empirically chosen for this edge and is maintained at all frames. The sum of squared differences (SSD) is applied for similarity measurement to align images based on the location of the myocardium. Although SSD was performed by searching though all pixels inside region of interest (brute force method) with integer shifting, this process does not consume much of the processing time.

2.2 Finite Element Warping

We use a finite element (FE) model of a 2D rectangular lattice constructed using bi-cubic Bezier basis functions with $\mathcal{C}(1)$ continuity to register an image at frame t (I_t) to a reference image I_0. This is similar to the commonly used B-spline free form deformation model, except with additional flexibility to change the basis functions and continuity constraints if desired. The FE model is defined by the deformation field $u : I_0 \rightarrow I_t$. After that, image warping is performed in the current image space by using the following equation

$$I_0^t(p) = I_t\left(\delta(p)\right), \text{ for } p \in I_0 \tag{1}$$

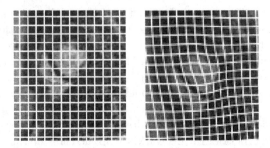

Fig. 1. An example of undeformed (left) and deformed (right) finite element model due to motion breathing

where p is a pixel and the current position δ is defined as

$$\delta(p) = p + u(p) \tag{2}$$

Within each element u is defined to be a function of finite element material coordinates ξ as

$$u(\xi) = \sum_n \Psi_n(\xi) \, U_n^e \tag{3}$$

where U_n^e are local element parameters and Ψ are element basis functions. There is a constant linear mapping between p and ξ for each element. The mapping from local element to global parameters is given by a general linear map G:

$$U^e = G \, U^g \tag{4}$$

This local-to-global map enables a flexible mechanism for incorporating a variety of continuity constraints. Figure 1 shows an illustration of warping an FE model between the reference and non-reference images from perfusion MRI.

3   Regularization

A non-rigid registration can be performed by minimizing the sum of squared pixel intensity differences

$$E_I = \sum_{p \in I_0} w^2(p) \left(I_0(p) - I_0^t(p) \right)^2 \tag{5}$$

where I_0^t denotes the registered image I_t onto I_0 as defined in (1). The coefficient w defines an image to locally control weighting in the image. The weight image is defined as an inverted and blurred version of the reference mask, which increases discrepancy errors far from the heart.

In practice, the image data and FE model are not sufficient to solve the problem, as it is ill-posed in the sense of Hadamard. We applied a Sobolev regularization to estimate the smoothing term:

$$E_S = \int_\Omega \alpha_1 \left\| \frac{\partial u}{\partial \xi_1} \right\|^2 + \alpha_2 \left\| \frac{\partial u}{\partial \xi_2} \right\|^2 + \beta_1 \left\| \frac{\partial^2 u}{\partial \xi_1^2} \right\|^2 + \beta_2 \left\| \frac{\partial^2 u}{\partial \xi_2^2} \right\|^2 + \beta_3 \left\| \frac{\partial^2 u}{\partial \xi_1 \partial \xi_2} \right\|^2 d\Omega$$

(6)

where $\alpha_1, \alpha_2, \beta_1, \beta_2, \beta_3$ are the smoothing weights. The smoothing terms E_S hence controls the rigidness of the allowed deformations. Using the Hessian filters and the smoothing terms, the objective function $E = E_I + E_s$ is optimized using the Levenberg-Marquardt algorithm [7].

3.1 Consecutive Frame Registration

The large variations in contrast between the blood pool and myocardium make registrations to a single reference frame prone to result in erroneous registrations. Instead registering into a pre-defined reference frame, we register an image to the previously registered image at the adjacent frame. Hence, if I_i is the reference frame, then image I_{i+1} and I_{i-1} are registered to I_i as I_i^{i+1} and I_i^{i-1}. Next, image I_{i+2} is registered to I_i^{i+1}, frame I_{i-2} is registered to frame I_i^{i-1}, until all frames are processed.

3.2 Validation Methods

Although manual drawing is a tedious and large task, we performed manual contouring on all unregistered frames in order to evaluate the quality of the registration method. We then applied the same transformations applied to the perfusion images to these manual mask contour images and were compared with the reference contour. The quality of the registered contours was quantified in terms of three quantities: 1) modified Hausdorff distance (MHD), 2) Jaccard index, and 3) horizontal and vertical movements. The MHD [3] measures a distance of two point sets C_1 and C_2 by the average of the minimum Euclidean distances between each point in C_1 and all points in C_2 or the reverse, whichever is greater,

$$H(C_1, C_2) = \max\left(d(C_1, C_2), d(C_2, C_1)\right)$$ (7)

$$d(X, Y) = \frac{1}{|X|} \sum_{x \in X} \min_{y \in Y} \|x - y\|$$ (8)

where $|\cdot|$ denotes the cardinality of a set.

The Jaccard index measures the amount of overlap of two point sets C_1 and C_2, i.e.,

$$J(C_1, C_2) = \frac{|C_1 \cap C_2|}{|C_1 \cup C_2|}$$ (9)

The third quantity is the measurement of contour shifting in horizontal and vertical directions. This is essentially a rigid body transformation with only a translation matrix to align two contour sets. By using least squares minimization, the translation error can be estimated by the centroid positions of the reference and registered current contour sets.

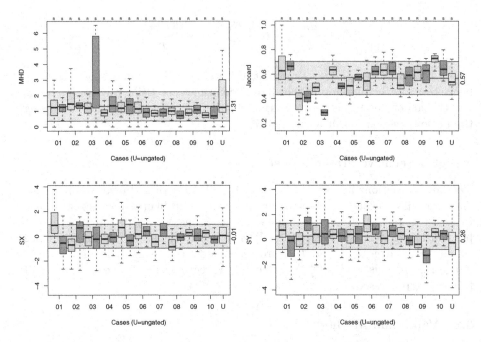

Fig. 2. Quantitative validations of the proposed method in terms of modified Hausdorff distances (top left), Jaccard indices (top right), horizontal shifting (bottom left) and vertical shifting (bottom right). Box plots are grouped into: rest (blue), Stress (red) and ungated (yellow) cases. Gray shaded areas denote mean ± stdev. The trends of MHD and Jaccard index values across the whole frames are given in Fig. 3.

The distribution of MHD, Jaccard, the horizontal and vertical shifting values are shown as boxplots in Fig. 2. The maximum MHD value was 6.49 pixel with the total average of 1.31 ± 0.93 pixels. The average of contour similarity indices were 0.57 ± 0.14. The maximum contour shifting was 4.5 pixels horizontally and 4 pixels vertically.

4   Experimental Results

The STACOM 2014 Motion Correction challenge data consists of 11 cases of dynamic contrast-enhanced MR perfusion acquisitions from a single mid-ventricular short-axis time series. Ten of them (case 1–10) contain two series each: acquisitions made during rest and adenosine induced stress. There are 50 frames in each series, except case 7 at rest (only 49 frames). Case 11 is an ungated stress perfusion sequence with a greater number of frames (130 frames) and the images contain more cardiac motion than the other ten ECG-gated cases. Reference contours were provided as mask images, where the frame number was determined a priori by the organiser.

We implemented the non-rigid registration algorithm in Matlab 7.14 running on an Intel Core Duo, at 1.83 GHz with 1.5 GB RAM. We determined a Region

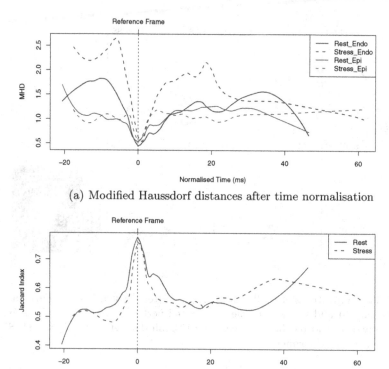

(a) Modified Haussdorf distances after time normalisation

(b) Jaccard indices after time normalisation

Fig. 3. Variations of MHD (top) and Jaccard indices (bottom) relative to the location of the reference frames. Lines were produced after local cubic polynomial regression fitting (LOESS) with smoothing parameter 0.2.

of Interest (ROI) area around the heart using the outer contours of the reference mask plus 15 pixels on either side, for the finite element warping. The smoothing weights were previously determined and set to $\alpha_1 = \alpha_2 = \beta_1 = \beta_2 = \beta_3 = 0.01$. For computational efficiency and reducing the risk of the optimization algorithm getting stuck in a local minimum, the algorithm was performed in multi-scale. A low-resolution step with nine elements across the ROI was applied for coarse alignment, followed by a higher resolution step using 25 elements.

Since the reference frame was used as the basis for non-rigid registration, we analysed how the registration method performed relative to the reference frame. Figure 3(a) shows the average MHD after the reference frames between cases were normalised. This was calculated by the absolute time of each frame relative to the acquisition time and then shifted to make the reference frame absolute time at $t = 0$. We can see how contours at both rest and stress were compared to the reference contour before and after the peak contrast ratio. Figure 3(b) shows the same plot but with the Jaccard index.

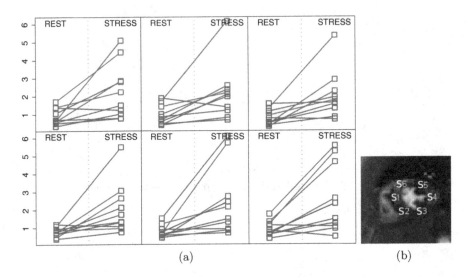

Fig. 4. Regional volume transfer coefficients (K_{trans}) after registration (a). Each case is paired between rest and stress from the ECG-gated perfusion data. Green lines are case 1–5 (NZ dataset) and red lines are case 6–10 (Utah dataset). S1, S2, S3, S4, S5 and S6 denote myocardial segments (b).

Perfusion values were measured based on regional volume transfer coefficients (K_{trans}), which were calculated from the two-compartment model script provided by the organiser. Six equiangular myocardial segments starting from anterior RV insertion point anti-clockwise were determined. Hence segment 1 and 2 are located in the septum, segment 3 at the inferior lateral, segment 4 and 5 are in the lateral wall and segment 6 is the anterior region. When we compared these values regionally and paired between rest and stress, the results are shown in Fig. 4.

5   Discussion

We have presented and tested our non-rigid registration method based on a finite element model on cardiac perfusion MRI. Since reference frames were defined at the adjacent frame (Section 3.1), initial coarse rigid registration did not give significant contribution to the final results. This initialisation step was performed to ensure large image shifting, which could also be caused by non-breathing movement, such as image scanning mis-alignment.

Based on quantitative registered contour measurements, our method achieved good results. Horizontal and vertical shifting variations from Fig. 2 are low with the average errors at -0.01 ± 0.97 and 0.26 ± 1.05 pixels, respectively. The maximum error shift in both direction was just less than 5 pixels. The amount of area overlap (Jaccard index) was moderate with the mean of 0.57 ± 0.14.

Jaccard indices were more varied across cases compared to other quantitative values, because it accounts the area of myocardium instead of the boundaries.

Small Haussdorf distances were achieved with small variation across all images, except in the ungated case and case 3 at stress (see Fig. 2). The noise level in the ungated case is more apparent than the other cases and since the ungated case has more frames, the errors were accumulated more in the subsequent frames due to the consecutive frame registration approach. The method had a difficulty to correct motion in case 3 at stress due to severe breathing and inaccurate triggering artifacts.

The effect of consecutive registration technique by using adjacent reference frames can be seen in Fig. 3. Small registration errors were maintained near the reference frame, but then fell off rapidly. As can be expected, the registration errors were higher in the pre-contrast frames compared to the washed-out frames. However, the method still could register low contrast frames with poor visibility of myocardium because the reference used was the adjacent frame which contains similar intensity profile. This would not be possible if we used the original reference frame. In Fig. 3(a), endocardial contours have larger MHD values compared to the epicardial contours. Figure 3 also shows the difficulty to register contours at stress, which is more visible in the endocardium than the epicardium.

Our method also produced sensible perfusion values, although we cannot validate them with a ground truth. From Fig. 4, the regional K_{trans} values were generally increased with varying degrees from rest to stress. Due to pharmacological stress, the perfusion bed is maximally dilated, resulting an increase of coronary flow circulation. The amount of K_{trans} changes from rest to stress can quantify the coronary flow reserve, which can indicate a coronary artery disease.

The two-compartment model fit has, to some extent, good tolerance for misregistered frames and corrupted perfusion values. The necessity to achieve perfect overlap in terms of the Jaccard index is disputable. After comparison with the ground truth data, a final conclusion can be drawn whether our algorithm was satisfactory in these cases.

The proposed method still needs more improvements to better overlap the reference myocardium, particularly for matching the endocardium. The finite element model was very simple in the current implementation, with a rectangular lattice configuration and constant stiffness (smoothing parameters) across the whole model. In the future, there is the possibility of varying the stiffness spatially so that myocardium has a different stiffness to lungs and liver, and the boundary between organs can be more flexible.

References

1. Canny, J.: A computational approach to edge detection. IEEE Trans. Pattern Anal. Mach. Intell. **8**(6), 679–698 (1986)
2. Coelho-Filho, O.R., Rickers, C., Kwong, R.Y., Jerosch-Herold, M.: MR myocardial perfusion imaging. Radiology **266**(3), 701–715 (2013)

3. Dubuisson, M.P., Jain, A.: A modified Hausdorff distance for object matching. In: Proceedings 12th IAPR International Conference on Pattern Recognition - Conference A: Computer Vision & Image Processing, vol. 1, pp. 566–568 (1994)
4. Gupta, V., Kirişli, H.A., Hendriks, E.A., van der Geest, R.J., van de Giessen, M., Niessen, W., Reiber, J.H.C., Lelieveldt, B.P.F.: Cardiac MR perfusion image processing techniques: a survey. Med. Image Anal. 16(4), 767–785 (2012)
5. Li, B., Liu, Y., Occleshaw, C.J., Cowan, B.R., Young, A.A.: In-line automated tracking for ventricular function with magnetic resonance imaging. JACC Cardiovasc Imaging 3(8), 860–866 (2010)
6. Li, B., Young, A.A., Cowan, B.R.: GPU accelerated non-rigid registration for the evaluation of cardiac function. Med. Image Comput. Comput. Assist. Interv. 11(Pt 2), 880–887 (2008)
7. Press, W.H.: Numerical recipes in C: the art of scientific computing, 2nd edn. Cambridge University Press, Cambridge (1992)

Deformable and Rigid Model-Based Image Registration for Quantitative Cardiac Perfusion

Devavrat Likhite, Ganesh Adluru, and Edward DiBella[✉]

UCAIR, Department of Radiology, University of Utah, Salt Lake City, USA
devavrat.likhite@utah.edu, gadluru@gmail.com,
Edward.DiBella@hsc.utah.edu

Abstract. <u>Background:</u> Inter-frame image registration is a major hurdle in accurate quantification of myocardial perfusion using MRI. The registration is not standard, in that changing contrast between frames makes it difficult to register the images automatically.

<u>Methods:</u> A multiple step approach was employed. First, a region around the heart was identified out automatically in order to focus the registration. Then we performed rigid shifts between frames with a cross correlation type of method, to obtain a coarse registration. Then we created model images from a two compartment model and an arterial input function from the RV blood pool of the images. These model images represent the uptake and washout of the contrast agent. However they do not contain any motion since the two compartment motion cannot explicitly model motion. These motion-free model images are used as reference images and each frame was registered to its associated model image. Rigid and deformable registration as implemented by ANTS. The entire process was automatic and required ~240 seconds.

This registration approach was tested on the 10 provided ECG-gated rest/stress datasets.

<u>Conclusion:</u> Rigid and deformable registration was performed on the provided datasets. The technique was found to perform better on datasets with higher signal to noise ratio and without sudden respiratory motions.

Keywords: Deformable registration · Rigid · Cardiac perfusion · Myocardial blood flow

1 Introduction

Quantification of myocardial blood flow using magnetic resonance imaging is useful for research and clinical studies, though would be used more widely if it was easier to perform and more standardized. Generally, myocardial perfusion is obtained from an ECG-gated T1 weighted imaging sequence that tracks the uptake and washout of a gadolinium based contrast agent. The time-series data is analyzed using semi-quantitative or quantitative methods. Approximately 30 seconds of data is required for quantitative analysis. This long of a breath-hold is not possible for many patients. Moreover, during a stress perfusion scan, it becomes difficult to maintain a steady

© Springer International Publishing Switzerland 2015
O. Camara et al. (Eds.): STACOM 2014, LNCS 8896, pp. 41–50, 2015.
DOI: 10.1007/978-3-319-14678-2_5

breath-hold. The presence of breathing motion makes it difficult to segment out the myocardium, which in turn makes quantification of myocardial blood flow difficult and prone to errors. In particular, breathing motion during the uptake of the contrast agent can give incorrect results.

One of the problems with registration of cardiac perfusion data is the changing contrast over time. This makes it difficult to automatically register all the frames in the series to a single frame in the data. Many different techniques have been proposed. These techniques involve for example iteratively updating a single reference image [1], or using statistical approach [2]. Adluru et al used model images created from fitting the data to a two compartment model to generate a reference image for each time point [3]. That method worked well for cardiac perfusion images, although only rigid shifts were used. In this article we evaluate the use of a deformable and rigid model based image registration for application to 5 gated stress/rest datasets from New Zealand and 5 from Utah.

One ungated perfusion dataset [4] that includes cardiac motion and has a higher temporal resolution is also included. The ungated acquisition has several advantages over conventional ECG-gated acquisitions, although the usability of the ungated technique for quantification depends on the robustness of the registration.

2 Methods

In this article we describe the use of deformable and rigid registration using the model images as the reference images. Each image in the time series is independently registered to its corresponding model image. Fig 1 lists the steps in the registration scheme used. The preprocessing step is a preliminary rigid registration step. The generation of model images follows. The model images are generated by fitting the data to a two-compartment model. These model images are then used as reference images for the deformable or rigid registration that follows. These steps are detailed below.

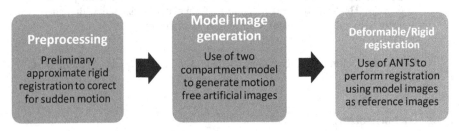

Fig. 1. Flowchart representing the flow of steps done during registration

Preprocessing

The images sometimes have substantial inter-frame respiratory motion. The presence of such large motion was found to generate erroneous model images. Hence a preliminary rigid registration is performed. The registration is done in a cropped region around the heart. This cropping is done automatically by detecting the approximate position of the left and right ventricle.

This preliminary registration makes use of neighboring frames to reduce motion. For each frame, its previous frame and next frame are averaged together to generate the reference image (which is typically blurry since the frames have different motion). Each image is then rigidly registered to its corresponding reference image by maximizing cross correlation. This registration corrects for sudden motion between frames. This preliminary method however does not correct for any drift seen in the position of the heart due to respiratory motion, and is only an approximate correction.

Generation of Model Images

After the preliminary registration step was used to reduce the respiratory motion to some extent, model images are created as described by Adluru et al in [3].

The idea behind model images is that when the images are perfectly registered and the signal intensity for each pixel is recorded over time, the signal intensity curves would be smooth and have no outliers. Conversely, if we have such smooth signal intensity curves, we can generate artificial images that that would reflect the change in contrast and have no motion.

As described in [3], the generation of model images was done by recording the signal intensities over time for every pixel in the image. These recorded curves were then approximated by a two-compartment model [5] widely used in DCE MRI.

$$C_{pix}(t) = C_{input}(t) * K^{trans}e^{-k^{ep}t} + v_p C_{input}(t) \tag{1}$$

The model requires Gd concentration, hence the recorded signal intensity curves at each pixel are converted to be proportional to Gd concentration curves by subtracting the precontrast signal from each curve. $C_{pix}(t)$ represents this signal difference curve. $C_{input}(t)$ is the input function from the right ventricular blood pool. The algorithm makes use of a routine that automatically finds the position of the left and right ventricle. Using the position of the right ventricle, a small region of interest is taken in the right ventricle to record the input function. K^{trans} and k^{ep} are the rate constants representing the exchange of contrast agent between plasma and extra cellular space. A delay term is inserted in eq. (1) to account for the time delay in input function. For speed, a linearized form of eq. (1) given by eq. (2) is used to perform the fitting operation.

$$C_{pix}(t) = (K^{trans} + k^{ep}v_p) \int_0^t C_{input}(\mu - \tau)d\mu$$
$$-k^{ep} \int_0^t C_{pix}(\mu)d\mu + v_p C_{input}(t - \tau) \tag{2}$$

The algorithm minimizes the chi-squared error between the fits and the recorded signal difference curves. The curves fits are then used to generate the model images, by replacing each signal curve by the corresponding curve fit. Fig 2 shows the model images for a few timeframes from different datasets. These model images are artificial images that have no respiratory or cardiac motion since the model does not support motion. These images typically preserve the change in contrast over time and structure seen in the acquired images fairly well. However the model images have enough artifacts that they are not a good choice to use directly to obtain perfusion values. As well, the use of the arterial input function from the right ventricle is not a good choice for the quantitation step, since the left ventricular tissue "sees" quite a significantly dispersed and delayed version of the right ventricle input function.

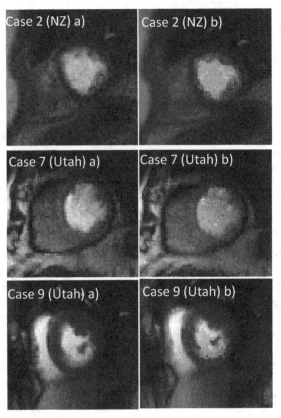

Fig. 2. Left column: Actual images (cropped manually). Right column: Corresponding model images (cropped manually). The model images have an artificial patchy appearance.

Registration Using Model Images

Deformable Registration

Deformable registration is performed using the generated model images as the reference images. Each image is registered independently to its corresponding model-based image. Deformable registration is done using Advanced Normalization Tools (ANTS) [6]. The technique uses a symmetric image normalization method that maximizes the cross correlation in the space of diffeomorphic maps [7]. The ANTS makes use of a multi-resolution framework and we used a 3 level resolution pyramid with a maximum of 100 iterations at the coarsest level, followed by 100 at the next coarsest and 10 iterations at full image resolution [8]. The set of parameters for ANTS were: step size for 2D symmetric image normalization transformation model=0.25, sigma for Gaussian regularizer on the deformation field=2 and sigma for Gaussian regularizer on the similarity gradient=10.

It was found that results of deformable registration of the heart were better when a region of interest was also supplied to ANTS. ANTS focuses the registration operation in the provided region of interest. To focus the registration on the heart, an algorithm was used to detect the position of the left and right ventricle automatically. Using this detected positions of the ventricles a binary mask with fixed size 60x80 pixels, centered on the heart, was generated and provided to ANTS.

Rigid Registration

Rigid registration was performed by using the same model images as the reference images. The registration was also performed using ANTS with the mutual information technique. The number of bins for mutual information registration was set to 32.The same binary mask as in the deformable registration was used to improve the accuracy of the registration process around the heart and to avoid focusing the registration efforts on registering the moving chest wall or other organs.

Quantification of Perfusion

The quantification of perfusion was done using the provided tool and the single frame manual segmentations provided with each dataset. The segmented myocardium was divided into six equiangular regions. The average signal intensity for the six regions was recorded over time. These are the tissue signal intensity curves. These tissue curves were then converted to be proportional to Gd concentration. The correct unsaturated arterial input function was provided as a separate file with each dataset. The tissue curves were then fit to a compartment model [5] and the resulting perfusion indices are reported.

Evaluation of Image Quality

Registration was seen to visually perform better on the Utah datasets compared to the New Zealand datasets. This may be due to the Utah datasets having less motion, and because they were found to have a higher blood signal to noise ratio (bSNR), defined as

$$bSNR = \frac{Mean\ signal\ in\ blood\ pool}{std.\ deviation\ of\ signal\ in\ blood\ pool}$$

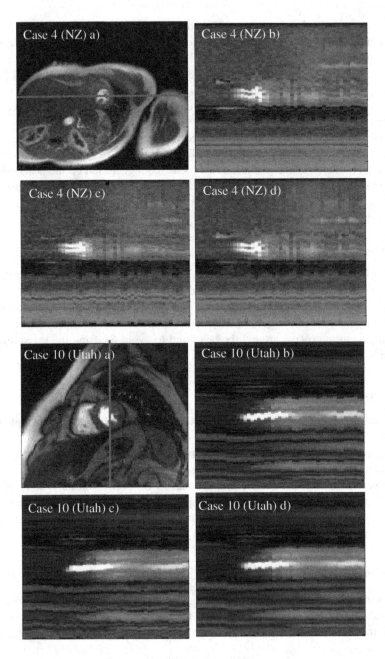

Fig. 3. A line profile through two datasets showing reduction in motion. a) Original image. Line profile through b) original image c) Image registered using deformable registration d) Image registered using rigid registration.

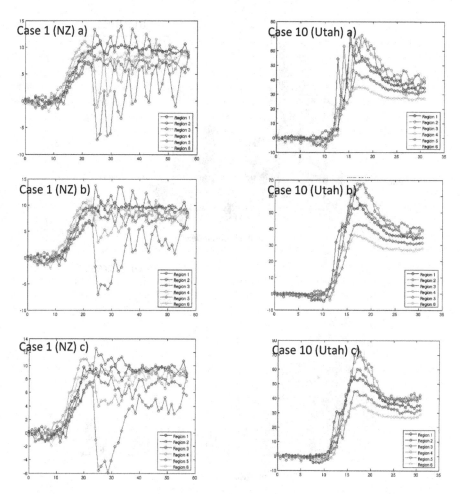

Fig. 4. Graphic showing the tissue curves before and after registration generated using the provided tool for two separate datasets NZ-Rest U- Stress. Tissue curves generated from a) original image b) Image registered using deformable registration c) Image registered using rigid registration.

Table 1. Estimate of the mean SNR and mean CNR for the two subset of datasets i.e. NZ-New Zealand dataset, U-Utah dataset

	SNR	CNR
NZ dataset	14.3	10.5
U dataset	31.3	25.9

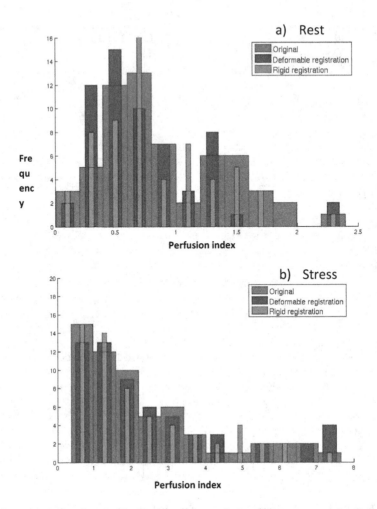

Fig. 5. Histograms showing the distribution of the perfusion indices reported for the provided datasets before and after registration

measured in the manually segmented frame that was provided for each dataset. Higher bSNR could help the registration method by providing better tracking of the blood pool feature.

Edge contrast to noise ratio (eCNR), a measure that estimates the endocardial edge contrast which also could aid the registration, was calculated as

$$eCNR = \frac{Difference\ in\ mean\ signal\ of\ the\ blood\ pool\ and\ myocardium}{std.\ dev\ of\ signal\ in\ blood\ pool}$$

3   Results

Deformable and rigid registration were performed on the provided datasets using the framework as described above. Figure 3 shows the line profile for two datasets before and after registration. It can be seen that the registration techniques were successful in suppressing the inherent motion present in the images. The tissue curves for six regions were also generated using software based on mpi2d [9], which was provided to participants in the challenge. Figure 4 shows the tissue curves before and after registration for a rest and stress dataset. The myocardial blood flow values were also generated using the provided tool. Figure 5 shows a histogram of the reported perfusion indices.

4   Discussion and Conclusion

Deformable and rigid registration was implemented using ANTS software as described in earlier sections. However deformable registration appeared visually to be superior to rigid registration in all cases. The results of registration were not as good without the preliminary registration step. The preliminary step helped the model images better represent the data. In the absence of the preliminary registration, the model images displayed a type of ghosting artifact in the presence of large motion. This in turn affected the accuracy of the deformable and rigid registration. Out of the given 10 datasets, the model-based registration technique used was found to work well on the Utah datasets (Utah). The results of registration on the New Zealand datasets (NZ) were comparatively poor. This difference in results was attributed to the difference in motion and to the higher bSNR and eCNR of the Utah datasets.

In conclusion, both the deformable and rigid registration were able to handle motion correctly in images with higher bSNR. Also the methods were found to handle shallow breathing motion better than a breath-hold followed by heavy breathing.

References

1. Bidaut, L.M., Vallee, J.P.: Automated registration of dynamic MR images for the quantification of myocardial perfusion. J. Magn. Reson. Imaging **13**, 648–655 (2001)
2. Gallippi, C.M., Kramer, C.M., Hu, Y.L., Vido, D.A., Reichek, N., Rogers, W.J.: Fully automated registration and warping of contrast-enhanced first pass perfusion images. J. Cardiovasc. Magn. Reson. **4**, 459–469 (2002)
3. Adluru, G., DiBella, E.V., Schabel, M.C.: Model-based registration for dynamic cardiac perfusion MRI. J. Magn. Reson. Imaging **24**(5), 1062–1070 (2006)
4. Harrison, A., et al.: Rapid ungated myocardial perfusion cardiovascular magnetic resonance: preliminary diagnostic accuracy. J. Cardiovasc. Magn. Reson. **15**(1), 26 (2013)

5. Tofts, P.S.: Modeling tracer kinetics in dynamic Gd-DTPA MR imaging. J. Magn. Reson. Imaging **7**(1), 91–101 (1997)
6. http://picsl.upenn.edu/software/ants/
7. Avants, B.B., et al.: Symmetric diffeomorphic image registration with cross-correlation: evaluating automated labeling of elderly and neurodegenerative brain. Med. Image Anal. **12**(1), 26–41 (2008)
8. Avants, B.B., et al.: Advanced Normalization Tools (ANTS), September 2011
9. Pack, N.A., Vijayakumar, S., Kim, T.H., McGann, C.J., DiBella, E.V.R.: A semi-automatic software package for analysis of dynamic contrast-enhanced MRI myocardial perfusion studies. Computers in Cardiology; S62-6, Park City, UT

Automatic Perfusion Analysis Using Phase-Based Registration and Object-Based Image Analysis

Lennart Tautz[✉], Teodora Chitiboi, and Anja Hennemuth

Fraunhofer MEVIS, Bremen, Germany
lennart.tautz@mevis.fraunhofer.de

Abstract. MRI perfusion imaging enables the non-invasive assessment of myocardial blood supply. The purpose of the presented work is to enable a quantitative assessment of the image sequences for clinical application. To this end an automatic preprocessing including ROI detection and outlier removal has been combined with a phase-based registration approach and an object-based myocardium segmentation. The suggested processing pipeline has been tested with 21 image sequences provided by the STACOM motion correction challenge. The corrected image sequences have been assessed by comparison with gamma variate curves fitted to the voxels intensity curves. The automatic segmentation could be compared with expert segmentations provided by the challenge organizers. The results indicate an improvement through the motion correction and a good agreement with the reference segmentation in most cases.

Keywords: Perfusion · Morphon · Registration · Quadrature filter · OBIA

1 Introduction

Magnetic resonance (MR) perfusion imaging provides non-invasive means for assessing the effect of coronary artery pathologies on the supplied heart muscle tissue. To analyze the local blood supply, image series showing the intensity variation induced by the wash-in and wash-out of an administered contrast agent are acquired in rest state as well as under pharmacologically induced stress.

The inspection of the myocardial perfusion is then based on the analysis of the time-intensity curves of image regions or single voxels, which results in parameters describing curve properties or derived physiological parameters such as the myocardial blood flow. To enable the extraction of these intensity curves from the image sequences, the motion induced through breathing and irregular myocardial contraction has to be compensated for. Because of the sparsity of the data, through-plane motion can not be corrected and thus it can be useful to exclude outliers from the analysis rather than considering intensity values from other tissue regions in the myocardial perfusion analysis. In-plane motion of the heart muscle can be discriminated into the movement through breathing and deformation

© Springer International Publishing Switzerland 2015
O. Camara et al. (Eds.): STACOM 2014, LNCS 8896, pp. 51–60, 2015.
DOI: 10.1007/978-3-319-14678-2_6

caused by the myocardial contraction. The joint compensation of these motion types is a challenging task.

An overview of existing approaches for image preprocessing and parameter extraction from time-intensity curves is given by Gupta et al. [7]. In the literature, this is either achieved through the identification of corresponding regions in every time frame using manual or automatic segmentation methods [9,16,17] or through time frame alignment followed by segmentation of the myocardium in one image that represents the corrected sequence [6,19].

In this paper we present an automatic processing pipeline for motion correction and segmentation of the myocardium. The approach consists of three processing steps, namely the removal of outliers, an in-plane motion correction with the intensity-invariant Morphon approach [18], and an automatic myocardium segmentation, which uses the temporal maximum intensity projection of the corrected image sequence. Because there is no ground truth data available to evaluate the results of the proposed methods, the validation method applied here compares the intensity curves of the processed image sequences against a fitted gamma variate curve, which is assumed to describe the typical intensity curve in tissue after contrast agent administration.

2   Materials and Methods

2.1   Image Data

The STACOM 2014 Motion Correction Challenge provided rest and stress perfusion image sequences for 10 patients (20 sequences total), and one image sequence of a new ungated acquisition. For the standard perfusion images, one expert contour at a reference time frame was also provided. The in-plane resolutions of the standard images vary between 1.875 and 2.344 mm, with a slice thickness of 8 mm. Each sequence consists of 50 time frames. The ungated image sequence has an in-plane resolution of 1.944 mm, a slice thickness of 8 mm and 130 time frames. The data was acquired at the University of Utah (Siemens Verio 3T and TrioTim 3T scanners) and at the University of Auckland (Siemens Avanto 1.5T). Four of the ten patients had a known coronary artery disease.

2.2   Preprocessing

As a first processing step, the location of the heart chambers in the image sequence is estimated. Existing approaches simply determine the right and left ventricle as blobs of high intensity in space and time [17]. However, high intensity changes occur also in aorta, kidney or moving fatty regions. Our method is thus based on the two assumptions that the contrast agent injection causes strong intensity changes over time during the contrast agent's first pass T_{circ} and that the heart is located in the center of the image. A weighted combination of the maximum standard deviation over time and the distance from the image border I_{dev} is thresholded with $I_{dev} + \alpha\sigma, \alpha \in [1,3]$, and the two bloodpool regions are detected via connected component analysis.

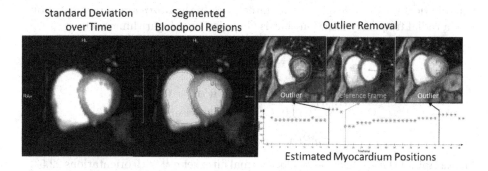

Fig. 1. ROI detection and outlier removal. The images show the preprocessing pipeline for the stress sequence of case 8. The bloodpool detection on the image I_{dev} is used to crop the image and place the *virtual navigator* for outlier detection (orange markers). The diagram on the right shows the estimated myocardium position per time frame, the circles mark the selected subsequence. The images above correspond to the reference frame as well as two removed outlier frames.

Based on this initial segmentation the region of interest can be restricted. Furthermore, the bloodpool centers are used to determine the orientations of *virtual navigators* as shown in Figure 1. The intensity changes along the *navigator* direction are used to split the image sequences into subsequences in order to exclude time frames with strong motion that can not be corrected in the subsequent registration step. To this end, a morphologic opening is applied to get rid of small vessels in the lung. Then a standard deviation filter is applied to detect the transitions between different regions and thereby find the myocardium border. In some sequences there are time frames with no intensity difference between myocardium and lung before contrast agent wash-in. These time frames are not removed because the subsequent intensity curve analysis requires a certain density of data sampling points. For the same reason the threshold applied for sequence splitting is iteratively increased until the sequence to process contains at least 50% of the original image sequence.

2.3 Motion Correction

The algorithm for the motion field calculation uses the local phase, which represents image features such as edges and lines but is invariant to their magnitude. The *Morphon* implementation by Tautz et al. is based on the Fourier Shift Theorem [11,18]. By estimating the voxel-wise difference in local phase between two images, the spatial difference can be determined. As proposed by Jepson and Fleet, the analytic signal is estimated by applying a quadrature filter, $q(x)$, which has a band-pass character that determines the scale of the structures or shifts of interest. The generalization of the analytic 1D signal to higher dimensions is achieved with a set of quadrature filters $q^{(i)}(\mathbf{x})$ with different orientations $\mathbf{n}_i$, and the generalized analytic signal in direction $\mathbf{n}_i$ for an image $I(\mathbf{x})$ is then obtained as $(I * q^{(i)})(\mathbf{x})$.

The spherically separable quadrature filters used in the *Morphon* implementation have a radial frequency function that is Gaussian on a logarithmic scale.

$$R_i(u) = e^{-\frac{4}{B^2 \ln 2} \ln^2\left(\frac{u}{u_i}\right)} \tag{1}$$

$$D_i(\hat{u}) = \begin{cases} \left(\hat{u}^T \hat{n}_i\right)^2 & \text{if } \hat{u}^T \hat{n}_i > 0, \\ 0 & \text{otherwise.} \end{cases} \tag{2}$$

$$q^{(i)}(\mathbf{u}) = R_i(\|\mathbf{u}\|) D_i(\hat{u}) \tag{3}$$

An example of the application of a log-normal filter set $q^{(i)}$ with orientations 22.5°, 67.5°, 112.5°, 157.5°, bandwidth $B = 1.5$, and center frequency u_i to two time frames of a perfusion sequence is shown in Figure 2. To capture the different types of motion that occur in perfusion sequences, the actual implementation of the *Morphon* uses a multi-resolution approach. The applied algorithm is described in detail in [18]. In the deformation field calculation, the displacement estimation as well as the certainty of the estimate are considered. Furthermore, it is assumed that plausible tissue deformations are relatively smooth. Therefore, spatial regularization is applied with a Gaussian kernel. The motion correction is started with one reference time frame, which is set to the image frame with the reference segmentation. Usually the intersection of right and left ventricular bloodpool time-intensity curves is chosen. The neighboring time frames are then successively warped onto their corrected predecessors by applying the deformation calculated with the *Morphon* algorithm. This means that registration errors will accumulate along the transformed time series and therefore the outlier removal has a strong impact on the final result of the registration approach.

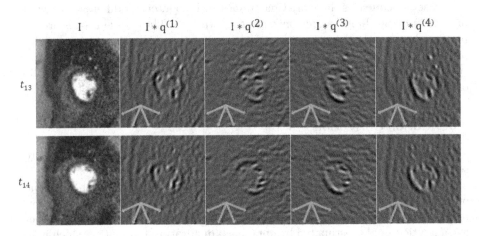

Fig. 2. Application of a set of log-normal filters $q^{(i)}$ with orientations 22.5°, 67.5°, 112.5°, 157.5° and bandwidth 1.5 to two successive time frames of a stress perfusion sequence (case 8)

2.4   Myocardium Segmentation

We consider the maximum intensity projection (MIP) of the motion corrected temporal perfusion image series, where both bloodpools and the myocardium are fully visible. The main challenge segmenting this image is to distinguish between the myocardium and neighboring tissue of similar intensity in situations where local contrast is poor. We apply an object-base image analysis segmentation approach proposed by Chitiboi et al. [3]. The image is initially partitioned into regions of about 5 mm^2, using a k-means clustering algorithm in three dimensions (X, Y, and intensity) called SLIC super-pixels [1]. The resulting regions (Figure 3, top left) are stored in an attributed relational graph and managed using a generic framework introduced by Homeyer et al. [8]. The image segments can be described by a custom set of properties regarding their intensity statistics, shape, and relation to other objects. The advantages of this image representation are the reduced sensitivity to noise of regions as opposed to individual pixels, as well as the possibility to directly use local context from the relational graph to infer the myocardial border where contrast is low.

The segmentation is started in the bloodpool, which is roughly estimated by iterative region growing on the object level starting from the bloodpool center using an adaptive threshold. A best fitting ellipse is computed using principal component analysis (PCA) and all neighboring objects more than 50% covered are also merged to account for partial volume effect, papillary muscles and texture along the endocardial wall (Fig. 3, top second, in orange).

Next, the myocardium is initialized by merging the first ring of image regions surrounding the bloodpool (Fig. 3, top third, in green) and gradually extends outwards to include neighboring image segments with similar intensity statistics. Then, the shape of the joint myocardium-bloodpool mask is similarly optimized using ellipse overlap and a minimal contour constraint. The coarse result obtained

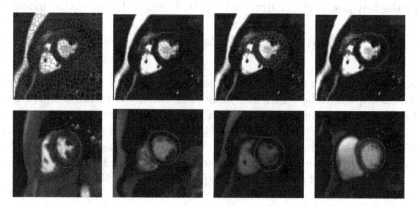

Fig. 3. Top (left to right): Initial image regions. Left ventricle bloodpool. Myocardium regions. Coarse segmentation of both ventricles and the myocardium. Bottom (left to right): Temporal MIP and automatic myocardium contours (after smoothing) for cases 1, 2, 5 and 8.

by the object-based segmentation is then locally refined using using morphological operations and smoothing to obtain the subpixel representation in Figure 3 (bottom row) [2].

3 Results

The often suggested assessment of the left ventricle's gravity center movement in the corrected sequence [14,18,20] is actually too coarse to provide information about the result's eligibility for a clinical interpretation. It is important that myocardial perfusion curves are not disturbed by voxels belonging to the blood-pool because a mixed curve could lead to wrong conclusions. Thus, some authors propose to calculate the overlap of the myocardium segmentation at different time frames or the distances of the segmented contours [12,20]. The result of this evaluation strongly depends on manual myocardium segmentations.

Because the actual interpretation of the perfusion sequence is based on the characteristics of the time-intensity curves of the myocardium, it is obvious to base the assessment of the motion correction on these curves. A quantitative curve assessment was introduced by Gupta et al. [5]. It assumes that the intensity curves are smooth and accumulates the deviations of intensity values from the mean intensity of their temporal predecessors and successors. Thus, peaks and valleys also contribute to the error measure.

Motion Correction. In order to provide a quantitative user-independent quality measure, our approach performs an automatic curve assessment. For all voxels in the region of interest, a gamma variate model curve is fitted. The deviation from this model curve is then used to assess the plausibility of the motion correction result. Based on indicator dilution theory, Thompsen et al. proposed to model tracer concentration curves through the gamma variate function [15], which was found to be suitable for modeling ventricular and myocardial time-intensity curves during the first pass of the contrast agent [10]. It can be formulated as follows:

$$C(t) = \begin{cases} s_0 + \gamma\,(t - t_0)^\alpha\, e^{-\frac{t-t_0}{\beta}} & \text{if } t > t_0 \\ s_0 & \text{if } t \le t_0 \end{cases} \tag{4}$$

Because compartments with different time-intensity curves, such as the left ventricular bloodpool, right ventricular bloodpool, the myocardium, lung, or liver, can be present in the inspected region of interest, fit parameters are estimated separately for every voxel. The end of the baseline t_0 as well as the mean baseline intensity s_0, the maximum intensity s_{max}, and the time frame of maximum intensity t_{max} are derived directly in a first curve analysis step. If α is also known, β and γ can be initialized as described in Equations 5 and 6 [13].

$$\beta = \frac{(t_{max} - t_0)}{\alpha} \tag{5}$$

$$\gamma = \begin{cases} (s_{max} - s_0)\left(\frac{e}{|\alpha - \beta|}\right)^\alpha & \text{if } t_{max} > t_0 \\ 0 & \text{if } t_{max} \le t_0 \end{cases} \tag{6}$$

The final parameters are calculated by means of least squares minimization with the *Minpack* library [4]. The gamma variate can only describe the first pass of the contrast agent and thus the fitting procedure only considers the first 25 seconds of the image sequence.

For this interval, the difference between original and fitted image is calculated and the mean difference between the original and the fitted voxel intensity curves is used as quality measure. Because of the differences in intensity encoding in MRI image data, errors are calculated relative to the intensity range in the image data. The maximum difference between the fitted curves and the intensity curves in the expert segmented myocardium was 2% before and 1% after motion correction. The mean error decreased for all sequences. Figure 4 shows the intensity values and fitted curves before and after motion correction for the points indicated by the markers in the corresponding image.

Segmentation. For the validation of the automatic segmentation, manually defined contours by experts have been provided by the STACOM 2014 organizers. Because the frames containing the expert contours have been used as reference frames for the motion correction, a direct comparison with the automatically detected contours is possible. The average Dice coefficient was 0.6 and ranged between 0.33 and 0.83. The Hausdorff distance was 2.2 mm on average and distance values ranged between 0 and 15 mm. Figure 4 shows the good agreement of the segmentation for the rest sequence of case 1 as well as the differences in the masks detected for the stress sequence of case 4.

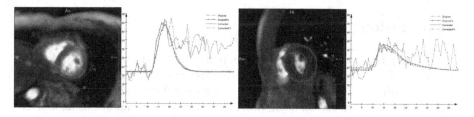

Fig. 4. Results for the stress sequences of case 4 and case 1. The green contours on the temporal maximum intensity projection images represent the reference segmentation, the orange contours depict the result of the automatic segmentation. Intensity curves before and after correction as well as the corresponding fitted curves are shown for the voxel location indicated by the asterisk marker on the image.

4   Discussion

The results showed that the suggested image processing pipeline delivered corrections and segmentations for all image sequences. The agreement of the automatic segmentation with the provided reference masks as well as the improvement of the intensity curves with regard to a plausible curve model indicate the potential of the suggested approach.

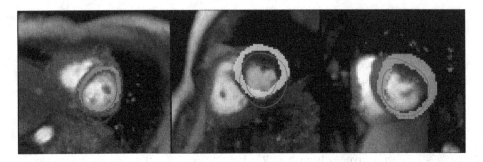

Fig. 5. Segmentation mismatch for the stress sequences of case 3, 4, and 5. The images show the temporal MIPs derived from the motion-corrected image sequences. The orange overlay represents the provided reference segmentation, the result of the presented processing approach is visualized via the blue and red contours.

The least segmentation overlap was achieved for the stress sequences of cases 3, 4, and 5. As shown in Figure 5, the temporal MIPs of the corrected sequences differ from the reference frame in such a way that no comparable segmentation can be achieved on these image data. The results showed a tendency of the segmentation to overestimate the myocardium region compared to expert delineation. This could generate misleading quantitative parameters in a per-segment analysis of myocardial perfusion, and the influence of this overestimation should be further investigated.

5   Conclusions

We presented a fully automatic approach for motion correction and automatic segmentation of the myocardium in MRI perfusion sequences. The described methods were successfully applied to 21 image sequences provided by the STACOM 2014 organizers. Plausibility checks using provided reference segmentations as well as comparisons with a fitted gamma variate curve model indicate that the provided segmentation pipeline could be used to preprocess and initialize a quantitative analysis of myocardial perfusion. The STACOM challenge evaluation will give further insights into the applicability towards the generation of clinically relevant quantitative parameters.

References

1. Achanta, R., Shaji, A., Smith, K., Lucchi, A., Fua, P., Süsstrunk, S.: Slic superpixels. EPFL Tech. Rep. 149300 (2010)
2. Chitiboi, T., Hennemuth, A., Tautz, L., Huellebrand, M., Frahm, J., Linsen, L., Hahn, H.: Context-based segmentation and analysis of multi-cycle real-time cardiac MRI. In: Proceedings of IEEE International Symposium on Biomedical Imaging, pp. 943–946 (2014)

3. Chitiboi, T., Hennemuth, A., Tautz, L., Stolzmann, P., Donati, O.F., Linsen, L., Hahn, H.K.: Automatic detection of myocardial perfusion defects using object-based myocardium segmentation. In: 2013 Computing in Cardiology Conference (CinC), pp. 639–642. IEEE (2013)

4. Cowell, W. (ed.): Sources and Development of Mathematical Software. Prentice-Hall Series in Computational Mathematics. Prentice-Hall, Upper Saddle River (1984)

5. Gupta, S., Solaiyappan, M., Beache, G., Arai, A., Foo, T.: Fast method for correcting image misregistration due to organ motion in time-series MRI data. Magn. Reson. Med. **49**(3), 506–514 (2003)

6. Gupta, V., Hendriks, E., Milles, J., van der Geest, R.J., Jerosch-Herold, M., Reiber, J., Lelieveldt, B.: Fully automatic registration and segmentation of first-pass myocardial perfusion MR image sequences. Acad. Radiol. **17**, 1375–1385 (2010)

7. Gupta, V., Kirisli, H., Hendriks, E., van der Geest, R., van de Giessen, M., Niessen, W., Reiber, J., Lelieveldt, B.: Cardiac MR perfusion image processing techniques: a survey. Med. Image Anal. **16**(4), 767–785 (2012)

8. Homeyer, A., Schwier, M., Hahn, H.: A generic concept for object-based image analysis. In: VISAPP, pp. 530–533 (2010)

9. Horkaew, P.: Analysis of CMR perfusion imaging based on statistical appearance models. In: KST, pp. 6–11 (2010)

10. Jerosch-Herold, M., Seethamraju, R., Swingen, C., Wilke, N., Stillman, A.: Analysis of myocardial perfusion MRI. J. Magn. Reson. Imaging **19**(6), 758–770 (2004). http://dx.doi.org/10.1002/jmri.20065

11. Knutsson, H., Andersson, M.: Morphons: segmentation using elastic canvas and paint on priors. In: Symposium on Image Analysis SSBA, vol. **2005**, pp. 73–76 (2005)

12. Li, C., Sun, Y.: Nonrigid registration of myocardial perfusion MRI using pseudo ground truth. In: Yang, G.-Z., Hawkes, D., Rueckert, D., Noble, A., Taylor, C. (eds.) MICCAI 2009, Part I. LNCS, vol. 5761, pp. 165–172. Springer, Heidelberg (2009)

13. Madsen, M.: A simplified formulation of the gamma variate function. Physics in Medicine and Biology **37**(7), 1597 (1992). http://stacks.iop.org/0031-9155/37/i=7/a=010

14. Milles, J., van der Geest, R., Jerosch-Herold, M., Reiber, J., Lelieveldt, B.I.: Fully automated motion correction in first-pass myocardial perfusion MR image sequences. IEEE Trans. Med. Imaging **27**(11), 1611–1621 (2008). http://dx.doi.org/10.1109/TMI.2008.928918

15. Mischi, M., den Boer, J., Korsten, H.: On the physical and stochastic representation of an indicator dilution curve as a gamma variate. Physiol. Meas. **29**(3), 281–294 (2008). http://dx.doi.org/10.1088/0967-3334/29/3/001

16. Santarelli, M., Positano, V., Michelassi, C., Lombardi, M., Landini, L.: Automated cardiac MR image segmentation: theory and measurement evaluation. Med. Eng. Phys. **25**(2), 149–159 (2003)

17. Spreeuwers, L., Breeuwer, M.: Automatic detection of myocardial boundaries in MR cardio perfusion images. In: Niessen, W.J., Viergever, M.A. (eds.) MICCAI 2001. LNCS, vol. 2208, pp. 1228–1231. Springer, Heidelberg (2001)

18. Tautz, L., Hennemuth, A., Andersson, M., Seeger, A., Knutsson, H., Friman, O.: Phase-based non-rigid registration of myocardial perfusion MRI image sequences. In: 2010 IEEE International Symposium on Biomedical Imaging: From Nano to Macro, pp. 516–519, April 2010

19. Weng, A., Ritter, C., Lotz, J., Beer, M., Hahn, D., Koestler, H.: Automatic postprocessing for the assessment of quantitative human myocardial perfusion using mri. Eur. Radiol. **20**(6), 1356–1365 (2010)
20. Xue, H., Guehring, J., Srinivasan, L., Zuehlsdorff, S., Saddi, K., Chefdhotel, C., Hajnal, J.V., Rueckert, D.: Evaluation of rigid and non-rigid motion compensation of cardiac perfusion MRI. In: Metaxas, D., Axel, L., Fichtinger, G., Székely, G. (eds.) MICCAI 2008, Part II. LNCS, vol. 5242, pp. 35–43. Springer, Heidelberg (2008)

LV Mechanics Challenge

Left Ventricular Diastolic and Systolic Material Property Estimation from Image Data

Adarsh Krishnamurthy, Christopher Villongco, Amanda Beck,
Jeffrey Omens, and Andrew McCulloch[✉]

Cardiac Mechanics Research Group, University of California,
San Diego, La Jolla, CA, USA
amcculloch@ucsd.edu

Abstract. Cardiovascular simulations using patient-specific geometries can help researchers understand the mechanical behavior of the heart under different loading or disease conditions. However, to replicate the regional mechanics of the heart accurately, both the nonlinear passive and active material properties must be estimated reliably. In this paper, automated methods were used to determine passive material properties while simultaneously computing the unloaded reference geometry of the ventricles for stress analysis. Two different approaches were used to model systole. In the first, a physiologically-based active contraction model [1] coupled to a hemodynamic three-element Windkessel model of the circulation was used to simulate ventricular ejection. In the second, developed active tension was directly adjusted to match ventricular volumes at end-systole while prescribing the known end-systolic pressure. These methods were tested in four normal dogs using the data provided for the LV mechanics challenge [2]. The resulting end-diastolic and end-systolic geometry from the simulation were compared with measured image data.

Keywords: Finite Element Method · Mesh generation · Parameter estimation · Unloaded geometry

1 Introduction

Cardiovascular simulations using patient-specific geometries of the ventricles are now possible with advances in computational modeling and medical imaging [3-8]. Such simulations can help researchers understand the mechanical behavior of the heart under different loading or disease conditions. However, to replicate the regional mechanics of the heart accurately, both the passive hyperelastic properties and the active tension developed during systole in the myocardium have to be correctly determined.

Using mathematical simulations of the cardiac cycle, it is possible to reverse engineer the mechanical properties of the heart by comparing the simulated material point displacements to image data. In this paper, we describe methods by which the passive material properties and the active systolic properties of the left ventricle can be optimized with the help of global ventricular measures such as cavity pressure and volume. High-resolution MRI data from four normal dogs, contributed from the National

© Springer International Publishing Switzerland 2015
O. Camara et al. (Eds.): STACOM 2014, LNCS 8896, pp. 63–73, 2015.
DOI: 10.1007/978-3-319-14678-2_7

Institutes of Health [2] defining the LV epicardial and endocardial surfaces, and muscle fiber orientations derived from *ex-vivo* diffusion tensor MRI and registered to the *in-vivo* geometry were used to test the models.

One of the requirements to determine regional material displacements accurately is a good estimate of the unloaded ventricular geometry for use as the stress-free reference state. Images obtained from animals or patients *in vivo* are always in some state of mechanical loading during the cardiac cycle. The geometry obtained at diastasis is also not stress-free since the cardiac pressure is not zero, and diastolic strains are near maximal. In this paper, we calculate the unloaded state from end-diastolic ventricular geometry making use of the pressure and volume measurements between diastasis and end-diastole, using the method developed by Krishnamurthy, et al. [9]. The resting material properties of the myocardium [10] and the unloaded geometry are optimized simultaneously to match the filling curve between diastasis and end-diastole.

To model the active contractile properties of the myocardium, we compared two different approaches. In the first method, the active contractile model of the ventricle was coupled to a three-element Windkessel model of the systemic arterial circulation. The parameters of a Hill-type contractile model [1] and the circulation model were adjusted to obtain ventricular systolic pressure and volume time-courses that are similar to the ones measured by cardiac catheterization. In the second method, the active forces developed were directly adjusted such that the ventricular volume in the model matches the measured end-systolic volume, at prescribed end-systolic pressure. The resulting end-systolic geometry from the model was then compared with the measured geometry at end-systole.

2   Methods

We make use of a cubic-Hermite finite element method to model the left ventricle of the dogs [11]. The finite element mesh is constructed from the surface data at end-diastole. A hyper-elastic constitutive relation [10] is used for the resting properties of the myocardium. In this section, we explain some of the methods that were developed to construct the geometric mesh and to estimate the material parameters of the model.

2.1   Geometry Fitting

To perform biomechanics simulations, a cubic-Hermite finite element mesh that matches the geometry of the left ventricle is constructed. The surface mesh for the epicardium and the endocardium are constructed by sampling points from the input data cloud (Fig. 1A). The surfaces are then fit to reduce the projected error between the data points and the mesh surfaces (Fig. 1C). Once the surfaces are fit separately, they are automatically combined to construct a linear hexahedral finite element mesh (Fig. 1D). This mesh is then successively subdivided twice (Fig. 1E, F) using the methods outlined in [12, 13], to estimate the cubic Hermite derivatives at the nodes. Finally, the 3D cubic-Hermite finite element mesh consisting of 28 elements and 66 nodes (1584 degrees of freedom) is constructed using the estimated derivatives (Fig. 1G).

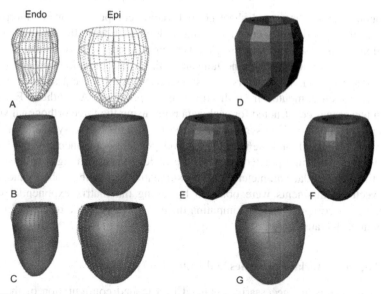

Fig. 1. Hexahedral mesh generation from input data. A linear surface mesh (A) is constructed separately for epicardial and endocardial data and is fitted to match the contours (B, C). A linear Hexahedral mesh is constructed from the surface meshes (D) and is subdivided twice (E, F) to obtain the final cubic-Hermite Hexahedral finite-element mesh (G).

2.2   Fiber Fitting

Canine myofiber vectors computed from diffusion-tensor MRI (DT-MRI), and registered to the geometry at diastasis were provided. This data is used to perform a volumetric fit to estimate the components of the fiber vector at the nodes of the finite element mesh. The cubic-Hermite finite element mesh at diastasis was constructed using the geometry fitting methods explained above from the diastasis surface data. Once this data is fitted to the dog ventricular geometry, it is interpolated using a log-Euclidean framework to estimate the fiber orientations within each element of the mesh (Fig. 2).

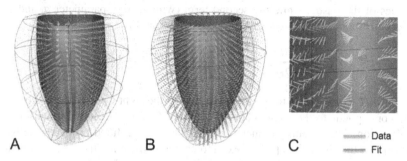

Fig. 2. Fiber orientation data from DT-MRI (A) registered to the geometry at diastasis. Diffusion tensors were fitted and interpolated using log-Euclidian metric (B). Comparison between the data and the fit (C) in a region of the ventricular mesh.

Orthogonal fiber, sheet, and sheet-normal vector components were interpolated throughout the ventricular geometry using a log Euclidean framework [9, 14]. Imbrication (transverse) and sheet angles were prescribed to be zero (the sheet and sheet-normal vectors are normal and tangent to the local epicardial and endocardial surfaces, respectively). The vectors corresponding to the sheet and sheet-normal directions were then computed from the fiber vector provided. A synthetic Euclidean diffusion tensor was constructed for each data point using the three orthogonal vectors and generic eigenvalues. The symmetric matrix logarithms of the synthetic diffusion tensors were computed, and the resulting six independent components of the log Euclidean tensors were interpolated between the nodes by performing a trilinear least squares fit of the nodal parameters. During simulations, the fiber, sheet, and sheet-normal vector components were obtained by taking the matrix exponential of the fitted log tensor components and computing the eigenvectors of the resulting Euclidean tensor at each Gauss point.

2.3   Passive Material Properties and Unloaded Geometry

The in-vivo images are necessarily obtained in a loaded configuration of the heart; often end-diastole or diastasis. However, an unloaded reference state is required to compute the stresses and strains correctly. This unloaded geometry, when loaded to the measured end-diastolic pressure, will deform to the measured end-diastolic geometry. Previous studies have used some simplifying assumptions for the unloaded geometry; these include using the end-systolic [15] or mid-diastolic [16] geometry as the unloaded state. Rajagopal, et al. [17] developed a method to estimate the unloaded geometry of human breasts that has been applied to heart modeling [18]. We make use of the method developed by Krishnamurthy, et al. [9], to estimate the unloaded geometry together with the passive material parameters.

The transversely-isotropic form of the constitutive model developed by Holzapfel and Ogden [10] is used to model the passive properties of the myocardium, In this model, the anisotropy in the fiber and cross-fiber directions of the myocardium is modeled using a separate exponential term with different exponents (Eq. 1). The first term (with scaling parameter a and exponent b) corresponds to the isotropic material properties of the tissue, while the second term (with scaling parameter a_f and exponent b_f) corresponds to the fiber direction passive properties.

$$\psi = \frac{a}{2b}e^{b(I_1-3)} + \frac{a_f}{2b_f}\left(e^{b_f(I_{4f}-1)^2} - 1\right) \tag{1}$$

In, Eq. 1, I_1 corresponds to the first invariant of the right Cauchy-Green strain tensor, I_{4f} corresponds to the components of the right Cauchy-Green strain tensor in the fiber direction. The default parameters of the model were fitted to match the biaxial tests [19] and the shear tests [20] of ex-vivo canine myocardial tissue. In the material parameter estimation, the ratio of the pressure scaling coefficients and the exponents were kept constant (same value as default) so as to maintain the anisotropy. This assumption results in two independent parameters that need to be adjusted to match the pressure-volume curve measured from diastasis to end-diastole.

2.4   Active Material Properties

We used two different methods to model systolic contraction in the ventricles. The first method makes use of a physiologically-based muscle contraction model [1] with length-tension and force-velocity relationships. It is coupled to a three-element Windkessel model to simulate ventricular ejection. The second method makes use of directly changing the active tension developed in the muscle to match the measured end-systolic ventricular volume while applying the measured end-systolic pressure as a boundary condition. In both methods, the active tension model used is transversely isotropic. The transverse direction active force was specified to be 70% of the fiber direction active force.

To determine the contractile parameters for the first method, the finite element model was iso-volumically contracted by activating the fibers and the resulting pressure time-course was compared with the measured catheter pressures. The parameters of the contractile model, specifically the active stress scaling coefficient (SfAct), activation rise time (tR), and activation decay time (tD), were adjusted to match the peak systolic pressure, dP/dt_{max}, and dP/dt_{min} respectively. The basal boundary conditions were not explicitly specified since the displacements at different time points of the cardiac cycle are not known. The finite element model was then coupled to the Windkessel model [21], whose parameters were then adjusted to match the volume time-course.

In the second method, the finite element model is first passively inflated to the end-systolic pressure. The active tension is then increased slowly in steps until the volume of the ventricle contracts to match the measured end-systolic volume. In addition, the basal epicardial displacements at end systole were directly specified from the available data. The resulting geometry is then used as the end-systolic geometry for comparison. This process can be repeated for each measured pressure and volume point pair in the cardiac cycle and the time-course of the active tension can be obtained. Thus, the time-varying elastance of the ventricles for the entire cardiac cycle can be estimated.

3   Results

The end-diastolic finite element mesh for each dog was fitted from the surface data clouds. This geometry was then used to estimate the unloaded reference geometry. The maximum RMS error between the fitted surfaces and the data points for different dogs is ~0.6mm (Table 1).

Table 1. RMS error (mm) between the surface data point cloud and the fitted surfaces for the different dogs, respectively

	Endocardial Surface (mm)	Epicardial Surface (mm)
D0912	0.53	0.61
D0917	0.48	0.48
D1017	0.60	0.65
D1024	0.43	0.46

The patient-specific parameters of the constitutive model were estimated together with the unloaded geometry. The estimated passive parameters are given in Table 2. The match between the simulated filling curves and the measured pressure-volume curves between diastasis and end-diastole is within 5% (Fig. 3). The pressure curve for dog D0917 was shifted up by 0.09kPa to make the pressure at diastasis zero.

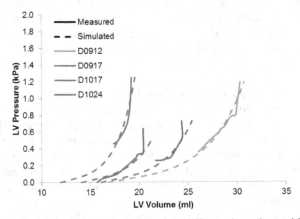

Fig. 3. Passive filling curves corresponding to the four different dogs along with their pressure-volume relation between diastasis and end-diastole. The unloaded volume varies depending on the stiffness of the ventricles for the individual dogs.

Table 2. Passive material parameters for the Ogden-Holzapfel constitutive relation

	a	a_f	b	b_f
D0912	0.760	0.560	9.726	15.779
D0917	0.988	0.728	14.589	23.669
D1017	0.988	0.728	14.589	23.669
D1024	0.760	0.560	19.452	31.558

The pressure and volume time-course for one of the dogs (D0912) is within 10% of their respective values using the first method of systolic contraction coupled to a Windkessel model (Fig. 4).

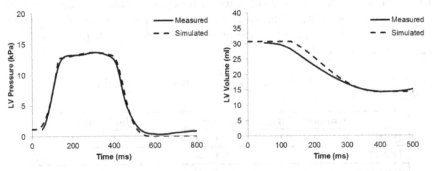

Fig. 4. Pressure and volume time courses during systole for one of the dogs (D0912). The active tension and the circulation parameters were adjusted to match these time-courses.

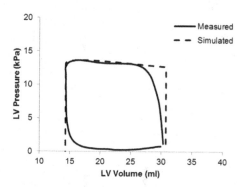

Fig. 5. Simulated PV loop using a circulation model during systole compared to the measured data for one of the dogs (D0912)

The end-systolic geometry from the two different systolic loading methods was compared to the geometry obtained from fitting the surfaces to end-systolic image data (Fig. 6). The epicardial and endocardial surfaces were within 10% of the measured data, with maximum deviation near the base for the method using the circulation model since the basal displacements were not specified. For the method where the displacements were specified, the deviations from the surface were smaller at the base. The end-systolic volumes for the cavity and wall obtained from the two different methods are within 10% of the measured data (Table 3).

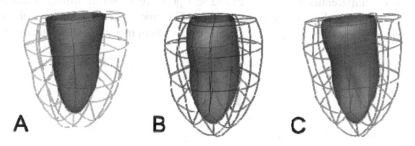

Fig. 6. End-systolic geometries for one dog (D0912) obtained from measured surfaces (A), from simulation using the circulation model (B), from simulation using prescribed pressure and volume (C)

Table 3. Comparison of end-systolic volume between the different methods

End-Systolic Volume (ml)	Measured	Circulation Model	Prescribed Pressure
LV Cavity	14.1	15.3	14.3
LV Wall	42.3	40.4	38.5

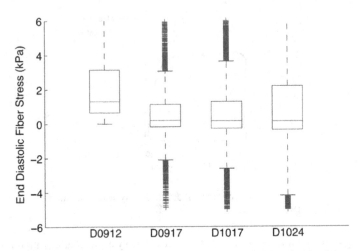

Fig. 7. Box plot of end diastolic fiber stress distribution for the 4 dogs

The fiber stresses at end-diastole (Fig. 7) and end-systole (Fig. 8) were computed by applying the appropriate pressure boundary conditions to the respective equilibrium geometries. The box-plots show the stress distribution with the 25th, 50th and 75th percentile shown as horizontal lines within the respective boxes. The resulting stress distribution shows that the fiber stresses are less than 3kPa at end-diastole similar to values of circumferential stress in a cylindrical pressure vessel of similar thickness and diameter at end-diastolic internal pressure. The fiber stresses at end-systole are higher due to active stresses generated by the myocardium that cause the contraction.

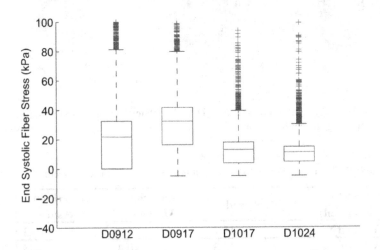

Fig. 8. Box plot of end systolic fiber stress distribution for the 4 dogs

4   Discussion

In reality, there are residual stresses present in the heart. The numerical method employed (finite elasticity) requires a reference state that is unstressed and unloaded, even in the case when residual stresses would have been included. However, the presence of residual stresses might change the displacements of the material points during systole. This might be one of the reasons for the discrepancy between the model and the measured images.

For passive material parameter estimation, we have assumed that the anisotropy of the material remains the same as it is during bi-axial testing. As a result, we kept the ratio of the stress scaling coefficients to the exponents the same. This reduces the number of parameters to be estimated and improves the confidence in the estimated parameters, especially when only global measurements such as pressure and volume are available. However, with the availability of 3D strain measurements *in-vivo*, it may be possible to separately estimate each of the parameters using the strain information from the fiber and cross-fiber directions.

For active material parameter estimation, having a physiological active force generation that includes length-tension relationship and the force-velocity relationship for cardiac muscles coupled to a circulation model could provide realistic pressure-volume curves. However, estimating the extra parameters might be difficult without prior knowledge of the behavior of these models. In the presence of pressure and volume data, directly prescribing the active force to obtain a geometry that matches the volume under prescribed pressure boundary conditions might provide a better estimate of the regional material point displacements and the overall contractility of the heart. This might be useful in certain disease conditions when the contractility of the heart changes.

Acknowledgements. The methods and simulations in this paper were performed using Continuity 6.4b (r8149). We would like to thank Jeff Van Dorn for providing us with technical support for the software.

References

1. Lumens, J., Delhaas, T., Kirn, B., Arts, T.: Three-wall segment (TriSeg) model describing mechanics and hemodynamics of ventricular interaction. Annals of Biomedical Engineering 37, 2234–2255 (2009)
2. Wang, V.Y., Lam, H.I., Ennis, D.B., Cowan, B.R., Young, A.A., Nash, M.P.: Modelling passive diastolic mechanics with quantitative MRI of cardiac structure and function. Medical Image Analysis 13, 773–784 (2009)
3. Trayanova, N.: Whole heart modeling. Circulation Research 108, 113–128 (2011)
4. Aguado-Sierra, J., Krishnamurthy, A., Villongco, C., Chuang, J., Howard, E., Gonzales, M.J., Omens, J., Krummen, D.E., Narayan, S., Kerckhoffs, R.C.P., et al.: Patient-Specific Modeling of Dyssynchronous Heart Failure: A Case Study. Progress in Biophysics and Molecular Biology (2011)

5. Niederer, S.A., Plank, G., Chinchapatnam, P., Ginks, M., Lamata, P., Rhode, K.S., Rinaldi, C.A., Razavi, R., Smith, N.P.: Length-dependent tension in the failing heart and the efficacy of cardiac resynchronization therapy. Cardiovascular Research **89**, 336–343 (2011)

6. Neal, M.L., Kerckhoffs, R.: Current progress in patient-specific modeling. Briefings in Bioinformatics **11**, 111 (2010)

7. Lumens, J., Blanchard, D.G., Arts, T., Mahmud, E., Delhaas, T.: Left ventricular underfilling and not septal bulging dominates abnormal left ventricular filling hemodynamics in chronic thromboembolic pulmonary hypertension. American Journal of Physiology-Heart and Circulatory Physiology **299**, H1083 (2010)

8. Sermesant, M., Peyrat, J.M., Chinchapatnam, P., Billet, F., Mansi, T., Rhode, K., Delingette, H., Razavi, R., Ayache, N.: Toward patient-specific myocardial models of the heart. Heart Failure Clinics **4**, 289–301 (2008)

9. Krishnamurthy, A., Villongco, C.T., Chuang, J., Frank, L.R., Nigam, V., Belezzuoli, E., Stark, P., Krummen, D.E., Narayan, S., Omens, J.H., McCulloch, A.D., Kerckhoffs, R.C.: Patient-Specific Models of Cardiac Biomechanics. Journal of Computational Physics **244**, 4–21 (2013)

10. Holzapfel, G.A., Ogden, R.W.: Constitutive modelling of passive myocardium: a structurally based framework for material characterization. Philosophical Transactions A **367**, 3445 (2009)

11. Costa, K., Hunter, P., Wayne, J., Waldman, L., Guccione, J., McCulloch, A.: A three-dimensional finite element method for large elastic deformations of ventricular myocardium: II—prolate spheroidal coordinates. Journal of Biomechanical Engineering **118**, 464 (1996)

12. Zhang, Y., Liang, X., Ma, J., Jing, Y., Gonzales, M.J., Villongco, C., Krishnamurthy, A., Frank, L.R., Nigam, V., Stark, P., Narayan, S.M., McCulloch, A.D.: An atlas-based geometry pipeline for cardiac Hermite model construction and diffusion tensor reorientation. Medical Image Analysis **16**, 1130–1141 (2012)

13. Gonzales, M.J., Sturgeon, G., Krishnamurthy, A., Hake, J., Jonas, R., Stark, P., Rappel, W.J., Narayan, S.M., Zhang, Y., Segars, W.P., McCulloch, A.D.: A three-dimensional finite element model of human atrial anatomy: new methods for cubic Hermite meshes with extraordinary vertices. Medical Image Analysis **17**, 525–537 (2013)

14. Arsigny, V., Fillard, P., Pennec, X., Ayache, N.: Log-Euclidean metrics for fast and simple calculus on diffusion tensors. Magnetic Resonance in Medicine: Official Journal of the Society of Magnetic Resonance in Medicine / Society of Magnetic Resonance in Medicine **56**, 411–421 (2006)

15. Walker, J.C., Ratcliffe, M.B., Zhang, P., Wallace, A.W., Fata, B., Hsu, E.W., Saloner, D., Guccione, J.M.: MRI-based finite-element analysis of left ventricular aneurysm. American Journal of Physiology-Heart and Circulatory Physiology **289**, H692 (2005)

16. Sermesant, M., Razavi, R.: Personalized computational models of the heart for cardiac resynchronization therapy. Patient-Specific Modeling of the Cardiovascular System, 167–182 (2010)

17. Rajagopal, V., Chung, J., Nielsen, P., Nash, M.: Finite element modelling of breast biomechanics: directly calculating the reference state. In: 28th Annual International Conference of the IEEE Engineering in Medicine and Biology Society, EMBS 2006, pp. 420–423 (2006)

18. Nordsletten, D.A., Niederer, S.A., Nash, M.P., Hunter, P.J., Smith, N.P.: Coupling multiphysics models to cardiac mechanics. Progress in Biophysics and Molecular Biology **104**, 77–88 (2011)

19. Yin, F.C.P., Strumpf, R.K., Chew, P.H., Zeger, S.L.: Quantification of the mechanical properties of noncontracting canine myocardium under simultaneous biaxial loading. Journal of Biomechanics **20**, 577–589 (1987)
20. Dokos, S., Smaill, B.H., Young, A.A., LeGrice, I.J.: Shear properties of passive ventricular myocardium. American Journal of Physiology-Heart and Circulatory Physiology **283**, H2650 (2002)
21. Kerckhoffs, R.C.P., Neal, M.L., Gu, Q., Bassingthwaighte, J.B., Omens, J.H., McCulloch, A.D.: Coupling of a 3D finite element model of cardiac ventricular mechanics to lumped systems models of the systemic and pulmonic circulation. Annals of Biomedical Engineering **35**, 1–18 (2007)

Evaluation of Personalised Canine Electromechanical Models

Sophie Giffard-Roisin[1]([✉]), Stéphanie Marchesseau[2], Loïc Le Folgoc[1], Hervé Delingette[1], and Maxime Sermesant[1]

[1] Inria, Asclepios Research Project, Sophia Antipolis, France
`sophie.giffard-roisin@inria.fr`
[2] Clinical Imaging Research Centre, NUS-ASTAR, Singapore, Singapore

Abstract. Cardiac modelling aims at understanding cardiac diseases and predicting cardiac responses to therapies. By generating the electrical propagation, the contraction and the mechanical response, we are able to simulate cardiac motion from non-invasive imaging techniques. Four healthy canine clinical data (left ventricles) were provided by the STACOM'2014 challenge. Our study is based on Bestel-Clement-Sorine mechanical modelling, while the electrophysiological phenomena is driven by an Eikonal model. Our model has been calibrated by a quantitative sensitivity study as well as a personalized automatic calibration. Results and comparison with clinical measures are shown in terms of left ventricular volume, flow, pressure and ejection fraction.

1 Introduction

Cardiac modelling aims at understanding cardiac diseases (such as heart failure, desynchronization or tachycardia) and predicting cardiac responses to treatment or therapies (as cardiac resynchronization therapy or radiofrequency ablation). The goal is to help cardiologists in detecting anomalies, planning interventions, and selecting suitable patients for a given therapy. Cardiac modelling is driven by the assumption that the electromechanical response of the heart can be simulated from anatomical and physiological data.

Heartbeat is initiated by an electrical wave that propagates through the myocardium, activating mechanical contraction at a microscopic scale. A suitable model needs to take into account the anatomical structure, the electrical propagation, as well as the mechanical function of the heart.

Our study is based on an Eikonal model [3] for the simulation of the electrophysiological system, while the active and passive mechanical behavior is defined by the Bestel-Clement-Sorine modelling as formulated in [1]. The latter ensures to take into account the microscopic scale phenomena of the contraction as well as laws of thermodynamics.

The coupled electro-mechanical simulation of the cardiac system is implemented within the SOFA platform[1]. The simulations were performed on healthy

---

[1] SOFA is an Open Source medical simulation software available at
http://www.sofa-framework.org

© Springer International Publishing Switzerland 2015
O. Camara et al. (Eds.): STACOM 2014, LNCS 8896, pp. 74–82, 2015.
DOI: 10.1007/978-3-319-14678-2_8

canine clinical data, provided by the STACOM'2014 challenge. They include Left Ventricular (LV) geometry, LV volume and LV pressure curves, as well as myocardial fibre directions.

2   Models and Methods

Canine and human hearts have close anatomical structures, that is why the canine heart is often used in pre-clinical studies. Both anatomies are composed of two ventricles, left (LV) and right (RV), and two atria. The heart function is mainly driven by the LV, acting like a pump to send the blood to the body. The system studied here is composed of a healthy canine left ventricle. In order to run the electrical and the mechanical cardiac models, input such as anatomical meshes and fibre directions have been processed.

2.1   Geometry Processing

Myocardial Mesh Generation. The myocardium mesh is generated using CGAL[2] meshing software, to create a tetrahedral mesh from medical image segmentations. The geometry is computed at end diastole (ED). The number of elements is roughly 50K, so that the average edge length is close to 1.5mm. This refinement ensures to have enough elements in the thickness of the muscle to describe the anisotropy (at least 5 layers transmurally) while limiting computation time.

In addition to the volumetric mesh segmentation, endocardial (inner lining) and epicardial (outer layer) surface zones are manually delineated, as illustrated in Fig. 1(a). These surface zones are useful for the electrical as well as for the mechanical simulations (Sec. 2.2).

For a single left ventricular model we consider that the contraction of the left ventricle does not depend on that of the RV as a first approximation. We depart from classic anatomical terminology in identifying the epicardium with the outer layer of the left ventricle segmentation.

Pericardium Surface Generation. Our model incorporates boundary conditions that faithfully replicate anatomical constraints on the motion of the heart. Specifically, the pericardial membrane is modelled as a fixed surface around the epicardium as in [2], and was obtained by dilating the segmentation from the diastasis phase of 1.5 mm, see Fig. 1(b)). The SOFA simulation platform allows for realistic collision constraints between the myocardium and the surrounding pericardium, which limits radial motion but also global translations. We model the presence of the RV as part of a pericardium membrane surrounding the LV. This is motivated by the fact that the pressure applied by the RV on the external wall of the LV could be approximated by a rigid constraint.

---

[2] CGAL is a Computational Geometry Algorithms Library, available at www.cgal.org.

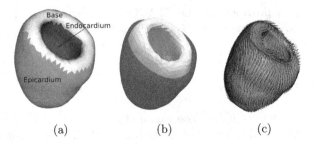

Fig. 1. Geometry and fibres processing: Identification of the surface zones of the LV myocardium mesh (a), pericardium surface membrane (b) and fibre directions from DTI imaging (c)

Fibre Directions. The myocardium is organized in muscle fibres which govern the electric propagation as well as the anisotropic contraction. The anisotropic tensor at each position can be measured via DTI imaging, and the principal directions (from eigen value decomposition) generate an approximation of the fibre directions. They are displayed in Fig. 1(c).

2.2 Electro-mechanical Modelling: SOFA Software

The pipeline efficiently couples the simulation of the electrophysiology and mechanics of the heart in the SOFA platform. The electrical wave propagation is simulated in the ED configuration, during the first step of the cardiac cycle. The mechanical contraction and relaxation of the myocardium are simultaneously computed from the depolarization times output by the electrical simulation, taking into account the different forces and boundary conditions. The pipeline is summarized in Fig. 2.

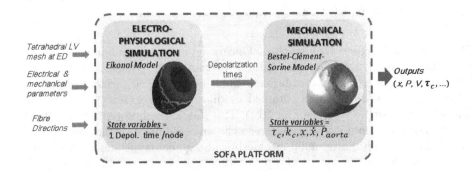

Fig. 2. Complete electromechanical pipeline. A single simulation computes simultaneously the electrical and the mechanical modellings.

Electrophysiological Simulation: Eikonal Model. The electrophysiological pattern of activity is simulated using an Eikonal model, describing the depolarization front propagation. The depolarization times T_d at each node of the mesh are estimated by solving the Eikonal equation $v\sqrt{\nabla T_d^t \mathbf{D} \nabla T_d} = 1$ using a Multi-Front Fast Marching Method [3]. v is the local conduction velocity, set here uniformly to 500 mm/s. D is the anisotropic tensor, with an anisotropic ratio of 0.1 between the fibre direction and the perpendicular directions, and with local fibre directions estimated according to section 2.1.

The initialization of the electric wave is set on the LV endocardial surface (see Fig. 1(a)), to simulate a simultaneous activation pattern of the endocardium from the extremities of the Purkinje network.

Mechanical Simulation: Bestel-Clement-Sorine Model. Our study is based on Bestel-Clement-Sorine (BCS) mechanical modelling as formulated by [1], improved and implemented on the SOFA platform by [2]. The BCS model is compatible with the laws of thermodynamics and it is based on the microscopic scale phenomena.

It is composed of a passive hyperelastic part described as a Mooney Rivlin material, that accounts for the elasticity. The stress along the cardiac fibres is decomposed into two parts. An active part models the contraction (binding/unbinding of actin-myosin filaments) together with an energy dissipation due to friction, and a parallel passive part corresponds to the elastic bound. The model is further improved by taking into account the circulation model representing the 4 phases of the cardiac cycle. Especially, the aortic pressure is modelled following a 2-parameter Winkessel model.

The BCS model is in particular able to capture the Starling effect (adaptation of the contraction enabling the stroke volume to compensate the end-diastolic volume) and the unbinding due to a too high relative speed between actin and myosin, with a constant α related to the cross-bridge release. For more details on the mechanical model, refer to [2].

3   Parameter Estimation

We use the approach described in [2] to estimate the parameters on canine hearts. Note that [2] was used to estimate parameters on human data and therefore cannot be applied as it is since the geometry, the cardiac period and the mechanical materials are different. A complete sensitivity study and a personalized calibration of the most relevant parameters have been performed.

3.1   Sensitivity Study

The parameters of the model are summarized in Tab. 1. The electrophysiological model is governed by a simple law, and has therefore mainly three parameters (once fibre directions and initial conditions are set), the local conduction velocity v, the anisotropic ratio A and the action potential duration ($APDs$).

For the mechanical part, the parameters can be separated in 3 groups: parameters related to the active contraction, parameters related to the passive material, and parameters related to the heamodynamic model.

Starting from the results of [2], a quantitative study has been performed in order to estimate the range of possible values of each parameter of Tab. 1. We used pressure and volume observations to control the simulation. Some parameters do not impact significantly the simulation, as the maximum stiffness k_0. Others are easily calibrated, because they are visually perceptible, as the APD.

Table 1. Parameters of the electro-mechanical model for the 4 cases

	Parameter Name	Unit	case 1	case 2	case 3	case 4
	A (Anisotropic Ratio)		0.1	0.1	0.1	0.1
Electric Part	v (Local Conduction Velocity)	$mm.s^{-1}$	500	500	500	500
	APD (Action Pot. Duration)	s	0.18	0.18	0.20	0.24
	σ_0 (Max Contraction)	MPa	30	29	20	21
	k_0 (Max Stiffness)	MPa	6	6	6	6
	k_{ATP} (Contraction Rate)	s^{-1}	40	40	40	40
	k_{RS} (Relaxation Rate)	s^{-1}	90	90	90	90
Contraction	E (Linear Modulus)	MPa	5	5	5	5
	α (Cross-bridges Unfasten Rate)		0.8	0.8	0.8	0.8
	μ (Viscosity)	$MPa.s$	0.32	0.32	0.5	0.49
	n_0 (Reduc. factor, Starling effect)		0.5	0.5	0.5	0.5
Passive Mat.	$c1, c2$ (Mooney-R. Modulus)	kPa	50	50	50	50
	K (Bulk Modulus)	MPa	1.7	1.7	2	1.9
Windkessel	Rp (Wind. Resistance)	$MPa.m^{-3}.s$	179	250	310	430
	τ (Wind. Charact. Time)	s	0.22	0.16	0.23	0.56

3.2 Mechanical Parameters Calibration: Unscented Transform Algorithm

The most influential and independent parameters identified as $[\sigma, \mu, K]$ have been calibrated for each heart using the Unscented Transform Algorithm [4]. The algorithm, derived from the Unscented Transform according to [2], calculates a set of n parameters of a nonlinear transformation that minimizes the difference between the measured observations and the predicted observations. Once having performed $2n+1$ simulations using some specific parameter values, the algorithm runs in one iteration. In our case, the observations are the minimal LV outgoing blood flow and the ejection fraction. LV outgoing flow is calculated as $-dV/dt$, with V the LV volume.

Independently, the Unscented Transform algorithm was used to calibrate the 2-parameter Windkessel model using the ground truth pressure curves.

4   Results

4.1   Clinical Data

The STACOM 2014 challenge revolves on data acquired on 4 healthy canine hearts. They include LV geometry and fibre directions. The 4 dogs were paced at 500ms basic cycle length. The tetrahedral mesh is constructed from binary images of the LV at ED.

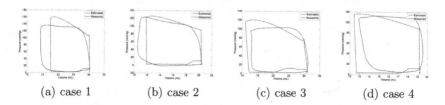

| (a) case 1 | (b) case 2 | (c) case 3 | (d) case 4 |

Fig. 3. Comparison between LV pressure volume diagrams computed from simulations (red) and ground truth measures (blue)

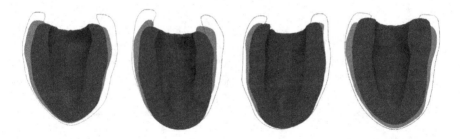

Fig. 4. Simulated end-systolic geometry (red) of the LV of the 4 cases and ground truth (blue). The dark blue line represents the initial position (ED).

4.2   Current Results

We give the results of the 4 canine simulations in terms of LV pressure volume diagrams (Fig. 3), LV volume, LV outgoing flow curves (Fig. 5) and ejection fractions (Tab.2). Comparison is made with the ground truth data, as LV volume and LV pressure curves were provided by the STACOM'2014 challenge for a complete cycle. We are displaying here the second cycle of the simulation, in order to avoid the wrong initial conditions.

The simulated geometry of the 4 cases at ES is shown in Fig. 4. The ground truth end-systolic position is shown in blue while red is the simulation. The dark blue line represents the initial position (ED).

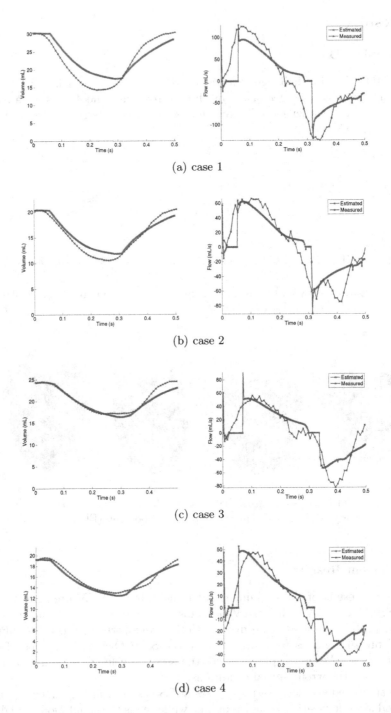

Fig. 5. Comparison between LV volume and outgoing flow (as $-dV/dt$) variations over one cardiac cycle computed from simulations (red) and ground truth measures (blue)

4.3   Discussion and Improvements

This first study shows promising results: the LV pressure volume diagrams and volume variations comparison indicate a realistic response of the model. Furthermore, the large variability of ejection fraction is reproduced in our results. We can also see from the slices of Fig. 4 that the modelled ventricle has a realistic movement (note the correct apico-basal shortening). However, the myocardium wall thickness variation is not completely reproduced, corresponding to a simulated muscle not incompressible enough.

Table 2. Comparison between ejection fractions computed from the simulations and the ground truth measures

Ejection fraction	case 1	case 2	case 3	case 4
Measured (%)	53	49	30	34
Estimated (%)	43	42	33	36

The calibration of a model of a standard case is the first step towards the prediction of its response to treatments and therapies. Since our model is driven by faithful anatomical constraints and mechanical laws, we are confident in the fact that such a model will be able to realistically simulate pathology cases and predict their responses to treatments.

5   Conclusions

In this paper we have adapted an electro-mechanical cardiac modelling to canine hearts. From the geometry of the left ventricle in end diastole and the heart period and the fibre directions, we are able to simulate heart movement over the whole cardiac cycle. The quantitative validation (results of the STACOM'2014 challenge) is comforting the tendency of the global indicators: the displacement fields obtained with the simulations and the displacement fields obtained by tagged MRI provided by the STACOM'2014 challenge are in good agreement.

Acknowledgments. The research leading to these results has received funding from the EU FP7 grants VP2HF (611823) and MedYMA (ERC 2011-291080). The authors would also like to thank Vicky Wang and the whole LV Mechanics challenge organization.

References

1. Chapelle, D., Le Tallec, P., Moireau, P., Sorine, M.: Energy-preserving muscle tissue model: formulation and compatible discretizations. International Journal for Multiscale Computational Engineering **10**(2) (2012)
2. Marchesseau, S., Delingette, H., Sermesant, M., Ayache, N.: Fast parameter calibration of a cardiac electromechanical model from medical images based on the unscented transform. Biomechanics and Modeling in Mechanobiology **12**(4), 815–831 (2013)
3. Sermesant, M., Konukoukoglu, E., Delingette, H., Coudière, Y., Chinchapatnam, P.P., Rhode, K.S., Razavi, R.S., Ayache, N.: An anisotropic multi-front fast marching method for real-time simulation of cardiac electrophysiology. In: Sachse, F.B., Seemann, G. (eds.) FIHM 2007. LNCS, vol. 4466, pp. 160–169. Springer, Heidelberg (2007)
4. Julier, S.J., Uhlmann, J.K.: A new extension of the Kalman filter to nonlinear systems. In: Int. Symp. Aerospace/defense Sensing, Simul. and Controls, vol. 3(26), p. 3.2, April 1997

Connection Forms for Beating the Heart
LV Mechanics Challenge (Methods)

Arthur Mensch[1], Emmanuel Piuze[1], Lucas Lehnert[1], Adrianus J. Bakermans[2], Jon Sporring[3], Gustav J. Strijkers[2], and Kaleem Siddiqi[1] (✉)

[1] School of Computer Science and Centre for Intelligent Machines,
McGill University, Montreal, Canada
siddiqi@cim.mcgill.ca
[2] Academic Medical Center,
University of Amsterdam Medical Center and Department of Biomedical Engineering,
Eindhoven University of Technology, Eindhoven, Netherlands
[3] Department of Computer Science, University of Copenhagen,
Copenhagen, Denmark

Abstract. We combine recent work on modeling cardiac mechanics using a finite volume method with the insight that heart wall myofiber orientations exhibit a particular volumetric geometry. In our finite volume mechanical simulation we use Maurer-Cartan one-forms to add a geometrical consistency term to control the rate at which myofiber orientation changes in the direction perpendicular to the heart wall. This allows us to estimate material properties related to both the passive and active parameters in our model. We have obtained preliminary results on the 4 canine datasets of the 2014 mechanics challenge using the FEBio software suite. In ongoing work we are validating and improving the model using rat heart (ex-vivo DTI and in-vivo tagging) MRI datasets, from which we have estimated strain tensors.

1 Introduction

A detailed understanding of cardiac mechanics is important for the evaluation of cardiomyopathy. In this paper we model heart wall mechanics by adopting the passive constitutive model in [1, 2] while incorporating a more recent active stress model [3] and augmenting this with a geometrical consistency term described using differential 1-forms. The geometrical term allows us to locally control the rate at which myofiber orientation changes in the direction perpendicular to the heart wall. The key idea is to control this rate so that the transmural fiber organization is approximately preserved through the beat cycle. Our approach is motivated by evidence that myofiber orientations lie on a minimal surface [4] and exhibit a particular volumetric geometry.

We have tested a preliminary version of these ideas using the FEBio software suite developed jointly by the University of Utah and Columbia University, which is made available to the public (see http://febio.org/febio/). Our simulations using the 4 canine datasets of the LV mechanics challenge yield plausible positional coordinates for the epicardium and the endocardium, left ventricular wall volumes

© Springer International Publishing Switzerland 2015
O. Camara et al. (Eds.): STACOM 2014, LNCS 8896, pp. 83–92, 2015.
DOI: 10.1007/978-3-319-14678-2_9

which approximately match the ground truth, and acceptable fiber stresses. In ongoing work we are further developing the model using the rat heart (DTI and tagging MRI) datasets of [4] from which we have estimated strain tensors.

We discuss our model of heart wall contraction in Sec. 2 and then describe the FEBio based simulation results in Sec. 3. We conclude with a brief presentation of the 2D tagging results in Sec. 4 which we are working on to improve the model.

2   Simulating Heart Wall Contraction

A model of the continuum mechanics of the heart wall should take into account various phenomena in heart tissue. During the half beat cycle (end-diastole to end-systole), heart fibers contract, and the myocardium reacts to this contraction according to its constitutive behavior, enforcing quasi-incompressibility. Moreover, geometrical constraints involving fiber orientation must be enforced for the movement to be coherent with geometrical modelling of the heart.

2.1   Numerical Methods

The continuum mechanics of the heart wall have been modeled ubiquitously using *finite element methods* (FEM) in a variety of applications [2,3,5]. However, finite element approaches, which essentially compute a discretised displacement that satisfies a variational principle, are mostly suited for static analysis of materials. For this reason, we apply *finite volume methods* (FVM) to simulate our material. This method, commonly used for fluid dynamics computation, has been applied to biomaterials in [6,7]. It simulates the movement of a mesh along time by computing forces applied to each vertex at each timestep, given the deformation map at the previous timestep. The FVM pipeline for simulation is described in Alg. 1, where we define time t, base configuration state $\boldsymbol{X}$, deformed state $\boldsymbol{x}(\boldsymbol{X}, t)$, spatial deformation gradient $\boldsymbol{F}(\boldsymbol{X}) = \frac{\partial \boldsymbol{x}}{\partial \boldsymbol{X}}$, and first Piola-Kirchhoff stress tensor $\boldsymbol{P} = \boldsymbol{P}(F)$.

2.2   Stress Calculation

We consider the heart wall to be hyper-elastic, which allows us to define a strain energy Ψ. In order to model passive behavior while enforcing geometric constraints on the heart displacement, we write :

$$\Psi_P = \Psi_H + \Psi_G \tag{1}$$

where Ψ_H models an hyper-elastic passive material and Ψ_G is a penalty term that forces the fibers to keep a certain structure. We then recall

$$\boldsymbol{P}_P = \frac{\partial \Psi_P}{\partial \boldsymbol{F}} \tag{2}$$

where $\boldsymbol{P}_P$ is the passive first Piola-Kirchhoff stress tensor. We then model active behavior using

$$\boldsymbol{P} = \boldsymbol{P}_P + \boldsymbol{P}_A = \boldsymbol{P}_H + \boldsymbol{P}_G + \boldsymbol{P}_A, \tag{3}$$

where $\boldsymbol{P}_A$ (which cannot be derived from a strain energy in general) represents the forces that are applied by the heart fibers to the heart tissue.

Algorithm 1. FVM simulation pipeline

Require: tetrahedral mesh of the heart, boundary conditions, initial transform F_0
  set boundary conditions on faces and vertices, for forces or displacement
  for all $T \in tetrahedrons$ **do**
      apply $F_0(T)$ to T
      update T.vertices
      update $F(T)$
  end for
  for t from t_{ED} to t_{ES} **do**
      for all $T \in tetrahedrons$ **do**
          $P \leftarrow P(F(T))$
          for all $v \in T.vertices$ **do**
              compute $f_{i,T}$ from P and boundary conditions
              update $f_{i,T}$ for physical coherence (incompressibility, collision detection)
          end for
      end for
      update $T.vertices$
      update $F(T)$
  end for

Passive Response. We use the state-of-the-art Holzapfel and Ogden [2] constitutive relation for the heart wall. This relation links Ψ_P to the right Cauchy-Green deformation tensor C and the local orientation of the fiber, given in original configuration by the vectors f_0, s_0, n_0, and models an orthotropic Neo-Hookean material. In this framework, it has been shown that Ψ_P can be written as a function of: $I_1 = tr(C)$, $I_{4i} = i_0 C i_0$ and $I_{8fs} = f_0 C s_0$. The explicit form of Ψ_H is then

$$\Psi_H = \frac{a}{2b} \exp(b\,(I_1 - 3)) + \sum_{i=f,s} \frac{a_i}{2b_i} \left(\exp\left(b_i\,(I_{4i} - 1)^2 \right) - 1 \right)$$
$$+ \frac{a_{fs}}{2b_{fs}} \left(\exp\left(b_{fs} I_{8fs}^2 \right) - 1 \right). \tag{4}$$

The following Cauchy stress defining an incompressible fibrous material is then used, with $i = F i_0$:

$$J\sigma_H = 2\Psi_1 B + 2\Psi_2 \left(I_1 B - B^2 \right) - pI + 2\Psi_{4f} f \otimes f + 2\Psi_{4s} s \otimes s$$
$$+ \Psi_{8fs} \left(f \otimes s + s \otimes f \right) + \Psi_{8fn} \left(f \otimes n + n \otimes f \right), \tag{5}$$

using the notation $\Psi_i \equiv \frac{\partial \Psi}{\partial I_i}$, and defining p as to preserve incompressibility of the material (we compute p within the pipeline described in Algorithm 1. This yields, as shown in [3]:

$$P_H = a\exp(b\,(I_1 - 3))F - pJF^{-T} + 2a_f\,(I_{4f} - 1) \exp\left(b_f\,(I_{4f} - 1)^2 \right) f \otimes f_0$$
$$+ 2a_s\,(I_{4s} - 1) \exp\left(b_s\,(I_{4s} - 1)^2 \right) s \otimes s_0$$
$$+ a_{fs} I_{8fs} \exp\left(b_{fs} I_{8fs}^2 \right) (f \otimes s_0 + s \otimes f_0). \tag{6}$$

Active Response. This involves the addition of contractive forces P_A to the passive P_P stress tensor, defined in (6), during the contraction period. The scale at which FVM computations are performed admits a simplification of these contractile forces; they can be formulated as a function of the deformation gradient F, and of the fiber direction f. We follow [3] and write the active stress tensor as:

$$P_A = T_a f \otimes f_0 \tag{7}$$

where T_a depends on contraction ratio λ and can be computed from various biochemical studies, including [8].

2.3   Geometrical Strain

Groups of muscle fibers are known to preserve certain local geometrical invariants during the beat cycle. For example, the total transmural change in the helix angle is approximately preserved while the heart wall thickens. Our goal is to reformulate such an invariant in such a way that it can be coupled with our FVM simulation.

Motivated by [9] and [4], the method of moving frames is applied to describe the local geometry of bundles of cardiomyocytes, shown to be consistent across different subjects and species. Let a point $x \in \mathbf{R}^3$ be expressed in terms of the natural frame field e_1, e_2, e_3, such that $x = \sum_i x_i e_i$. A differential orthonormal frame field embedded in $\mathbf{R}^3$ will be denoted as $(f_1, f_2, f_3) : \mathbf{R}^3 \to \mathbf{R}^3$, where $f_i \cdot f_j = \delta_{ij}$, and $f_1 \times f_2 = f_3$, and where $\cdot$ is the inner product, δ_{ij} is the Kronecker delta, and $\times$ is the 3-dimensional cross product. A frame field can be expressed as a rotation of the natural frame field, $f_i = \sum_j a_{ij} e_j$, where the attitude matrix $A = \{a_{ij}\}$ is a differentiable matrix field such that $a_{ij} : \mathbf{R}^3 \to \mathbf{R}$ are differentiable functions,

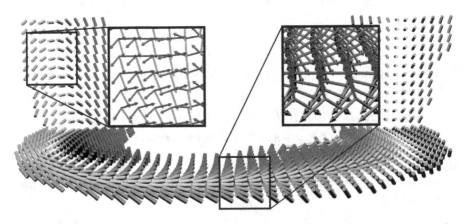

Fig. 1. Principal fiber direction and cardiac frame field f_1 (red), f_2 (green), and f_3 (blue) for a rat's heart from [4]. Here, the base is located upwards and the apex downwards. Color coding indicates the helix angle of the fiber direction, from $-90°$ (green) to $+90°$ (red).

and $\boldsymbol{A}^{-1} = \boldsymbol{A}^T$. Since each $\boldsymbol{e}_i$ is constant, the differential geometry of the frame field is completely characterized by the attitude matrix $\boldsymbol{A}$. Its differential structure yields [9] $\mathrm{d}\left[\boldsymbol{f}_1\ \boldsymbol{f}_2\ \boldsymbol{f}_3\right]^T = (\mathrm{d}\boldsymbol{A})\,\boldsymbol{A}^{-1}\left[\boldsymbol{f}_1\ \boldsymbol{f}_2\ \boldsymbol{f}_3\right]^T$ where d is the differential operator, and $(\mathrm{d}\boldsymbol{A})\,\boldsymbol{A}^{-1}$ is the Maurer-Cartan matrix of connection forms. The Maurer-Cartan matrix is skew symmetric, such that it has at most 3 independent, non-zero elements c_{12}, c_{13}, and c_{23} which express the initial rate of turn of the frame vector $\boldsymbol{f}_i$ towards $\boldsymbol{f}_j$ when moving in a general direction of $\boldsymbol{v}$. A linear model for the motion of a frame vector, when considering neighboring frames, can thus be expressed as a Taylor series

$$\boldsymbol{f}_i(\boldsymbol{x}_0 + \boldsymbol{v}) = \boldsymbol{f}_i(\boldsymbol{x}_0) + \mathrm{d}\boldsymbol{f}_i\langle\boldsymbol{v}\rangle + \mathcal{O}(\|\boldsymbol{v}\|^2), \tag{8}$$

where the differential $\mathrm{d}\boldsymbol{f}_i$ is taken at $\boldsymbol{x}_0$. Expressing the direction of motion as $\boldsymbol{v} = \sum_k v_k \boldsymbol{f}_k$, we have $\mathrm{d}\boldsymbol{f}_i\langle\boldsymbol{v}\rangle = \sum_{j\neq i} \boldsymbol{f}_j \sum_k v_k c_{ijk}$, using the short hand notation $c_{ijk} = c_{ij}\langle\boldsymbol{f}_k\rangle$. Since only 3 unique non-zero combinations of i, j are possible there are only 9 unique non-zero combinations of c_{ijk} possible. The contraction operation $c_{ij}\langle\boldsymbol{v}\rangle$ can be written to first order as $c_{ij}\langle\boldsymbol{v}\rangle = \nabla_v \boldsymbol{f}_i \cdot \boldsymbol{f}_j\big|_{\boldsymbol{x}}$, where $\boldsymbol{x} \in \mathbf{R}^3$ is the center of computation and $\nabla_v \boldsymbol{f}_i$ is the covariant derivative of $\boldsymbol{f}_i$ in the direction $\boldsymbol{v}$. In the case where $\boldsymbol{v} \equiv \boldsymbol{f}_k, k = 1, 2, 3$, we thus have

$$c_{ijk} \equiv c_{ij}\langle\boldsymbol{f}_k\rangle = \boldsymbol{f}_j^T\,\mathcal{J}_{\boldsymbol{f}_i}(x_1, x_2, x_3)\,\boldsymbol{f}_k, \tag{9}$$

where $\mathcal{J}_{\boldsymbol{f}_i}(x_1, x_2, x_3)$ is the Jacobian matrix of $\boldsymbol{f}_i$ in x_1, x_2, x_3.

We use a smooth and consistent choice of a local frame field throughout the heart wall. The first frame axis $\boldsymbol{f}_1$ corresponds to a clockwise turning of the local fiber orientation $\boldsymbol{u}_1$ with respect to the centroid of the left ventricle using the signed function $\nu(\boldsymbol{x}, \boldsymbol{u})$, where $\boldsymbol{x}$ is a point in the heart wall. We then estimate a transmural direction $\hat{\boldsymbol{f}}_3$ from the gradient of a distance transform produced as follows: a) the binary image (mask) of the heart is closed using mathematical morphological operations, b) the euclidean distance to the heart wall is evaluated at every point to both the epicardium and endocardium, and c) the endocardium gradient is negated and the average of the two gradients is then computed. The normals $\hat{\boldsymbol{f}}_3$ are then aligned to point from outer to inner wall. With $\boldsymbol{f}_1$ and $\hat{\boldsymbol{f}}_3$, a local frame is specified at $\boldsymbol{x}$,

$$\boldsymbol{f}_1 = \frac{\nu(\boldsymbol{x}, \boldsymbol{u}_1)\boldsymbol{u}_1}{\|\boldsymbol{u}_1\|}, \quad \boldsymbol{f}_3 = \frac{\left(\hat{\boldsymbol{f}}_3 - (\hat{\boldsymbol{f}}_3 \cdot \boldsymbol{f}_1)\boldsymbol{f}_1\right)}{\|\hat{\boldsymbol{f}}_3 - (\hat{\boldsymbol{f}}_3 \cdot \boldsymbol{f}_1)\boldsymbol{f}_1\|}, \quad \boldsymbol{f}_2 = \boldsymbol{f}_3 \times \boldsymbol{f}_1, \tag{10}$$

where $\boldsymbol{f}_3$ is the part of $\hat{\boldsymbol{f}}_3$ orthogonal to $\boldsymbol{f}_1$. Fig. 1 shows a sample of this frame field within two cross-sectional cardiac slices.

Figure 2 illustrates the behavior of the frame field for a selection of connection forms. One-form contractions c_{ijk} can be interpreted as the amount of turning of $\boldsymbol{f}_i$ towards $\boldsymbol{f}_j$ in the direction $\boldsymbol{f}_k$. For example, c_{123} describes a transmural rotation of $\boldsymbol{f}_1$ towards $\boldsymbol{f}_2$ when moving towards $\boldsymbol{f}_3$, as shown in Fig. 2b.

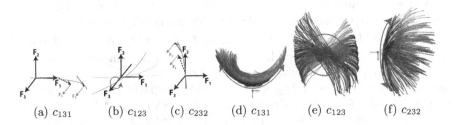

(a) c_{131} (b) c_{123} (c) c_{232} (d) c_{131} (e) c_{123} (f) c_{232}

Fig. 2. Examples of the geometry expressed by the connection forms c_{ijk}

Geometrical Energy. We use $\boldsymbol{f}_1$ as the local fiber direction and $\boldsymbol{f}_3$ as the local heart wall direction. Based on empirical studies, we find the total change of the transmural helix angle remain approximately constant at 120° during systole [10]. Locally, along a small distance dl, transmural helix angle α can be written [9] as $\alpha = c_{123}\,dl$. Therefore, we must have, for any transmural infinitesimal vector $\boldsymbol{v}(t) = l_3(t)\boldsymbol{f}_3$ at time t:

$$c_{123}(t + dt) \times l_3(t + dt) = c_{123}(t) \times l_3(t) \tag{11}$$

where $\boldsymbol{v}(t + dt) = \boldsymbol{F}\boldsymbol{v}(t)$. Differentiating this expression yields

$$d(\ln c_{123}) = -\frac{dl_3}{l_3} \tag{12}$$

Using the Green-Lagrange tensor $\boldsymbol{E} = \dfrac{1}{2}(\boldsymbol{F}\boldsymbol{F}^T - \boldsymbol{I})$, we reduce the right term of Eq. 12 and yields the constraints, using Eq. 9

$$0 = d(\ln c_{123}) + \boldsymbol{f}_3 \boldsymbol{E}\boldsymbol{f}_3, \text{ i.e.}$$
$$0 = d(\ln(\boldsymbol{f}_2^T \boldsymbol{J}_{\boldsymbol{f}_1}\boldsymbol{f}_3)) + \boldsymbol{f}_3 \boldsymbol{E}\boldsymbol{f}_3 \tag{13}$$

writing $\boldsymbol{J}_{\boldsymbol{f}_1}$ the spatial derivative (i.e. Jacobian matrix) of vector field $\boldsymbol{f}_1$.

Energy term. Following the classical way of pseudo enforcing a constraint with a Lagrangian multiplier penalty, we write

$$\Psi_{123} = \alpha_{123}(d(\ln(\boldsymbol{f}_2^T \boldsymbol{J}_{\boldsymbol{f}_1}\boldsymbol{f}_3)) + \boldsymbol{f}_3^T \boldsymbol{E}\boldsymbol{f}_3) \tag{14}$$

where α_{123} is a scalar measuring the amount of force that this energy will generate. We compute $d(\ln(\boldsymbol{f}_2^T \boldsymbol{J}_{\boldsymbol{f}_1}\boldsymbol{f}_3))$ by a finite difference of the term at $t + dt$ and the term at t. The energy term Ψ_{123} will only restrict motion in the local normal direction. It will effectively push against an excessive volumetric deformation, so as to ensure that transmural helix angle remains constant. Other geometrical energy terms could also be formulated in this fashion. For now, we set $\Psi_G = \Psi_{123}$.

3   Application to the LV Mechanics Challenge

The four canine datasets provided to participants of the challenge include material point positions (mesh node coordinates) at diastasis (DS), ex-vivo fiber orientations obtained using DTI registered to the DS volume, and ground truth node positions for 4 material points at the base of the heart along with pressure values within the left ventricle for about 40 frames covering the period from DS to end diastole (ED) to end systole (ES) (see Fig. 3). We have been working to implement the models described in the previous section within the framework of FEBio, a software suite developed jointly by the University of Utah and Columbia University, for finite element simulation of biomaterials: http://febio.org/febio/. The results we present here are preliminary and are based on a different model, the transversely-isotropic Mooney-Rivlin constitutive model, along with an active stress component. It also remains to examine the effect of the geometrical consistency term via simulation.

To set up the simulation within FEBio we took as input data the material node positions at DS, along with the fiber orientations registered to that volume as inputs. We also fed in the left ventricular cavity pressure values specified at each frame

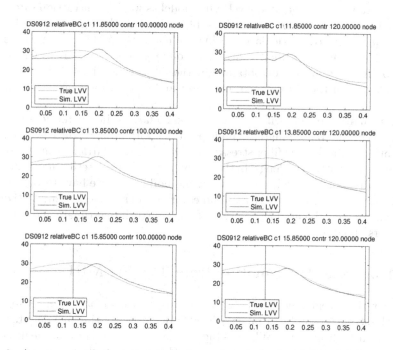

Fig. 3. A comparison of ground truth (green) and simulated (blue) left ventricular volumes for canine dataset 0912 for $c1$ stiffness parameters 11.85, 13.85 and 15.85 (rows 1 to 3) and contraction curve scaling parameters 100 and 120 (columns 1 and 2). The y-axis in each plot is the left ventricular volume in ml and the x-axis is time in seconds ($0s$ = DS; $0.13s$ = ED; $0.41s$ = ES). The plots show a qualitative agreement between the volume curves particularly during the contraction phase (ED $\rightarrow$ ES) over this range of parameters.

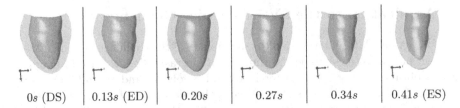

| 0s (DS) | 0.13s (ED) | 0.20s | 0.27s | 0.34s | 0.41s (ES) |

Fig. 4. Frames of the simulation for canine dataset 0912 corresponding to the parameters in the bottom left plot of Fig. 3. The frames illustrate the contraction of the left ventricle from ED to ES accompanied by the thickening of the myocardium, the lifting of the apex and the corresponding decrease in left ventricular volume.

of the heart beat cycle and the positional coordinates of the 4 points at the base of the left ventricle as fixed parameters to this model. The ground truth displacements were interpolated around the outer ring of points at the base, corresponding to the epicardium at that slice. The motion of all the other points was derived by the FEBio simulation. Our simulations showed that over a range of choices for stiffness parameters to the Mooney-Rivlin model as well as contraction rates, the left ventricular volumes were relatively stable and matched the given ground truth volumes qualitatively, particularly during the contraction phase from ED to ES (Fig. 3). The ground truth left ventricular volumes were used only to gauge the fidelity of the ejection fraction obtained by the simulation. Fig. 4 shows frames of the simulation for the stiffness parameter set at 15.85 with a contraction rate of 100.

Our simulation results will be discussed and analyzed in greater detail with a comparison of the tracked material node positions with ground truth as well as an examination of the derived fiber stresses at ED an ES, in an article being prepared by the organizers of the challenge. In the following section we describe another ongoing effort where, using the local frequency method of [11], we have recovered the (2D) deformation tensor in short-axis planes for a set of rat cine-tagging MRI data. The strain map can be used as a notion of ground truth to estimate and tune the parameters of our model.

4   Myocardial Deformation from Tagging MRI

We review the recent method of [11] for recovering the deformation tensor and from it the strain tensor, by estimating local frequencies from independent tagging sequences on rat heart data. Whereas tagging data is not provided in the mechanics challenge, this analysis can be used independently to tune the parameters of the model so that its behaviour is consistent with expected material properties.

In our case the tagging is in (2D) short axis planes, and we have two orthogonal tagging directions. The 2D Gabor transform in the continuous case is defined as [11]

$$G(\mathbf{p}, \omega) = \int_{\mathbb{R}^2} f(\mathbf{q})\overline{\psi(\mathbf{q} - \mathbf{p})}e^{-2\pi i(\mathbf{q} - \mathbf{p})\omega}d\mathbf{q}. \tag{15}$$

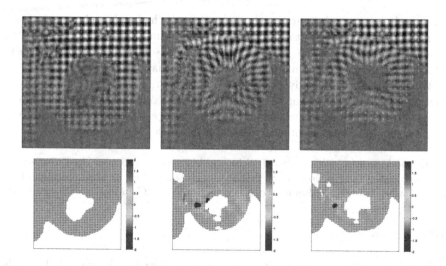

Fig. 5. Recovered deformation tensors applied to the horizontal (cyan) and vertical (yellow) tagging directions, with the corresponding strain tensors (relative to frame 1) shown below each frame. Frames 1 (0 ms), 9 (65 ms) and 17 (130 ms) are shown from top left to top right. See text for a discussion. (Best viewed by zooming in on the electronic version.)

Here f is the 2D tagging image, ψ is a windowing function with $\overline{\psi}$ denoting its complex conjugate, $\mathbf{p}, \mathbf{q}$ are position and ω is a frequency vector. The Gabor transform gives a spectrum for a neighborhood of each pixel. Since the tagging pattern deforms over time, the idea is to detect the most dominant non-zero frequency in the spectrum of each pixel and then track this frequency in time.

Once the most dominant frequency vector $\omega_t(i, j)$ is determined for each pixel (i, j) and each frame, the deformation tensor $\mathbf{F}$ is calculated. The deformation tensor relates to the frequency vector via

$$\omega_{t+1}(i, j) = \omega_t(i, j)\mathbf{F}^{-1}. \tag{16}$$

For smoothness we assume a symmetric deformation tensor and use the two orthogonal tagging sequences to solve for the three entries of $\mathbf{F}$ using GMRES [12]. As an initial guess the deformation tensor is set to the identity matrix (no deformation). To further improve the quality of the deformation tensor field and to account for noise (created by large deformations and tag fading) each entry of $\mathbf{F}$ was smoothed spatially using a Gaussian filter with $\sigma = 1$ and temporally with a Gaussian filter with $\sigma = 2.0$. Using the smoothed deformation tensor field, the Green Lagrange-Strain tensor can be calculated for every frame at every pixel location via $\mathbf{E} = \frac{1}{2}(\mathbf{F}^{\top}\mathbf{F} - \mathbf{I})$.

Fig. 5 shows tagging results on a rat data set from [4]. The recovered deformation tensor is applied to the horizontal (cyan) and vertical (yellow) tagging directions, which are then overlaid on the superposition of the two tagged images.

Below each tagging sub-figure we show the trace of the local strain tensor. Each strain map is relative to the tissue configuration in frame 1 and not to the previous frame. Regions with positive strain are in red, regions with negative strain are in blue and regions of low strain are in green (see colormap).

We intend to use the analysis above to tune the parameters of the model developed in Section 2. The essential idea is that in 2D axial slices the strain tensors resulting from the constitutive model with its passive, active and geometrical components, should be consistent with those obtained from tagging data.

Acknowledgments. We thank Jeff Weiss and his research group at the University of Utah for sharing the FEBio suite as well as providing guidance on the implementation of new material models within it. We are grateful to NSERC and FRQNT for support.

References

1. Wang, V.Y., Lam, H., Ennis, D.B., Cowan, B.R., Young, A.A., Nash, M.P.: Modelling passive diastolic mechanics with quantitative mri of cardiac structure and function. Medical Image Analysis **13**(5), 773–784 (2009)
2. Holzapfel, G.A., Ogden, R.W.: Biomechanical Modelling at the Molecular, Cellular, and Tissue Levels, vol. 508. Springer (2009)
3. Rossi, S., Ruiz-Baier, R., Pavarino, L.F., Quarteroni, A.: Orthotropic active strain models for the numerical simulation of cardiac biomechanics. International Journal for Numerical Methods in Biomedical Engineering **28**(6–7), 761–788 (2012)
4. Savadjiev, P., Strijkers, G.J., Bakermans, A.J., Piuze, E., Zucker, S.W., Siddiqi, K.: Heart wall myofibers are arranged in minimal surfaces to optimize organ function. Proc. Natl. Acad. Sci. USA **109**(24), 9248–9253 (2012)
5. Wang, H., Gao, H., Luo, X., Berry, C., Griffith, B., Ogden, R., Wang, T.: Structure-based finite strain modelling of the human left ventricle in diastole. International Journal for Numerical Methods in Biomedical Engineering **29**(1), 83–103 (2013)
6. Irving, G., Schroeder, C., Fedkiw, R.: Volume conserving finite element simulations of deformable models. ACM Transactions on Graphics (TOG) **26**, 13 (2007)
7. Sifakis, E., Barbic, J.: Fem simulation of 3d deformable solids: a practitioner's guide to theory, discretization and model reduction. In: ACM SIGGRAPH 2012 Courses, p. 20. ACM (2012)
8. Niederer, S., Hunter, P., Smith, N.: A quantitative analysis of cardiac myocyte relaxation: a simulation study. Biophysical Journal **90**(5), 1697–1722 (2006)
9. Piuze, E., Sporring, J., Siddiqi, K.: Moving frames for heart fiber geometry. In: Gee, J.C., Joshi, S., Pohl, K.M., Wells, W.M., Zöllei, L. (eds.) IPMI 2013. LNCS, vol. 7917, pp. 524–535. Springer, Heidelberg (2013)
10. Streeter, D., Bassett, D.: An engineering analysis of myocardial fiber orientation in pig's left ventricle in systole. The Anatomical Record **155**(4), 503–511 (2005)
11. Bruurmijn, L.C.M., Kause, H.B., Filatova, O.G., Duits, R., Fuster, A., Florack, L.M.J., van Assen, H.C.: Myocardial deformation from local frequency estimation in tagging mri. In: Ourselin, S., Rueckert, D., Smith, N. (eds.) FIMH 2013. LNCS, vol. 7945, pp. 284–291. Springer, Heidelberg (2013)
12. Golub, G.H., Van Loan, C.F.: Matrix Computations, 3rd edn. Johns Hopkins University Press, Baltimore (1996)

Patient–Specific Parameter Estimation for a Transversely Isotropic Active Strain Model of Left Ventricular Mechanics

Sjur Gjerald, Johan Hake, Simone Pezzuto[✉], Joakim Sundnes, and Samuel T. Wall

Simula Research Laboratory, 1235 Lysaker, Norway
simonep@simula.no

Abstract. Computational models are valuable tools for understanding the mechanical function of the heart. In particular, the prospect of doing patient–specific simulations of heart function may have a significant impact on clinical practice. However, patient–specific simulations give rise to severe challenges related to model choices, parameter fitting and model validation. In this study we investigate parameter variability in a model of left ventricular mechanics applied to four different canine heart cases. The mechanics is modeled by a transversely isotropic active strain model, with two parameters adjusted to fit end diastolic and end systolic pressures and volumes. The chosen model is able to accurately reproduce these data, and enables very efficient parameter fitting. Visual inspection of the resulting deformed geometries also shows a reasonable match with the image based reference.

1 Introduction

Understanding the mechanical function of the heart is important for effective treatment of challenging clinical conditions such as heart failure. Computational models based on detailed anatomical and physiological descriptions of the heart are a promising tool for increasing our understanding of the complex phenomena underlying the pumping function of the heart. Generic heart models focusing on qualitative phenomena have been developed for decades, as well as more specific models matched to data from *in vivo* and *in vitro* experiments. In recent years, a number of research groups are moving towards patient specific models of heart electrophysiology and mechanics [1,14], with the aim of building models that can predict clinical outcome of therapeutic interventions on the level of the individual patient.

The high potential of patient specific simulations of mechanical function is paired with considerable challenges in their use. Even if restricting attention to the passive mechanical properties of the tissue, the material behaviour is highly complex, with strong non–linearity and high anisotropy [11,18]. Choosing the right model, and fitting model parameters based on limited data available, is a substantial challenge [9]. Validation of the computational models is also associated with numerous open questions.

© Springer International Publishing Switzerland 2015
O. Camara et al. (Eds.): STACOM 2014, LNCS 8896, pp. 93–104, 2015.
DOI: 10.1007/978-3-319-14678-2_10

In this paper we explore parameter variability in a set of simplified models of passive and active heart mechanics. Four canine left ventricular models are reconstructed from high–resolution MR images, for which passive mechanics is described by a hyperelastic model based on invariants of the right Cauchy–Green tensor [8], while an active strain approach [15] is used to describe the contraction of the muscle. Material parameters are adjusted to match measured pressure–volume relations, and the resulting models are visually compared to image based reference models.

The paper is organised as follows. In Section 2 we present the techniques used to reconstruct the geometry, as well as the details of the mechanical model and the numerical solution strategy for solving the equations and fitting model parameters. A summary of the results is presented in Section 3, while Section 4 gives a critical discussion of our findings.

2   Methods

2.1   Preprocessing of the Geometry and Microstructure

The data provided for the challenge includes, for each of the 4 cases, a high resolution DT–MRI scan, a hexahedral mesh on top of which an interpolated fibre field is available, and 6 points clouds for the endocardium and epicardium respectively at diastasis (DS), end–diastole (ED) and end–systole (ES) points of the the cardiac cycle.

For sake of simplicity the DT–MRI data has not been used by the present study. Indeed, the DS stage provides a reasonable approximation of a stress–free reference configuration. Moreover, the fibre field can be interpolated from the hexahedral mesh.

The meshing procedure, briefly sketched in Figure 1, has been implemented as a PYTHON script. The main steps are as follows:

A. Triangularization of the raw points dataset for the endocardium and the epicardium. The hole at the apex is closed with an additional point obtained by extrapolating the hole's boundary points.

B. Construction of the ventricle base, defined as the least–squares fitting plane of the points belonging to the basal boundaries of endocardium. These points are then projected onto the plane and eventually all the three surfaces (endocardium, epicardium and base) are rotated and translated in order to have the base to correspond to the yz–plane at $x = 0$.

C. Meshing of the volume enclosed by the 3 aforementioned surfaces with the open–source software GMSH [7]. The quality of the mesh is improved by re-parametrising the endocardium and the epicardium using the "compound geometry" feature [16] of GMSH.

D. Roto–translation (with the same map used for B.), interpolation and normalisation of the fiber field at the mesh nodes and quadrature points.

It is worth to remark that the above procedure is fully automatic and generic with respect to the case and the cardiac stage. In this respect, we generated meshes for all the stages and cases $(3 \cdot 4 = 12$ in total) to better compare simulations results to the target geometries.

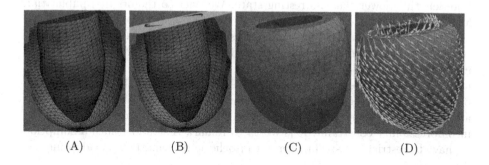

(A)   (B)   (C)   (D)

Fig. 1. The epicardial and endocardial surfaces were given as point clouds that were triangularized (A). One node was added at the apex to cover the apical hole. A plane was fitted to the base of the endocardium by a least squares method (B). The basal nodes of both endocardium and epicardium were projected into this plane, and the heart was moved and rotated so that the plane coincided with the yz–plane at $x = 0$. Then the cardial wall was tetrahedralized with GMSH (C). Fiber orientations were provided and interpolated at the nodes and integration points of the final mesh (D).

2.2   The Mechanical Model

A configuration of a continuum body $\mathcal{B}$ is a function χ from $\mathcal{B}$ to $\mathbb{R}^3$. Given two configurations, a reference and an actual one, respectively denoted by χ_0 and χ, a deformation φ maps a point $\mathbf{X} \in \chi_0(\mathcal{B}) \equiv \Omega_0$ onto a point $\mathbf{x} \in \chi(\mathcal{B}) \equiv \Omega$. The gradient of this map is the deformation gradient tensor

$$\mathsf{F}(\mathbf{X}) := \frac{\partial \varphi}{\partial \mathbf{X}},$$

in terms of which the right Cauchy–Green tensor is defined as $\mathsf{C} = \mathsf{F}^{\mathsf{T}}\mathsf{F}$.

Myocardium is generally modelled as an orthotropic material, with two preferential directions described by the fibres field $\mathbf{f}_o(\mathbf{X})$ and the sheets field $\mathbf{s}_o(\mathbf{X})$. While the role of fibres is known to be fundamental, the role of the sheets, as well as their distribution across the tissue, is still under debate. For the present study the fibre fields were provided for all four test cases, while the sheet fields were not available. We have therefore adopted a transversely isotropic material model, where the strain energy function is defined through the first and fourth invariants of the right Cauchy-Green tensor:

$$\mathcal{I}_1 = \mathrm{tr}\mathsf{C}, \quad \text{and} \quad \mathcal{I}_{4,\mathbf{f}_o} = \mathbf{f}_o \cdot (\mathsf{C}\mathbf{f}_o).$$

The strain energy density function, adapted from [8], reads

$$W(C) = \frac{a}{2b}\left(e^{b(\mathcal{I}_1 - 3)} - 1\right) + \frac{a_f}{2b_f}\left(e^{b_f(\mathcal{I}_{4,f_o} - 1)_+^2} - 1\right), \tag{1}$$

where $(\mathcal{I}_{4,f_o} - 1)_+ := \max\{\mathcal{I}_{4,f_o} - 1, 0\}$, hence this term is set to zero if the local fibre length is lower than its resting state. We refer to the original publication for details.

The tissue is assumed fully incompressible, i.e. $J := \det(F) = 1$. This constraint is (weakly) enforced in a standard manner by introducing a Lagrange multiplier p, see e.g. [5]. It is worth noting that the total wall volume, computed for each case at different stages (see Table 2) is not constant: this could be due to blood perfusion or segmentation uncertainty. Nonetheless, the wall volume variation is limited (below 5% in most of the cases) so it is reasonable to keep the incompressibility constraint. It is worth to remark that under such assumption we have to restrict the strain–energy to isochoric deformations by adopting:

$$\widehat{W}(C) := W(C_{iso}) = W(J^{-\frac{2}{3}}C).$$

The activation of the muscle is achieved by means of the active strain approach, which is based on a multiplicative decomposition of the deformation gradient tensor,

$$F = F_e F_a,$$

where F_a is the active deformation induced by cell contraction, and F_e is purely elastic deformation, see [13, 15] for details. The specific form of F_a relies on the assumptions that there is a shortening in the fiber direction f_o and that the active contraction is volume preserving. By introducing a single activation parameter γ, which represents relative local active fibre shortening, we get

$$F_a = (1 - \gamma)f_o \otimes f_o + \frac{1}{\sqrt{1 - \gamma}}\left(I - f_o \otimes f_o\right). \tag{2}$$

The active deformation F_a doesn't store elastic energy, so that only the elastic portion F_e contributes to the strain energy in (1). We have

$$\widetilde{W}(C_e) = \widehat{W}(F_a^{-T} C_{iso} F_a^{-1}). \tag{3}$$

We are interested in controlling the cavity volume V_{inner}, defined by the endocardial surface. For this purpose we introduce an additional Lagrange multiplier p_{inner}, which can be shown to be the endocardial pressure [17]. This formulation is useful when a specific volume is targeted, while the inner pressure is unknown. The resulting Lagrangian reads:

$$\mathcal{L}(\varphi, p, p_{inner}; \gamma, V_{inner}) := \int_{\Omega_0} \widehat{W}(F_a^{-T} C_{iso} F_a^{-1}) \det F_a \, dV$$

$$- \int_{\Omega_0} p(J - \det F_a) \, dV - p_{inner}\left(\mathcal{V}(\varphi) - V_{inner}\right), \tag{4}$$

where V_{inner} is given and $\mathcal{V}(\varphi)$ is the inner cavity volume computed for a specific deformation φ from the endocardial surface Γ_{endo}:

$$\mathcal{V}(\varphi) := \int_{\Gamma_{endo}} \varphi \cdot (\operatorname{cof} F) N \, dA,$$

where N is the outward unit normal of Γ_{endo} and $\operatorname{cof} F$ is the cofactor of the tensor F.

In a similar fashion, when an inner pressure p_{inner} is prescribed, while the volume is computed afterwards, it is enough to remove p_{inner} from the list of the unknowns and add it to the list of the parameters:

$$\mathcal{L}(\varphi, p; \gamma, p_{inner}) := \int_{\Omega_0} \widehat{W}(F_a^{-T} C_{iso} F_a^{-1}) \det F_a \, dV$$

$$- \int_{\Omega_0} p(J - F_a) \, dV - p_{inner} \mathcal{V}(\varphi). \quad (5)$$

The volume is then $V_{inner} = \mathcal{V}(\varphi)$.

Along with the inner pressure, the only other boundary condition imposed is a zero normal displacement of the base. This implies that the mechanical solution is defined up to a rotation around the ventricle axis and a translation in the yz–plane. Thus three additional constraints are imposed in order to obtain a solution with no superimposed rigid motions. This is clearly a rough approximation of the mechanics at the base; on the other hand, it guarantees that the whole deformation is only dictated by the strain–energy and the inner load, without being affected by other external sources.

The mechanical model is discretized with quadratic finite elements for the displacement and linear finite elements for the pressure, leading to a stable discretization [4]. The non–linear problem is solved by the quasi–Newton's method, i.e. we recompute the Jacobian for the tangent problem only when strictly necessary, with an incremental strategy for parameter continuation. The tangent problem is solved by using the direct solver MUMPS [3]. The solver, fully parallelised, is based on the open–source framework FEniCS [12], and the source code is fully available[1]. The computational effort required to solve these problems is very low: a modern laptop/desktop computer is enough to obtain a whole pV–loop in less than 10 minutes with the coarsest mesh (around 5000 elements) and about 2 hours on the finest mesh (20 000 elements), with 4 MPI processes.

2.3   Parameter Estimation and Sensitivity Analysis

The full problem has six parameters in total: four for the passive mechanics, namely a, b, a_f and b_f in (1), one for the activation, i.e. γ in (2), and one which can be either p_{inner} or V_{inner}, depending on the specific formulation, (5) or (4).

Since the problem depends continuously on each parameter, we can argue that within a physiological range of the parameters the solution depends as well

---

[1] The download link is https://bitbucket.org/peppu/lvchallenge.

continuously on each parameter. This suggests a homotopy argument: starting from a given stage, say the end–systolic point, computed with the initial set of parameters, we can track the solution when one parameter changes without recomputing the whole pV–loop, but by simply following the curve implicitly defined by the solution with respect to the parameter.

The numerical approximation is therefore based on a simple continuation algorithm [10]: we start from a point on the solution curve, then the next point along the curve is first predicted using the tangent, and then corrected by the Newton's method. It is worth noticing that thanks to this strategy we do not recompute the entire pV–loop during the fitting procedure and sensitivity analysis. This significantly reduce the computational cost.

The fitting procedure aims to match the measured volumes and pressures. Indeed, the only data available for the fitting was the pressure and corresponding volume at two distinct points in the cardiac cycle, which is obviously not enough to determine all material parameters uniquely. This is a common situation for models of this kind, in particular when aiming for image based patient specific simulations. With limited data available, we are left to make reasonable *a priori* choices based on values from the literature for some parameters, and fit the remaining to match the given pressures and volumes.

In order to have better overview on how the solution depends on the parameters, we first performed a sensitivity analysis for the end–diastolic stage. We analysed the sensitivity of the inner volume, the ventricle total length and the average thickness just below the base, with respect to the passive material parameters a, b, a_f and b_f.

3   Results

The sensitivity analysis has been performed in detail for case **1024**. More precisely, the above mentioned quantities of interest have been tracked both by varying one parameter at a time while holding the others at their reference value, and by varying two parameters simultaneously. The analysis exhibited respectively a very weak impact of b_f, a modest impact of b and an apparent effect of a and a_f on all the quantities of interest.

Hence, for the end–diastolic stage, we chose to fix $b = 10.810$ and $b_f = 14.154$, i.e. to their reference values, and then further analyse the simultaneous sensitivity to a and a_f. The result is depicted in Figure 3. The black line in each plot represent the target value for the corresponding quantity. For instance, concerning the inner volume, there is an implicit curve $g(a, a_f) = 0$ on which the inner volume is always captured. On the other hand, the optimal pair (a, a_f) can be also selected to better match other quantities such as wall thickening or lengthening of the ventricle. A good compromise for this specific case is to choose $a \lesssim 20$ kPa and $a_f \lesssim 100$ kPa.

The results of the parameter fitting that matched end–diastolic and end–systolic volumes and pressures are shown in Table 1. We see that there is considerable variability in the parameters. For the **0912** case we had to adjust the

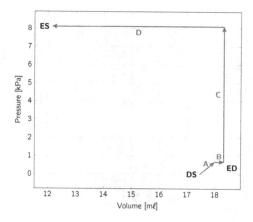

Fig. 2. Parameter fitting procedure (1024 case). The ventricle is first passively inflated, by means of model (5) with $\gamma = 0$, to the given target pressure (A). Then a_f is iteratively adjusted until the volume matched the target volume (B). To reach the end–systolic point, we hold the volume constant by means of (4), at the ED value, while we increase γ until the target ES pressure is reached (C). We eventually keep the pressure constant, using (5), while increasing γ further until the volume also matched the target ES value (D).

parameters a from our *a priori* values, as we were otherwise unable to reach the target volume for end–diastole. Apart from this we see that cases **0917** and **1017** are fairly similar, while case **1024** is characterised by high stiffness. These values appear to be consistent with the provided end–diastolic and end–systolic pressures and volumes.

The active contraction parameter γ for cases **1017** and **1024** is consistent with the values reported in the literature and obtained by fitting experimental data from muscular thin films [2,6,15], while for the other two cases is slightly higher.

Simulation results obtained with the fitted parameters are shown in Figure 4. All four cases are displayed, for end–diastole (ED, left column) and end–systole (ES, right column), and compared with the surfaces extracted from the points clouds. The solid red surfaces show the result of the model, while the transparent surfaces are based on the points clouds. We see that there is some variation in how well the geometries match, both for ED and ES, but all the model results are visually similar to the image based reference. Note that the model parameters are fitted only to match the provided pressures and volumes, and have not been tuned further to make the geometries match.

The geometric data pictured in Figure 4 is quantified in Table 2 to compare how well the fitting method matched other global geometric measures besides the extracted volumes. We show good agreement in wall thickness and its change between diastole and systole, as well as the change in length of the ventricles for the diastole, and a modest mismatch for the systole. There is no observed

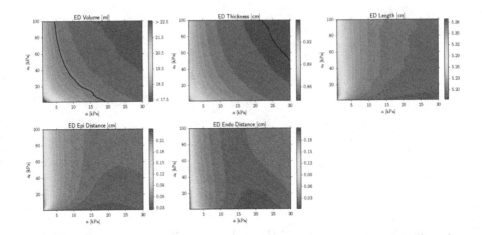

Fig. 3. Sensitivity to a and a_f parameters for the end–diastolic point of case **1024**. On top we show the end–diastolic volume [mℓ], the length of the ventricle [cm] and the average thickness [cm] just below the base. The bottom row show the Hausdorff distance between the computed endocardial (resp. epicardial) surface and the given one. The black line is the corresponding target value.

pattern in the change in wall volume in the target simulations, with some cases decreasing and other increasing, but very small changes are observed in either direction, indicating our assumption of incompressibility is not far off. The calculated Hausdorff distance, or greatest deviance between the two data sets, is in the range of 2 - 4 mm indicating that the geometries are reasonably well watched at the simulated points in the cardiac cycle.

Figure 5 and shows the fibre Cauchy stress both in diastole and in systole. Excluding some artefacts around the base and the apex, the range of the values is consistent with those reported in the literature.

The average strain and the stress in the fibre direction over the whole tissue is reported in Table 3. The invariant $\mathcal{I}_{4,f_o}$ is comparable to γ, which means that the residual stress is relatively low. The computed stress is not uniform in the transmural direction, with a higher value attained around the midwall and decreasing towards the epicardium and the endocardium. The standard deviation for the stress in also rather high, being generally greater than 0.5 kPa at end–diastole and greater than 15 kPa at end–systole, which highlights the heterogeneous distribution of the stress across the tissue (not shown).

4   Discussion

We have presented that by adjusting two different parameters we were able to provide a good fit to end–diastolic and end–systolic pressures and volumes for four different test cases. This result is not very surprising, since the parameters

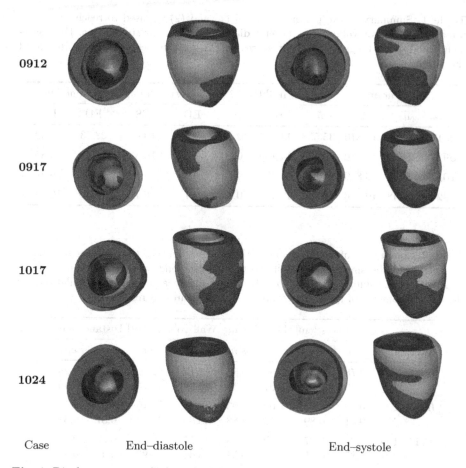

| Case | End–diastole | End–systole |

Fig. 4. Displacements applied to the DS geometry, read solid surfaces, from the four cases (0912, 0917, 1017, 1024) and two stages (ED, ES) are compared with the epi/endo triangulation, transparent surfaces, of the given point cloud for each stage/case

we adjust directly affect the stiffness and contractility of the ventricle, and are therefore well suited for matching the pressure–volume relation. With only pressure and volume available, and only at two distinct points, the chosen model and fitting strategy appears to be well suited for matching the measured results. As evident from Figure 4 and the data in Table 2, the deformed geometries are also fairly similar to the image based references, although the fit is not perfect.

There exist a large number of alternative models for describing active and passive heart mechanics. The most common approach for active-passive coupling is to introduce an additive decomposition of the stress tensor, the so-called active stress approach. We chose the active strain formulation primarily because of its attractive mathematical properties, and the ease by which we could introduce the activation parameter γ to control the end–systolic volume. However, it is

Table 1. Summary of the parameters from (1) and (2) we used to reach the target pressure and target volume for the end–diastolic and end–systolic stage. For convenience we report the given target pressures and target volumes which were used to fit the parameters.

	Parameters (a and a_f in [kPa])					Pressure [kPa]		Volume [mℓ]	
Case	a	b	a_f	b_f	γ	ED	ES	ED	ES
0912	1.181	10.810	35.558	14.154	0.213	0.7	10.8	28.83	13.59
0917	2.362	10.810	20.103	14.154	0.202	0.6	10.3	19.56	10.85
1017	2.362	10.810	25.815	14.154	0.157	0.6	8.8	23.25	16.29
1024	9.448	10.810	32.191	14.154	0.155	0.7	8.1	18.32	12.14

Table 2. Comparison of global geometrical quantities between the reference (or target) geometry and the simulation for all the cases at the end–systolic and end–diastolic stages. The last columns represents the Hausdorff distance between the simulation and the target geometry of the endocardium and the epicardium respectively.

		Thickness [cm]		Length [cm]		Wall volume [mℓ]		Distance [cm]	
Case	Stage	*ref*	*sim*	*ref*	*sim*	*ref*	*sim*	*endo*	*epi*
0912	ED	0.78	0.81	5.56	5.54	44.15	42.70	0.31	0.26
	ES	1.03	1.04	5.01	5.38	42.60	42.70	0.58	0.45
0917	ED	0.70	0.75	5.09	5.03	33.28	31.16	0.27	0.25
	ES	0.81	0.89	4.55	4.88	30.35	31.16	0.37	0.38
1017	ED	0.78	0.77	5.59	5.58	40.57	39.97	0.35	0.32
	ES	0.87	0.85	5.11	5.51	35.68	39.97	0.43	0.45
1024	ED	0.98	0.97	5.25	5.30	41.77	41.66	0.06	0.07
	ES	1.10	1.08	4.77	5.37	38.15	41.66	0.72	0.62

likely that a simple active stress model, with a single parameter controlling the developed tension at end systole, would yield very similar results. The use of a transversely isotropic material law may also have affected the results. Heart tissue is known to be orthotropic, although the significance of the sheets for intact ventricle mechanics is debated. While some studies have shown very low sensitivity of global deformation measures to the stiffness in the sheet direction, others have reported its significance for measures such as wall thickening and rotation and shortening of the ventricle. It is possible that including some of these quantities in our parameter fitting, as well as an orthotropic passive and/or active material law, would further improve the model results shown in Figure 4.

However, it is likely that any significant improvement of the model results would require more data available for the fitting. For instance, estimating strains from ultrasound speckle-tracking or tagged MR images would give much more

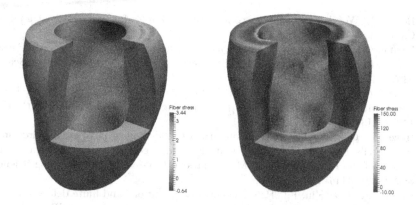

Fig. 5. Fibre stress (in kPa) for case **1024** at diastole (left) and systole (right)

Table 3. Summary of average value of the fourth invariant $\mathcal{I}_{4,f_o}$ and Cauchy stress (in kPa) in the fibre direction over the whole tissue, for end–diastole and end–systole stages and different patients

Case	Avg. $\mathcal{I}_{4,f_o}$		Avg. stress	
	ED	ES	ED	ES
0912	1.03	0.76	1.80	36.41
0917	1.03	0.80	1.29	32.68
1017	1.02	0.85	1.20	21.92
1024	1.01	0.85	0.90	25.43

detailed and local information on material properties. This information would probably allow us to include and fit more parameters in the material law, which would potentially improve the quality of the final result.

References

1. Aguado-Sierra, J., Krishnamurthy, A., Villongco, C., Chuang, J., Howard, E., Gonzales, M.J., Omens, J., Krummen, D.E., Narayan, S., Kerckhoffs, R.C.P., McCulloch, A.D.: Patient-specific modeling of dyssynchronous heart failure: A case study. Progress in Biophysics and Molecular Biology **107**(1), 147–155 (2011)
2. Alford, P.W., Feinberg, A.W., Sheehy, S.P., Parker, K.K.: Biohybrid thin films for measuring contractility in engineered cardiovascular muscle. Biomaterials **31**(13), 3613–3621 (2010)
3. Amestoy, P.R., Duff, I.S., L'Excellent, J.-Y., Koster, J.: MUMPS: a general purpose distributed memory sparse solver. In: Sørevik, T., Manne, F., Gebremedhin, A.H., Moe, R. (eds.) PARA 2000. LNCS, vol. 1947, pp. 121–130. Springer, Heidelberg (2001)
4. Arnold, D.N., Brezzi, F., Fortin, M.: A stable finite element for the stokes equations. Calcolo **21**(4), 337–344 (1984)

5. Bonet, J., Wood, R.: Nonlinear continuum mechanics for finite element analysis. Cambridge University Press (1997)
6. Feinberg, A.W., Feigel, A., Shevkoplyas, S.S., Sheehy, S., Whitesides, G.M., Parker, K.K.: Muscular thin films for building actuators and powering devices. Science **317**(5843), 1366–1370 (2007)
7. Geuzaine, C., Remacle, J.-F.: Gmsh: A three-dimensional finite element mesh generator with built-in pre- and post-processing facilities. Int. J. Numer. Meth. Eng. **11**(79), 1309–1331 (2009)
8. Holzapfel, G.A., Ogden, R.W.: Constitutive modelling of passive myocardium: a structurally based framework for material characterization. Philosophical Transactions of the Royal Society A: Mathematical, Physical and Engineering Sciences **367**(1902), 3445–3475 (2009)
9. Humphrey, J.D., Yin, F.C.P.: On constitutive relations and finite deformations of passive cardiac tissue: I. a pseudostrain-energy function. Journal of Biomechanical Engineering **109**(4), 298–304 (1987)
10. Kuznetsov, Y.: Elements of applied bifurcation theory, vol. 112. Springer (1998)
11. LeGrice, I., Hunter, P., Young, A., Smaill, B.: The architecture of the heart: a data-based model. Philosophical Transactions of the Royal Society of London. Series A: Mathematical, Physical and Engineering Sciences **359**(1783), 1217–1232 (2001)
12. Logg, A., Mardal, K.-A., Wells, G.N., et al.: Automated Solution of Differential Equations by the Finite Element Method. Springer (2012)
13. Nardinocchi, P., Teresi, L.: On the active response of soft living tissues. Journal of Elasticity **88**(1), 27–39 (2007)
14. Niederer, S.A., Plank, G., Chinchapatnam, P., Ginks, M., Lamata, P., Rhode, K.S., Rinaldi, C.A., Razavi, R., Smith, N.P.: Length-dependent tension in the failing heart and the efficacy of cardiac resynchronization therapy. Cardiovascular Research **89**(2), 336–343 (2011)
15. Pezzuto, S., Ambrosi, D., Quarteroni, A.: An orthotropic active-strain model for the myocardium mechanics and its numerical approximation. European Journal of Mechanics-A/Solids (2014)
16. Remacle, J.-F., Geuzaine, C., Compère, G., Marchandise, E.: High-quality surface remeshing using harmonic maps. International Journal for Numerical Methods in Engineering **83**(4), 403–425 (2010)
17. Rumpel, T., Schweizerhof, K.: Volume-dependent pressure loading and its influence on the stability of structures. International Journal for Numerical Methods in Engineering **56**(2), 211–238 (2003)
18. Streeter, D.D., Spotnitz, H.M., Patel, D.P., Ross, J., Sonnenblick, E.H.: Fiber orientation in the canine left ventricle during diastole and systole. Circulation Research **24**(3), 339–347 (1969)

Estimation of Diastolic Biomarkers: Sensitiviy to Fibre Orientation

Sander Land[1], Steve Niederer[1], and Pablo Lamata[1,2]([⊠])

[1] Department of Biomedical Engineering, King's College London, London, UK
pablo.lamata@kcl.ac.uk
[2] Deptartment of Computer Science, University of Oxford, Oxford, UK

Abstract. An accurate estimation of myocardial stiffness and decaying active tension is critical for the characterization of the diastolic function of the heart. Computational cardiac models can be used to analyse deformation and pressure data from the left ventricle in order to estimate these diastolic metrics. The results of this methodology depend on several model assumptions. In this work we reveal a nominal impact of the choice of myocardial fibre orientation between a rule-based description and personalised approach based on diffusion-tensor magnetic resonance imaging. This result suggests the viability of simplified clinical imaging protocols for the model-based estimation of diastolic biomarkers.

Keywords: Cardiac computational physiology · Diastolic biomarkers · Model personalization · Fibre orientation

1 Introduction

Heart failure (HF) is a major public health issue that affects over 23 million worldwide, and rising. The lifetime risk of developing HF is one in five, and this disease represents a considerable burden to the healthcare system. HF with preserved ejection fraction (HF-PEF), also known as diastolic HF, accounts for nearly half of patients with HF. The prognostic outlook of HF-PEF is similar to that of HF with reduced ejection fraction, and its study has recently sparked research interest, focusing on the diastolic dysfunction as a dominant contributor to symptoms [11].

Despite this recognised importance, it is difficult to understand and characterise diastolic dysfunction, even with advanced imaging modalities. An increased stiffness of the walls of the ventricular cavity is one of the causes of an impaired filling, and it is thus a relevant biomarker of HF-PEF. Nevertheless, current diagnostic guidelines are based on indirect surrogates, and there is a need for a reliable and clinically relevant methodology to characterise myocardial stiffness [11]. The general hypothesis that motivates this work is that the combination of advanced imaging and modelling technologies can fulfil this need.

The model-driven extraction of a biomarker can be simply described as the process of finding the best set of model parameters that explain the observed

© Springer International Publishing Switzerland 2015
O. Camara et al. (Eds.): STACOM 2014, LNCS 8896, pp. 105–113, 2015.
DOI: 10.1007/978-3-319-14678-2_11

data. Current imaging technologies provide with a reasonable estimation of cardiac deformation, and catheterised sensors record the pressure inside the ventricular cavity. The task that remains is now to find the stiffness of the myocardium that best explains the interplay between these two variables, the amount of cavity dilation driven by the increment of pressure. The simplest solution is driven by a data fitting process, where the relationship pressure vs. volume data during filling is described as an exponential line. This method is currently adopted in the clinical arena, and has demonstrated its relevance in characterising HF-PEF [18]. More complex solutions use 3D computational mechanical models of the left ventricle [13–17]. This approach has recently shown fundamental advantages, including its ability to automatically decouple the effects of the increased stiffness and the slower relaxation of the myocytes [17], and the better robustness to noise in pressure data [16].

Nevertheless, the use of 3D computational models is also limited by their additional complexity and associated uncertainty to components or parameters that are not observed in the clinical data. This work addresses the study of the level of anatomical detail, the amount and resolution of clinical images needed for an accurate estimation of myocardial stiffness. Specifically, we quantify the error incurred by an assumption in the spatial organization of myocardial fibres.

2   Methods

2.1   Data

High resolution MRI data from four normal dogs was contributed by The National Institutes of Health [15]. Data was processed by organisers of STACOM challenge in order to provide binary masks defining the LV geometry and muscle fibre orientations. The DT-MRI data have already been registered to the in-vivo geometry. Geometries and in-vivo left ventricular pressures were available at two states in the cardiac cycle: stress free (diastasis - DS), and end of inflation (end-diastole - ED). These geometries only reflect the location of the epicardial and endocardial surfaces – they do not encode material point displacements.

2.2   Model Components and Construction

The left ventricle is represented with a finite element model, non-linear elasticity governed by an exponential transversely isotropic material constitutive law (The "Guccione law", with parameters re-formulated as C_1, α, r_3, r_4, as described in [17]).

The computational domains describing the left ventricle at DS and ED in each case are built from their segmentations, using a fully automatic web-service that works with C1 continuous meshes [5,8]. Fibre orientation is defined at DS, either extracted from the DT-MRI data and then projected into the computational mesh using the methods described in [6], or by using the conventional rule of +60 to -60 degrees from endocardial to epicardial surface.

2.3   Parameter Estimation Process

The computational model simulates diastolic filling by a passive inflation of the ventricle at DS (starting with null pressure) adding the difference in pressure recorded between DS and ED (around 0.7 kPa in all four cases). Dirichlet boundary conditions are applied to all nodes of the base, with the amount of displacement of each node determined by the difference between ED and DS configurations after correspondences are set through a common mesh personalization methodology.

The optimisation functional, the comparison between the model result and the data, is defined by the volume reached at ED. Only α, one of the four constitutive parameters, is estimated. Due to the simplicity of the functional space, a parameter sweep with α ranging from 10 to 50 in each case (up to 150 in case 4), fixing C_1, r_2, r_3 and r_4 to 1.66, 0.51, 0.24 and 0.25 (values obtained by linear combination of parameters previously reported in the literature [13–15]). We used a highly optimized mechanical simulation code [9, 10] running on a Linux virtual machine with 4 cores using the cloud infrastructure of VPH-Share (http://www.vph-share.eu). Each simulation took around 3.5 minutes.

3   Results

3.1   Computational Meshes

Ventricular anatomy was represented with cubic meshes with 144 elements and 219 nodes, see Fig. 1. The mesh generation tool reported an average fitting residual (distance from mesh to the centre of the voxel) of 0.14 ± 0.002 mm, well below the voxel size of 0.325mm. Meshes had a Jacobian ratio, a metric of the quality, of 0.37 ± 0.02 (with a worst-case of 0.33), which are values within the expected range for meshes with collapsed elements [7].

3.2   Stiffness Constitutive Parameters

The results of fitting α are reported in Table 1, showing nominal changes with the choice of fibre field by chosen functional (see Fig. 3). A personalised fibre field resulted in softer (Case 1) or stiffer (Cases 2-4) material properties. The corresponding relationship between pressure and volume transient is illustrated in Fig. 4.

Cases 1 to 3 reported stiffness values very close to previous studies done *in-vivo* through medical imaging, both with rule-based [14] and DT-MRI fibre fields [15], see Table 1, and case 4 was stiffer than any other reported in the literature (3 times stiffer than [12] accordingly to the product $C_1 \cdot \alpha$).

4   Discussion

Our results in four cases indicate that the estimation of myocardial stiffness has a nominal dependence on the accuracy of the fibre orientation. This suggests

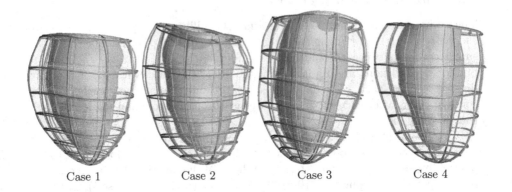

Case 1   Case 2   Case 3   Case 4

Fig. 1. Computational meshes at diastasis (red) and end diastole (gold) in the four cases, illustrating the amount of deformation experienced by the ventricle. Note that any material point correspondence between these two configurations is the result of using the same mesh personalization process [8].

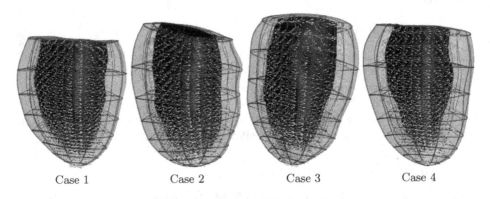

Case 1   Case 2   Case 3   Case 4

Fig. 2. Computational meshes at diastasis (DS) after personalization of the fibre orientation from PC-MRI data in the four cases

Table 1. Myocardial constitutive parameters (C_1, α) of the reformulated Guccione law [17] in this study (Case 1 to 4) and in the literature ([12–15])

	Case 1	Case 2	Case 3	Case 4	[13]	[12]	[14]	[15]
C_1	1.66	1.66	1.66	1.66	1.2	0.5	1.8	1.7
α, Rule-based	21.6	13.3	19.3	103.8	43.4	112.8	18.5	
α, DT-MRI	22.0	13.0	19.2	102.4				19.6

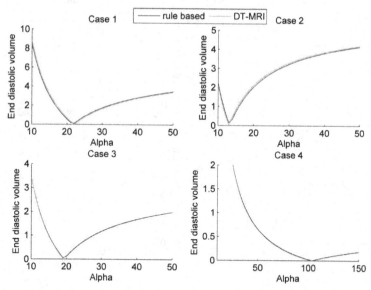

Fig. 3. Fitting functional based on the difference between simulated and measured end diastolic volume, in the four cases

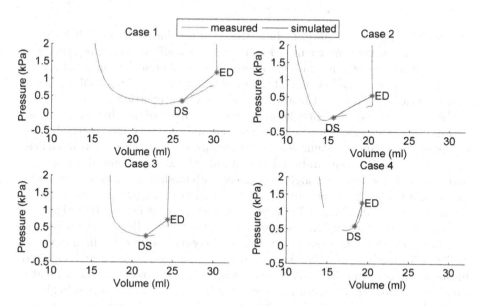

Fig. 4. Pressure-Volume (PV) plot by experimental and simulated (with rule-based fibres and optimal α) data. The results illustrate the consequence of fitting material parameters by comparison between diastasis (DS) to end diastole (ED).

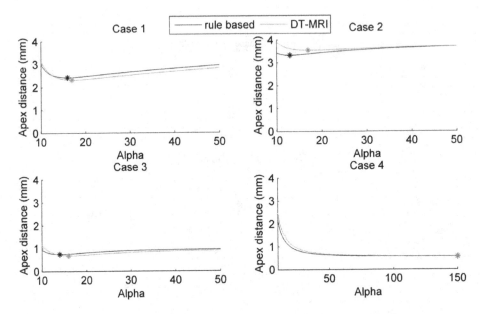

Fig. 5. Fitting functional based on the distance between apical mesh points in simulated and measured end diastolic meshes, in the four cases. Note that Case 4 did not find the minimum in the physiological range of parameters explored, but that the two lines almost overlap in this case.

that the identification of diastolic biomarkers for the diagnosis of HFPEF, based in a functional comparing volume, does not require additional imaging studies to capture patient-specific information about the spatial organization of myocytes.

The choice of a simple volume functional is a cause of the nominal impact of fibre orientation in the identification of the material properties. The comparison of the volume of the left ventricle minimises the impact of imaging (data) errors and model assumptions. An imaging protocol able to track the material point correspondence, and to estimate accurate strains, is a hard endeavour in clinical practice. A cardiac computational model able to exactly mimic deformations and myocardial strain is strongly dependent on boundary conditions and model assumptions. The use of currents [4] for the functional is an intermediate solution between using volume and deformations that needs to be further investigated.

In order to further explore the generalizability of our findings, we explored the behaviour of another functional, the distance between the apical points, reported in Fig. 5. This is motivated by the fact that boundary conditions were prescribed in the entire base, and the apical location will be then the most challenging material point to predict. Furthermore, the material point correspondence, achieved implicitly by an automatic mesh personalization process, may be considered more accurate in this anatomical region without circumferential symmetry and with the biggest curvature, a local feature that will constrain better the problem of image registration used. Changes in α with the choice of the fibre field are now slightly larger, but these are still small. Moreover, a personalised fibre field does not always lead to a better prediction of deformation, as shown by the results of case 2.

Material parameters were only constrained by a single observation, the change of volume from DS to ED. Optimising only for α, after fixing C_1, is a strategy taken in this work justified by the "quasi linear behaviour" observed at the physiological range of diastolic filling, which leads to a coupling between the linear and exponential coefficients of the constitutive law, as reported in human cases [16,17]. Using more observations, more diastolic frames, is known to better constrain the parameter space, and could be used to optimise also for C_1. The abrupt transition in the PV line shown in the data (see cases 1-3, Fig. 4) suggest the recruitment of some active forces, rather than a passive behaviour. Nevertheless, case 4 shows a more plausible smooth transition of the PV line, which suggests that the assumption of a 'quasi linear passive behaviour' is not always valid. In any case, the addition of more frames to the functional could lead to a change in material parameters as discussed, but we would not expect it to change the nominal dependence on fibre orientation observed.

The comparison of our results to the literature is limited by scope, since previous works have focused in the complete cardiac cycle [1–3]. The fibre model (the choice of maximum helix angle and of the coefficient modulating the transmural variation) has been shown to have an impact in bulk metrics like ejection fraction, wall thickening and cavity shortening [1]. On the contrary, the passive inflation in our experiments introduced nominal changes in cavity volume (see Fig. 3), and a change in lengthening only noticeable in one case (case 2, see Fig. 5). This can be explained by the smaller difference in fibre distribution than in previous studies, and by the less relevant contribution of the passive inflation in the overall mechanics of the cardiac cycle.

5 Conclusion

A personalised description of fibre orientation is not a critical component of a computational analysis for the estimation of diastolic biomarkers.

Acknowledgments. Authors acknowledge the support from the European Comission (Project FP7-ICT-269978), from the National Institute for Health Research Biomedical Research Centre at Guy's and St Thomas' National Health Service Foundation Trust and King's College London, and support from the Centre of Excellence in Medical Engineering funded by the Wellcome Trust and EPSRC (Grant WT 088641/Z/09/Z). PL holds a Sir Henry Dale Fellowship funded jointly by the Wellcome Trust and the Royal Society (grant no. 099973/Z/12/Z).

References

1. Carapella, V., Bordas, R., Pathmanathan, P., Lohezic, M., Schneider, J.E., Kohl, P., Burrage, K., Grau, V.: Quantitative study of the effect of tissue microstructure on contraction in a computational model of rat left ventricle. PLoS ONE **9**(4), e92792 (2014)
2. Geerts, L., Kerckhoffs, R., Bovendeerd, P., Arts, T.: Towards patient specific models of cardiac mechanics: a sensitivity study. In: Magnin, I.E., Montagnat, J., Clarysse, P., Nenonen, J., Katila, T. (eds.) FIMH 2003. LNCS, vol. 2674, pp. 81–90. Springer, Heidelberg (2003)
3. Gil, D., et al.: What a difference in biomechanics cardiac fiber makes. In: Camara, O., Mansi, T., Pop, M., Rhode, K., Sermesant, M., Young, A. (eds.) STACOM 2012. LNCS, vol. 7746, pp. 253–260. Springer, Heidelberg (2013)
4. Imperiale, A., Routier, A., Durrleman, S., Moireau, P.: Improving efficiency of data assimilation procedure for a biomechanical heart model by representing surfaces as currents. In: Ourselin, S., Rueckert, D., Smith, N. (eds.) FIMH 2013. LNCS, vol. 7945, pp. 342–351. Springer, Heidelberg (2013)
5. Lamata, P., Niederer, S., Nordsletten, D., Barber, D., Roy, I., Hose, D., Smith, N.: An accurate, fast and robust method to generate patient-specific cubic hermite meshes. Medical Image Analysis **15**(6), 801–813 (2011)
6. Lamata, P., Niederer, S., Plank, G., Smith, N.: Generic conduction parameters for predicting activation waves in customised cardiac electrophysiology models. In: Camara, O., Pop, M., Rhode, K., Sermesant, M., Smith, N., Young, A. (eds.) STACOM 2010. LNCS, vol. 6364, pp. 252–260. Springer, Heidelberg (2010)
7. Lamata, P., Roy, I., Blazevic, B., Crozier, A., Land, S., Niederer, S., Rod Hose, D., Smith, N.: Quality metrics for high order meshes: Analysis of the mechanical simulation of the heart beat. IEEE Transactions on Medical Imaging **32**(1), 130–138 (2013)
8. Lamata, P., Sinclair, M., Kerfoot, E., Lee, A., Crozier, A., Blazevic, B., Land, S., Lewandowski, A., Barber, D., Niederer, S., Smith, N.: An automatic service for the personalization of ventricular cardiac meshes. Journal of the Royal Society Interface **11**(91) (2014)
9. Land, S., Niederer, S., Lamata, P., Smith, N.: Improving the stability of cardiac mechanical simulations. IEEE Transactions on Biomedical Engineering (2015, in press)
10. Land, S., Niederer, S., Smith, N.: Efficient computational methods for strongly coupled cardiac electromechanics. IEEE Transactions on Biomedical Engineering **59**(5), 1219–1228 (2012)
11. Mcmurray, J., et al.: Esc guidelines for the diagnosis and treatment of acute and chronic heart failure 2012. European Journal of Heart Failure **14**(8), 803–869 (2012)
12. Okamoto, R.J., Moulton, M.J., Peterson, S.J., Li, D., Pasque, M.K., Guccione, J.M.: Epicardial suction: a new approach to mechanical testing of the passive ventricular wall. J. Biomech. Eng. **122**(5), 479–487 (2000)
13. Omens, J.H., MacKenna, D.A., McCulloch, A.D.: Measurement of strain and analysis of stress in resting rat left ventricular myocardium. Journal of Biomechanics **26**(6), 665–676 (1993)
14. Usyk, T., Mazhari, R., McCulloch, A.: Effect of laminar orthotropic myofiber architecture on regional stress and strain in the canine left ventricle. Journal of Elasticity and the Physical Science of Solids **61**(1–3), 143–164 (2000)

15. Wang, V.Y., Lam, H., Ennis, D.B., Cowan, B.R., Young, A.A., Nash, M.P.: Modelling passive diastolic mechanics with quantitative mri of cardiac structure and function. Medical Image Analysis **13**(5), 773–784 (2009)
16. Xi, J., Shi, W., Rueckert, D., Razavi, R., Smith, N., Lamata, P.: Understanding the need of ventricular pressure for the estimation of diastolic biomarkers. Biomechanics and Modeling in Mechanobiology **13**(4), 747–57 (2014)
17. Xi, J., Lamata, P., Niederer, S., Land, S., Shi, W., Zhuang, X., Ourselin, S., Duckett, S.G., Shetty, A.K., Rinaldi, C.A., Rueckert, D., Razavi, R., Smith, N.P.: The estimation of patient-specific cardiac diastolic functions from clinical measurements. Medical Image Analysis **17**(2), 133–146 (2013)
18. Zile, M., Baicu, C., Gaasch, W.: Diastolic heart failure - abnormalities in active relaxation and passive stiffness of the left ventricle. New England Journal of Medicine **350**(19), 1953–1959+2018 (2004)

Fully-Coupled Electromechanical Simulations of the LV Dog Anatomy Using HPC: Model Testing and Verification

Jazmin Aguado-Sierra[1]([✉]), Alfonso Santiago[1], Matias I. Rivero[1],
Mariña López-Yunta[1], David Soto-Iglesias[2], Lydia Dux-Santoy[2],
Oscar Camara[2], and Mariano Vazquez[1]

[1] Barcelona Supercomputing Centre, Barcelona, Spain
jazmin.aguado@bsc.es
[2] PhySense, DTIC, Universitat Pompeu Fabra, Barcelona, Spain

Abstract. Verification of electro-mechanic models of the heart require a good amount of reliable, high resolution, thorough in-vivo measurements. The detail of the mathematical models used to create simulations of the heart beat vary greatly. Generally, the objective of the simulation determines the modeling approach. However, it is important to exactly quantify the amount of error between the various approaches that can be used to simulate a heart beat by comparing them to ground truth data. The more detailed the model is, the more computing power it requires, we therefore employ a high-performance computing solver throughout this study. We aim to compare models to data measured experimentally to identify the effect of using a mathematical model of fibre orientation versus the measured fibre orientations using DT-MRI. We also use simultaneous endocardial stimuli vs an instantaneous myocardial stimulation to trigger the mechanic contraction. Our results show that synchronisation of the electrical and mechanical events in the heart beat are necessary to create a physiological timing of hemodynamic events. Synchronous activation of all of the myocardium provides an unrealistic timing of hemodynamic events in the cardiac cycle. Results also show the need of establishing a protocol to quantify the zero-pressure configuration of the left ventricular geometry to initiate the simulation protocol; however, the predicted zero-pressure configuration of the same geometry was different, depending on the origin of the fibre field employed.

Keywords: High-Performance Computing (HPC) · Electromechanical simulations · Canine model · Ground-truth data · Verification

1 Introduction

Biophysical models of the heart have significantly improved their realism during the last years by incorporating patient-specific geometries and boundary conditions obtained from processing multimodal images and signals. In addition, continuous improvements in hardware and infrastructure computing facilities,

© Springer International Publishing Switzerland 2015
O. Camara et al. (Eds.): STACOM 2014, LNCS 8896, pp. 114–122, 2015.
DOI: 10.1007/978-3-319-14678-2_12

specially in High-Performance Computing (HPC) and Graphical Processing Units (GPU) are dramatically reducing computational costs associated to these tools. These are steps required for translating these biophysical models into clinical routine and develop simulation-based pipelines that can help on the management of a patient.

Nevertheless, electromechanical simulations of the heart remain a computational challenge extremely difficult to properly validate and verify. This is due to the complexity of the heart's physiology where multiple physical phenomena are tighly coupled at a different spatial and temporal scales, hampering the acquisition of complete sets of measurements to be used as reliable ground-truth data. Furthermore, detailed biophysical models including different spatial scales have a large amount of parameters that often are tuned based on limited experiments. Therefore, substantial effort is still required on performing sensitivity analysis of these parameters, verification studies to assess the appropriateness of the developed solvers and validation experiments to compare simulations with observations.

The majority of biophysical models of the heart were usually tuned to replicate observations obtained in laboratory experiments (e.g. patch clamp) that allowed to estimate some parameters. More recently some pioneering modelling work aimed at using patient-specific heart geometries derived from imaging and estimated some parameters comparing clinical measurements with electromechanical simulations [1–3]. Nevertheless, clinical measurements from humans are often incomplete and sparse, then not quite appropriate for exhaustive validation and verification of the electromechanical solvers. More controlled gold-standard electrophysiological data, derived either synthetically [4] or with experimental models [5], has been used in some simulation benchmarks to verify, customize, validate and integrate different cardiac electrophysiological solvers. A challenge organized in STACOM'11 aiming at validating myocardial tracking and deformation algorithms applied to image sequences [6], but, to our knowledge, there has not been yet a challenge for assessing simulated deformation fields provided by electromechanical models of the heart.

The STACOM'14 workshop included a challenge precisely aiming at evaluating electromechanical solvers of the heart using ground-truth data obtained from tag-MRI of experimental dog models. In this paper we make use of this data to test and verify the electromechanical simulations that have been developed over the last years at the *anonymized centre*. These simulations have been implemented to make use in the most efficient way high-performance computational resources, with a massively parallel implementation, an explicit formulation and a tight coupling between the electrical and mechanical solvers.

2   Methods

The software used for this study is an in-house, finite-element, multi-physics, High-Performance Computing (HPC) software. The experimental data, which is fully described described in [7], was kindly provided by the University of Auckland as part of the mechanical challenge at the STACOM'14 workshop.

2.1   Use of Experimental Data

High resolution Magnetic Resonance Imaging (MRI) data from one of the four datasets of normal dogs were used. The point clouds defining the LV geometry at diastasis, were used to generate the mesh employed as the starting point of our simulation protocol. Two more left ventricular geometries were provided for each dog at two hallmark times of the cardiac cycle: end of filling (end-diastole) and end of contraction (end-systole). Left ventricular volume and pressure were measured experimentally at several time points when the animals were being paced at 500 ms. The hemodynamic information was used to setup the appropriate boundary conditions during the cardiac cycle. They were also used to approximately tune some electric propagation information like total activation time, and action potential duration/repolarization.

2.2   Mathematical Description of the Anatomy

The provided endocardial and epicardial point clouds at diastasis were used to generate the mesh. Two meshes of different resolution were built using an in-house volume mesh generation and visualization code called Iris. One of the resulting left ventricular mesh has $19,591$ regular tetrahedral elements ($4,835$ nodes). The average element volume is $2.7e - 03$ cm^3, so that the average side lengths of the elements are 0.2874 cm. The second left ventricular mesh has $226,079$ regular tetrahedral elements ($46,401$ nodes). The average element volume is $0.191204e - 03$ cm^3, so that the average side lengths of the elements are 0.11 cm. Note that the framework used in this work uses CGS system of units (centimetre-gram-second). Note that the same mesh is used to solve both electrophysiology and biomechanics problems. Material parameter calibration was performed in the lowest resolution mesh.

2.3   Fibre Orientation Description

Muscle fibre orientations were derived from ex vivo diffusion tensor MRI available from the dog experiments. They were provided as raw DTI data regularly sampled at a grid of points, already been registered to the in-vivo geometry in diastasis, and as fibres post-processed and interpolated at the nodes of an hexahedral mesh of $9,225$ nodes. As part of our protocol, we generated a field of fibres as described by Streeter [8] at ± 60 degrees to compare and analyse the impact on the electromechanics given the use of different fibre fields: Streeter and the given DTI.

2.4   Electromechanical Framework

No measurements were provided from the dog experiments to adapt the electrical part of the solver, therefore two different assumptions on the behaviour of the left ventricle of a healthy dog were made to simulate electrical wave propagation:

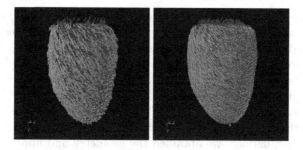

Fig. 1. Left: Synthetic fibre orientation generated using the model of Streeter et al. Right: Post-processed DTI fibres (at 9925 points) and interpolated into the high resolution, tetrahedral mesh using a closest neighbor interpolation.

- All of the myocardium was stimulated at the same time. This assumption holds if we assume a dense Purkinje system, an infinite conductivity and a synchronous activation of the whole myocardium.
- The activation occurs in the endocardium at the same time. This assumption holds if we assume a dense Purkinje fibre system. Conductivity was approximated by the knowledge of a "healthy, normal" ECG of a dog paced at a basic cycle length of 500 ms.

Electrophysiology. Ion concentration gradients across the myocyte cell membrane determine the electrical action potential that triggers contraction. To simulate the electrical activity, we solve a reaction-diffusion equation in our finite element mesh. We employ the monodomain formulation, solved explicitly [9]. The tissue is considered anisotropic to the fibre orientation. For this paper, we have employed the ionic cell models by Fitzhugh [10]. Conductivity in the fibre direction for the Fitzhugh-Nagumo model is 0.007 mS/cm in the fibre direction and 0.0023 mS/cm in the transverse directions. The conductivity was setup so that the total activation time occurs within 50 ms.

2.5 Biomechanics

The mechanical deformation part is solved at the same resolution of the electrophysiology mesh, thus avoiding any type of errors induced by interpolation between different meshes used for different physical solvers. The myocardial constitutive model employed in this study is a transversally isotropic version of the Holzapfel and Ogden [12] model. Therefore, the myocardium is considered as a non-homogeneous, non-linearly elastic, slightly compressible material [13].

In this study, the phase of diastasis can be considered to be a stress-free state. However, pressure in diastasis is low, but not zero. To obtain accurate results in the computational simulations, the zero-pressure configuration must be the starting point of the simulations. A deflation protocol was established, to obtain the stressed geometry at the time of diastasis.

Zero-Pressure Configuration Protocol. The first step is to "collapse" the geometry to a zero pressure state, in which the internal stresses of the solid can be assumed to be zero. The measured pressure in diastasis for the data in this simulation was 0.36 kPa. To deflate the geometry, we applied an equal, but opposite pressure to the endocardial walls of the left ventricular mesh. The resulting configuration is shown in figure 2. The mesh was allowed to deflate until a steady state was reached, at a V_0 of 16.3 ml for the DTI fibre mesh. Instead, for the mesh with the Streeter fibres, the V_0 was 16.7 ml. When volume was constant for each of the simulations, we obtained the geometry and fibre orientations in the assumed zero-pressure configuration and re-inflated the geometry to the pressure in diastasis. This process is iteratively done to recover the geometry in diastasis and is also used to calibrate the passive material parameters to obtain the pressure-volume relationship at the time of end diastole.

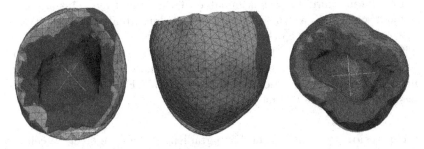

Fig. 2. Zero-pressure configuration of the LV geometry with DTI fibres in blue, compared to the initial geometry in white. Right: Zero pressure configuration of the DTI fibre mesh in blue; Streeter fibre mesh is shown in red.

2.6   Excitation Contraction Coupling

The electrophysiology model triggers the myocardial contraction using the model published by Hunter et al.[14], where a synthetic calcium transient is generated for the Fitlzhugh-Nagumo electrophysiology model as:

$$Ca_i(t) = Ca_0 + (Ca_{max} - Ca_0)\frac{t}{\tau_{Ca}}e^{1-t/\tau_{Ca}} \tag{1}$$

Where the parameters were modified to represent the calcium transient of a dog heart beat at a 500 ms basic cycle length, obtained using a detailed model of the dog M cell[15] (Fig. 3). Furthermore, the force-calcium relationship used was adapted from the model published by Hunter et al to generate the simulation in this study.

2.7   Boundary Conditions

A left ventricular pressure waveform was provided for this study. The pressure was applied normal to the endocardial walls throughout the cardiac cycle.

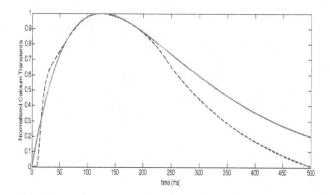

Fig. 3. Normalised Calcium Transients. Solid line indicates the Calcium Transient function used in the simulations. The dotted line indicates the calcium transient obtained from a detailed single M cell model of a dog.

The basal nodes were fixed to prevent them from moving in the longitudinal direction, but were allowed to move freely in the crossectional direction. The basic cycle length was 500 ms. The timings of the pressure waveform protocol were synchronized with the pacing stimuli of the electromechanical problem, since no hemodynamic model exists in our implementation at the moment (Fig. 4).

2.8   Simulation Protocol

The simulation protocol follows the time sequence in figure 4. Briefly, the simulations initiated from the zero-pressure configuration, and were allowed to reach steady state before the initiation of the protocol. The mesh is inflated to the pressure in diastasis. The course of the cardiac cycle initiates at that point. The mesh is allowed to passively inflate up to the pressure in end diastole. Slightly before the end of diastole, the electrical stimuli are triggered (at 95 ms). The stimulation protocol includes a simulation where all the myocardium is activated synchronously, and using endocardial stimuli (see Table 1).

Table 1. Simulations

Number	fibres	Synchronous EP Stimuli	EP Model
1	DTI fibres	All myocardium	FHN
2	Streeter fibres	Endocardial	FHN
3	DTI fibres	Endocardial	FHN

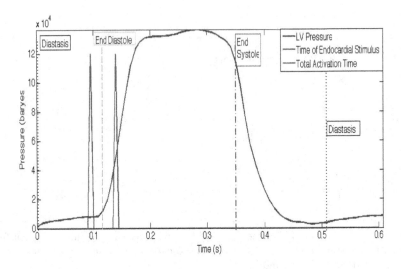

Fig. 4. Pressure time course as boundary conditions normal to the endocardium. Marked are the three defined cardiac cycle hallmarks: Diastasis in black, End Diastole in cyan and End Systole in green. Time of the start of the electrical stimuli is shown in magenta while the total time of activation is shown in orange.

3   Results

3.1   Electrical Activation: Whole vs. Partial Endocardial Activation

Assuming that the electrical activation occurs simultaneously throughout the whole myocardium creates a non-physiological timing of the events on the cardiac cycle. Peak of contraction occurs 90 ms after electrical activation, which corresponds to a just a few milliseconds after valve opening. For this reason, the use of simultaneous stimuli throughout the myocardium was deemed non-physiological for our methodology. In the other hand, synchronizing the electro-mechanic events to the hemodynamics, creates more physiological responses.

3.2   Fibre Orientation: Streeter vs. DTI

DT-MRI is not always available for implementing electro-mechanical simulations, particularly when creating patient-specific simulations. One of the most popular ways to generate a fibre field is to apply the transmural dispersion as measured experimentally. One of such models was proposed by D. Streeter. The purpose of these simulations is to quantify the influence of the fibre orientation to the electro-mechanics of each model and to verify the error when compared with ground truth data. An important observation, is that the predicted zero-pressure configuration of the same geometry was influenced by the fibre field used for each of the simulations.

4 Conclusions

Establishing a more physiological electrical activation sequence provides more realistic timings of the mechanic and hemodynamic events in the cardiac cycle. fibre orientation swiftly modifies the electric activation sequence and the breakthrough of the electric propagation, however more data would be necessary to verify the electrophysiology. Fibre orientation also has an impact on the zero-pressure configuration of the model. Zero-pressure volumes differ depending on the fibres employed, which will have an impact on the overall parameter estimation and the geometrical deformation of the LV.

Acknowledgments. This work has been done with the support of the grant SEV-2011-00067 of Severo Ochoa Program, awarded by the Spanish Government to the Barcelona Supercomputing Center. Part of the research leading to these results has received funding from the Seventh Framework Programme (FP7/2007-2013) under grant agreement n 611823. It has also been partially funded from the by the Spanish Ministry of Economy and Competitiveness (TIN2011-28067).

References

1. Sermesant, M., Moireau, P., Camara, O., Sainte-Marie, J., et al.: Cardiac function estimation from mri using a heart model and data assimilation: advances and difficulties. Medical Image Analysis **10**(4), 642–656 (2006)
2. Kerckhoffs, R., McCulloch, A., Omens, J., Mulligan, L.: Effects of biventricular pacing and scar size in a computational model of the failing heart with left bundle branch block. Medical Image Analysis **13**(2), 362–369 (2009)
3. Trayanova, N., Constantino, J., Gurev, V.: Electromechanical models of the ventricles. American Journal of Physiology **301**, 279–286 (2011)
4. Niederer, S., Kerfoot, E., Benson, A., Bernabeu, M., et al.: Constitutive modelling of passive my- ocardium: a structurally based framework for material characterization. Philosophical Transactions of the Royal Society A: Mathematical, Physical and Engineering Sciences **369**(1954), 4331–4351 (2009)
5. Camara, O., Sermesant, M., Lamata, P., Wang, L., et al.: Inter-model consistency and complementarity: learning from ex-vivo imaging and electrophysiological data towards an integrated understanding of cardiac physiology. Progress in Biophysics and Molecular Biology **107**(1), 122–133 (2011)
6. Tobon-Gomez, C., Craene, M.D., McLeod, K., Tautz, L., et al.: Benchmarking framework for myocardial tracking and deformation algorithms: an open access database. Medical Image Analysis **17**(6), 632–648 (2013)
7. Wang, V., Lam, H., Ennis, D., Cowan, B., Young, A., Nash, M.: Modelling passive diastolic mechanics with quantitative MRI of cardiac structure and function. Med. Image Anal. **13**(5), 773–784 (2009)
8. Streeter, D.: Gross morphology and fibrous structure of the heart. In: Handbook of Physiology: The Cardiovascular System, vol. 1, pp. 61–112. Oxford University Press (1979)
9. Vázquez, M., Arís, R., Houzeaux, G., Aubry, R., et al.: A massively parallel computational electrophysiology model of the heart. International Journal for Numerical Methods in Biomedical Engineering **27**(12), 1991–1929 (2011)

10. Fitzhugh, R.: Impulses and physiological states in theoretical models of nerve membrane. Biophysical Journal **1**, 445–466 (1961)
11. ten Tusscher, K.H.W.J., Panfilov, A.V.: Alternans and spiral breakup in a human ventricular tissue model. Am. J. Physiol. Heart Circ. Physiol. **291**(3), H1088–H1100 (2006)
12. Holzapfel, G., Ogden, R.: Constitutive modelling of passive myocardium: a structurally based framework for material characterization. Philosophical Transactions of the Royal Society A: Mathematical, Physical and Engineering Sciences **367**(1902), 3445–3475 (2009)
13. Lafortune, P., Arís, R., Vázquez, M., Houzeaux, G.: Coupled electromechanical model of the heart: parallel finite element formulation. International Journal for Numerical Methods in Biomedical Engineering **28**, 72–86 (2012)
14. Hunter, P., McCulloch, A., ter Keurs, H.: Modelling the mechanical properties of cardiac muscle. Progress in Biophysics and Molecular Biology **69**(2), 289–331 (1998)
15. Flaim, S.N., Giles, W.R., McCulloch, A.: Contributions of sustained ina and ikv4.3 to transmural heterogeneity of early repolarization and arrhythmogenesis in canine left ventricular myocytes. Am. J. Physiol. Heart Circ. Physiol. **291**, H2617–H2629 (2006)

STACOM Challenge: Simulating Left Ventricular Mechanics in the Canine Heart

Liya Asner[✉], Myrianthi Hadjicharalambous, Jack Lee, and David Nordsletten

Department of Biomedical Engineering, King's College London, London, UK
`liya.asner@kcl.ac.uk`

Abstract. In this paper we outline our approach for creating subject-specific whole-cycle canine left-ventricular models, as part of the 2014 STACOM Challenge. Each canine heart was modeled using the principle of stationary potential energy, with the myocardium treated as a nearly incompressible hyperelastic material. Given incomplete data on the motion and behavior of each canine heart, we decreased model complexity by employing reduced–parameter constitutive laws. Additionally, base plane motion and left ventricular volume input data were integrated into the cardiac cycle model through the inclusion of novel external energy potentials (using Lagrange multipliers), which allow for relaxed adherence to the constraints and minimize spurious energy modes stemming from model simplification and data noise. Subsequently, using the available data we employ the reduced-order unscented Kalman filter (ROUKF) approach to estimate the myocardial passive parameters and active tension. Finally, along with model predictions for each canine, we assess the spatial convergence and robustness of our model.

Keywords: Cardiac mechanics · Canine heart · Parameter estimation · Data assimilation

1 Introduction

Aspects of left ventricular mechanics – including motion, constitutive relations, microarchitecture and contractile function – have been the focus of intense research. Complementing this effort, the mathematical modeling of the full cycle mechanics has become well–established [13], incorporating varying degrees of the inherent physiological complexity into passive and active tissue constitutive models [9] as well as advanced physiological boundary conditions [4]. While these models are idealised, they provide a platform for assessing patient-specific myocardial function as well as prediction through tuning a series of model parameters. The model-tuning process has raised interest in inverse problems in whole heart mechanical modelling, and currently a range of tractable methods to quantify the parameters underpinning function have been proposed [1,5,11]. This approach has been applied within the cardiac modelling community to estimate both passive and active mechanical parameters [4,11,14,15].

© Springer International Publishing Switzerland 2015
O. Camara et al. (Eds.): STACOM 2014, LNCS 8896, pp. 123–134, 2015.
DOI: 10.1007/978-3-319-14678-2_13

Various inverse estimation techniques have been proposed in the literature to date, including sequential quadratic programming, which has roots in nonlinear optimisation [1,14], the unscented transform algorithm [11] and families of data assimilation methods including Kalman filter-based sequential assimilation, and adjoint-based variational assimilation [5], although a systematic comparison of the techniques is currently lacking. Further to the estimation methodology used, the accuracy and quality of prediction is clearly limited by the selected models, their construction as well as the data available for parameterization. For a unique parameterization, the well-posedness and conditioning of the problem is critical, requiring careful selection of the appropriate forward model so available input data may be judiciously integrated. The common approach in the literature has been to limit the number of parameters estimated and use a much richer set of image data that covers the full spatial and temporal extent of the pertinent cardiac phases to constrain the parameterization process [7]. For instance, full Lagrangian displacement field extracted from tagged MRI has been the basis for estimating 4 parameters [14,15], while the surface motion derived from cine MRI has been used for estimation of 4 parameters [11], or 1 parameter in 6 different regions of myocardium [4].

In this paper we employ these developed approaches for constructing canine left ventricular models as part of the 2014 STACOM Challenge. The problem is a challenging one due to its underconstrained nature, whereby the input data consists of the surface geometry provided at three time points and a pressure-volume loop. Accordingly, to produce accurate deformation, the solution approach requires a corresponding increase in the "regularisation" – this may be provided by further reduction of model complexity to prevent over-fitting and sensibly-posed boundary conditions to constrain the motion of the ventricle to be physiological. Our approach employs a reduced-parameter constitutive law adapted from the literature, and a generic strain-dependent active law. For each of the cases the models are personalised based on the available data. The methods used are described in Section 2, and the results are shown in Section 3. We were able to match pressure-volume loops, compute displacements and stresses through the cycle, and ascertain that numerical convergence was achieved in these variables.

2   Methods

2.1   Cardiac Mechanics Model

The mechanical deformation and pressure (u, p) in the canine left ventricle were modeled using the principle of stationary potential energy which minimizes a free energy functional, Π [2]. Momentum in the heart was neglected due to the dominance of mechanical stresses through the cycle. The myocardial muscle was modeled as a hyperelastic material, as described by equation (1). The strain energy comprised passive and active terms (subscript p and a, respectively). Viscoelastic effects were also neglected due, in part, to the lack of validated material models. As the myocardial volume was observed to change up to 12%

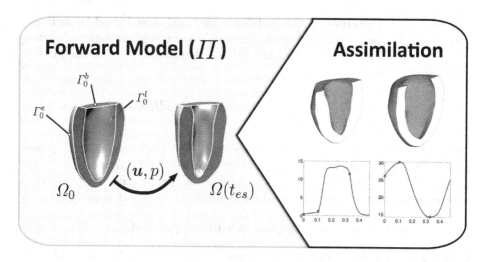

Fig. 1. Schematic of the forward model and given data for STACOM 2014

through the cardiac cycle (percentage volume change between end–diastole and end–systole was 3.6%, 8.9%, 12.0% and 8.3% for the four cases), the material was modeled as nearly incompressible (with bulk modulus κ) as shown in equation 1.

$$W(\boldsymbol{u}, p) = W_p(\boldsymbol{C}) + W_a(\boldsymbol{C}) + p\left(J - 1 - \frac{p}{2\kappa}\right) \qquad (1)$$

Here $\boldsymbol{C}$ and J denote the right Cauchy Green strain and the Jacobian respectively [2]. The passive strain energy W_p was modeled using a reduced form of the Holzapfel-Ogden model [7,8] characterized by two scaling parameters $\{a_1, a_2\}$ and two exponential parameters $\{b_1, b_1\}$, with indices 1 and 2 corresponding to the fibre and the cross-fibre terms:

$$W_p(\boldsymbol{C}) = \frac{a_1}{2b_1}\{\exp[b_1(I_{\boldsymbol{C}_f} - 1)^2] - 1\} \;+\; \frac{a_2}{2b_2}\exp[b_2(I_{\hat{\boldsymbol{C}}} - 3)].$$

The active generation of internal energy was modeled via a simple time-dependent scaling: $W_a(\boldsymbol{C}) = \alpha(t)(I_{\boldsymbol{C}_f} - 1)$.

Both the passive and the active strain energy functions are directly dependent on fibre strains, and therefore on the choice of the fibre distribution in the myocardium. The use of DTI-based fibres provided for the four cases consistently led to non-physiological lengthening of the ventricle in systole, even with a uniform relaxation (see Figure 6). Instead we have constructed idealised fibre fields based on the geometries, with the angles between sheet planes and fibre vectors varying linearly in the transmural direction between $-80°$ and $80°$ from epi- to endocardium. As shown in Section 3, this distribution allowed us to simulate long axis shortening of the LV, which is normally observed in systole.

From the definition of the strain energy given by equation (1), the energy functional Π can be written as the sum of the internal energy and external (boundary-based) energies. Additional Lagrange multipliers $\boldsymbol{\lambda}^b$ and λ^l are introduced along the base plane and lumen surfaces respectively to ensure adherence of the model to base plane motion and volume change data, as discussed in the following sections.

$$\Pi(\boldsymbol{u}, p, \boldsymbol{\lambda}^b, \lambda^l) := \int_{\Omega_0} W(\boldsymbol{u}, p) \, d\boldsymbol{X} - \sum_{k=b,l} \Pi_k^{ext}(\boldsymbol{u}, \lambda^k), \tag{2}$$

where Π_b^{ext} denotes the base plane energy, and Π_l^{ext} the lumen wall boundary energy. The final solution for any point in time $t \in [0, T]$ in the heart cycle is determined as the saddle point of the free energy functional Π, ensuring adherence to boundary conditions whilst minimizing the internal energy, i.e.

$$\Pi(\boldsymbol{u}, p, \boldsymbol{\lambda}^b, \lambda^l) = \inf \{ \sup \{ \Pi(\boldsymbol{v}, q, \boldsymbol{q}, \mu), \ (q, \boldsymbol{q}, \mu) \in \boldsymbol{X} \}, \ \boldsymbol{v} \in \boldsymbol{U} \} \tag{3}$$

Here $\boldsymbol{U}$ is the space of admissible displacement solutions and $\boldsymbol{X} = W \times \gamma_b \boldsymbol{U} \times \mathbb{R}$ the space of Lagrange multipliers, with W being the space of hydrostatic pressure solutions, and $\gamma_b \boldsymbol{U}$ the trace space of $\boldsymbol{U}$ on the base plane (see Figure 1).

2.2 Base Plane and Endocardial Boundary Energies

In our model the specific external energy terms were applied on the boundaries to enable assimilation of the data provided. To ensure proper base plane motion of the model Π_b^{ext} was selected as,

$$\Pi_b^{ext}(\boldsymbol{u}, \boldsymbol{\lambda}^b) := \int_{\Gamma_0^b} \boldsymbol{\lambda}^b \cdot \left(\boldsymbol{u} - \boldsymbol{u}_d(t) - \frac{1}{2} \boldsymbol{K}(t) \boldsymbol{\lambda}^b \right) d\boldsymbol{X}, \tag{4}$$

where $\boldsymbol{u}_d(t)$ is the displacement of the base plane and $\boldsymbol{K}(t)$ a constraint relaxation matrix. The motion of the base plane was given through the position of four points in space $\boldsymbol{X} = (\boldsymbol{x}_1, \boldsymbol{x}_2, \boldsymbol{x}_3, \boldsymbol{x}_4)$ at three points in time (DS, ED and ES). Therefore the displacement fields $\boldsymbol{u}_d(t)$ applied on the whole base through the cycle had to be interpolated. Specifically we used singular value decompositions to construct affine mappings $\boldsymbol{A}_{(DS \text{ to } ED)}$ and $\boldsymbol{A}_{(ED \text{ to } ES)} \in \mathbb{R}^3$ that accommodated the given transformation of points $\boldsymbol{X}$, i.e.

$$\boldsymbol{A}_{(DS \text{ to } ED)} \, \boldsymbol{X}_{DS} = \boldsymbol{X}_{ED},$$
$$\boldsymbol{A}_{(ED \text{ to } ES)} \, \boldsymbol{X}_{ED} = \boldsymbol{X}_{ES},$$

The mappings were then applied on the whole set of base points $\boldsymbol{x}^b$:

$$\boldsymbol{x}_{ED}^b = \boldsymbol{A}_{(DS \text{ to } ED)} \boldsymbol{x}_{DS}^b,$$
$$\boldsymbol{x}_{ES}^b = \boldsymbol{A}_{(ED \text{ to } ES)} \boldsymbol{x}_{ED}^b = \boldsymbol{A}_{(ED \text{ to } ES)} \boldsymbol{A}_{(DS \text{ to } ED)} \boldsymbol{x}_{DS}^b.$$

At any time during the heart cycle $[0, T]$ (with $t_{DS} = 0$) the displacement of the base points can be linearly interpolated in time using the DS, ED and ES values:

$$t \in [0, t_{ED}] : \quad \boldsymbol{u}_d(t) = \frac{t}{t_{ED}} \left(\boldsymbol{x}_{ED}^b - \boldsymbol{x}_{DS}^b \right),$$

$$t \in [t_{ED}, t_{ES}] : \quad \boldsymbol{u}_d(t) = \frac{t - t_{ED}}{t_{ES} - t_{ED}} \left(\boldsymbol{x}_{ES}^b - \boldsymbol{x}_{ED}^b \right) + \boldsymbol{x}_{ED}^b - \boldsymbol{x}_{DS}^b,$$

$$t \in [t_{ES}, T] : \quad \boldsymbol{u}_d(t) = \frac{T - t}{T - t_{ES}} \left(\boldsymbol{x}_{ES}^b - \boldsymbol{x}_{DS}^b \right).$$

Strict adherence to the interpolated base condition gives rise to unphysiological stress / strain distributions. The additional term $-\frac{1}{2}\boldsymbol{K}(t)\boldsymbol{\lambda}^b$ in the base boundary energy expression (4) allowed us to relax the constraint and lower the artificially induced boundary stresses. The matrix was chosen as $\boldsymbol{K} = \varepsilon(\boldsymbol{I} - \mathbf{n}_b(t) \otimes \mathbf{n}_b(t))$ with $\mathbf{n}_b$ denoting the base plane normal through time, so that $(\boldsymbol{u} - \boldsymbol{u}_d) \cdot \mathbf{n}_b(t) = 0$ (i.e. translation of the base plane is exact), while $(\boldsymbol{u} - \boldsymbol{u}_d - \varepsilon\boldsymbol{\lambda}^b) \cdot \boldsymbol{v} = 0$ for any vector $\boldsymbol{v}$ in the plane (i.e. in-plane motion is relaxed). Sending $\varepsilon \to \infty$ requires no adherence to the in-plane motion, while sending $\varepsilon \to 0$ requires strict adherence ($\varepsilon \sim 10^{-7}$ m/Pa was used).

Incorporation of the lumen volume data was achieved using the boundary energy term Π_l^{ext} given as,

$$\Pi_l^{ext}(\boldsymbol{u}, \lambda^l) := \lambda^l \left(\frac{1}{3} \int_{\Gamma^l} \boldsymbol{x} \cdot \mathbf{n} \, d\boldsymbol{x} + \frac{1}{3} \int_{\Gamma^{lb}} \boldsymbol{x} \cdot \mathbf{n}_b(t) \, d\boldsymbol{x} - V(t) \right), \quad (5)$$

where $V(t)$ is the given volume data and Γ^{lb} is the base plane area at the top of the lumen, completing the boundary integral over the LV cavity. By divergence theorem,

$$\frac{1}{3} \int_{\Gamma^l} \boldsymbol{x} \cdot \mathbf{n} \, d\boldsymbol{x} + \frac{1}{3} \int_{\Gamma^{lb}} \boldsymbol{x} \cdot \mathbf{n}_b(t) \, d\boldsymbol{x} = \frac{1}{3} \int_{\Gamma^{lv}} \boldsymbol{x} \cdot \mathbf{n} \, d\boldsymbol{x} = \frac{1}{3} \int_{\Omega_{lv}} \nabla \cdot \boldsymbol{x} \, d\boldsymbol{x} = V(t),$$

with Ω_{lv} the corresponding LV cavity volume domain and Γ^{lv} the corresponding LV cavity boundary. Equation (5) enforces strict adherence of the model to the given data as any deviation sends $\Pi \to \infty$.

Dependence on Γ^{lb} in equation (5) can be removed by introducing the matrix $\boldsymbol{I}_b(t) = (1/2)(\boldsymbol{I} - \mathbf{n}_b(t) \otimes \mathbf{n}_b(t))$. As $\boldsymbol{I}_b \mathbf{n}_b = \mathbf{0}$, by divergence theorem,

$$\boldsymbol{I}_b(t) : \int_{\Gamma^l} \boldsymbol{x} \otimes \mathbf{n} \, d\boldsymbol{x} = \boldsymbol{I}_b(t) : \int_{\Gamma^{lv}} \boldsymbol{x} \otimes \mathbf{n} \, d\boldsymbol{x} = \int_{\Omega_{lv}} \nabla \cdot (\boldsymbol{I}_b(t)\boldsymbol{x}) \, d\boldsymbol{x}$$

$$= (\boldsymbol{I}_b(t) : \boldsymbol{I})V(t) = V(t), \quad (6)$$

providing a means for measuring volume without requiring base plane area (even when base plane translation / rotation is observed).

2.3   Finite Element Solution

The solution to equation (3) was approximated using the finite element method (see [6] for discussion). Specifically $\mathbb{Q}^2 - \mathbb{Q}^1$ Taylor-Hood element [3] interpolation was used for $u_h - p_h$, as well as surface $\mathbb{Q}^2$ for λ_h^b and a single constant for λ^l. Taking the directional derivatives of equation (3) with respect to all state variables gives the following form of the minimization problem:

$$D_{u_h} \Pi[v_h] + D_{p_h} \Pi[q_h] + D_{\lambda_h^b} \Pi[q_h] + D_{\lambda^l} \Pi[\mu] = 0 \quad \forall \, (v_h, q_h, q_h, \mu) \in U^h \times X^h.$$

The final model solution at any time point is given as the $(u_h, p_h, \lambda_h^b, \lambda^l) \in U^h \times X^h$ which satisfies,

$$\int_{\Omega_0} \nabla_F W(u_h, p_h) : \nabla_X v_h \; + \; q_h(J_h - 1) \, dX$$

$$- \lambda^l \int_{\Gamma^l} v_h \cdot \mathbf{n} \, dx \; - \; \mu \left(I_b(t) : \int_{\Gamma^l} x \otimes \mathbf{n} \, dx - V(t) \right)$$

$$- \int_{\Gamma_0^b} \lambda_h^b \cdot v_h \, dX \; - \; \int_{\Gamma_0^b} q_h \cdot \left(u_h - u_d(t) - K(t)\lambda_h^b \right) \, dX = 0,$$

$$\forall \, (v_h, q_h, q_h, \mu) \in U^h \times X^h \tag{7}$$

Equation (7) was solved for each load state through the cardiac cycle enabling the reconstruction of the myocardial motion.

2.4   Passive and Active Material Parameter Estimation

In order to simulate the cycle for each of the cases we required a suitable set of constitutive law parameters. These parameters were estimated using the reduced-order unscented Kalman filter (ROUKF) [4,12]. The method is particularly efficient since the number of parameters is low, and consequently few forward model runs are required in the estimation process. Assimilation was based on pressure observations through the whole cycle.

We first considered the passive stage independently. This was taken to start at the points marked in the PV loop as DS, and end at or just before ED. The available pressure-volume data was normalised and coarsely fit to the experimental results presented in Klotz [10]. The parameters $b_1 = b_2 = 5.0$ were chosen so that inflation of an idealized LV of average size (tuning cross-sectional area, long axis length and wall thickness) across the group produced the degree of exponential growth observed. More comprehensive estimates of $\{b_1, b_2\}$ were not made due to their coupling with outer stiffness parameters $\{a_1, a_2\}$. The nature of this coupling meant that adjusting $\{a_1, a_2\}$ for any *reasonable* pair $\{b_1, b_2\}$ allowed a good fit to the data. In the purely passive stage of the cycle (DS-ED), the absence of the W_a term in the total strain energy meant that the remaining passive parameters $\{a_1, a_2\}$ could be estimated. All diastolic pressures were observed simultaneously in a ROUKF iteration, and the estimation was repeated with updated states and covariance matrices until convergence was achieved (as measured by the closeness of the determinant of the background error covariance matrix to 1). In some cases the fitting process highlighted pressure outliers at or before ED, which were treated as containing some active tension.

In the second stage of the cycle (ED-DS) the passive parameters were fixed, and the magnitude of the active tension was estimated as a time-varying scalar $\alpha(t)$, $t \in [t_{ed}, T]$. A number of models (quadratic, cubic Hermite and $\tanh^2$) were evaluated as possible parametrisable expressions for the active tension, but neither of these gave a reasonable fit to the pressure-volume data. We have therefore made no assumptions on the functional form of $\alpha(t)$, and estimated it as a piecewise constant in time. Two ROUKF iterations were run per time step to ensure filter convergence, and the initial guess for each step was updated based on the estimate at the previous time step.

All of the parameters were estimated globally in space, since no localised data could be used in the estimation process. For each case the final simulation results were computed using the estimates for a_1, a_2 and $\alpha(t)$.

3   Results

The computed deformation of meshes consisting of 4608 quadratic hexahedral elements for all cases is illustrated by Figure 2. Characteristic twist and shortening are observed in systole.

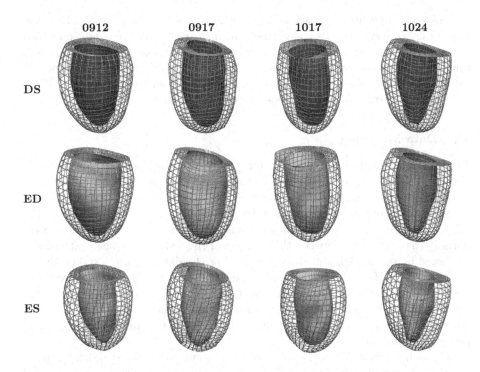

Fig. 2. LV configurations for all cases at DS, ED and ES. The endocardial surface is coloured by magnitude of displacement from DS. The colour is scaled from blue to red per row, with the highest ED value being 3.7 mm and the highest ES value 8.9 mm. Mesh lines are shown on the epicardial surface to illustrate deformation directions.

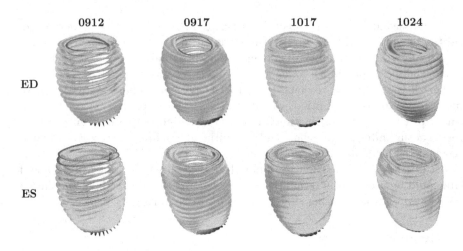

Fig. 3. Fibre stresses σ_f for all cases at ED and ES. The surfaces are coloured by the value of the stress from blue (0 kPa) to red (4 kPa at ED and 40kPa at ES).

The computed fibre stresses at ED and ES are shown in Figure 3. Extreme values were observed on the base plane, which suggests that the condition which propagates motion of four epicardial points to the whole of the base surface could be introducing inaccurate displacements. Even though the magnitude of the stresses on the base was reduced through the use of the relaxed condition, this region still exhibited likely non-physiological stresses.

3.1   Data Matching

The pressure-volume loops obtained on meshes are shown in Figure 4. Volumes were prescribed through the model, and were matched exactly. Only minor pressure errors are present, mostly at the corners of the loops.

Since surface data was not used for estimation in the current setup, the process could not fully account for local effects in deformation. However, a comparison was performed between the location of the endo- and epicardial surfaces predicted by the model, and those provided as the data. Figure 5 shows several views of the surfaces in the original image coordinates ES for the case 0912. High-error regions are located either near the points of attachment between the left and the right ventricles, or on the septal wall. This suggests that including the right ventricle or a corresponding boundary condition in the model has the potential to improve the results.

Figure 6 illustrates the effect of fibre orientations on myocardial deformations at ES, as discussed above. The DTI fibres provided, as well as the commonly used −60° to 60° distribution resulted in non-physiological and non-data-compliant lengthening of the ventricle in systole.

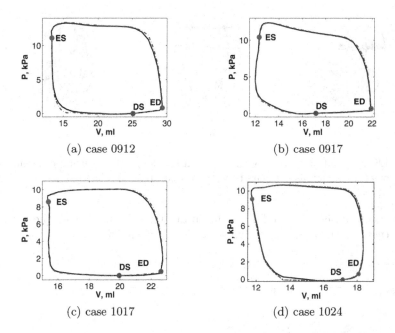

(a) case 0912

(b) case 0917

(c) case 1017

(d) case 1024

Fig. 4. Pressure-volume loops: data in solid, and simulation in dash-dotted line

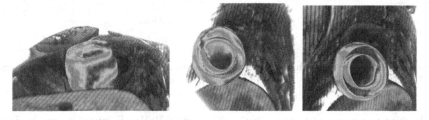

Fig. 5. Deformation of endo- and epicardial surfaces of the mesh for case 0912, shown in image coordinates at ES. Colour marks distances to nearest points on the data surfaces (0..4 mm from purple to red).

3.2 Verification

In order to assess the reliability of the method in modelling left ventricular mechanics we performed a number of additional tests.

Mesh convergence of the solutions was studied on a series of uniform refinements of a coarse quadratic hexahedral mesh: mesh 1 was composed of 72 elements, mesh 2 of 576, mesh 3 of 4608, and mesh 4 of 36864. In the absence of a ground truth solution, simulation results on mesh 4 were taken as reference. This allowed us to compute relative errors in the main problem variables:

$$e = \|\boldsymbol{v} - \boldsymbol{v}_{\text{ref}}\|/\|\boldsymbol{v}_{\text{ref}}\|, \quad \boldsymbol{v} = \boldsymbol{u}, p, \boldsymbol{\sigma}_{\boldsymbol{f}}.$$

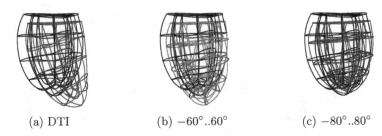

(a) DTI   (b) −60°..60°   (c) −80°..80°

Fig. 6. ES deformation of the LV mesh for case 0912 produced using different fibre orientations (in colour), as compared to DS configuration (in black).

The errors on meshes 1, 2 and 3 are shown in Figure 7. In all cases the error on mesh 3 (used as the challenge submission) is less than 5%.

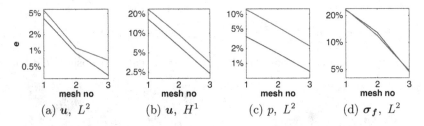

(a) u, L^2 (b) u, H^1 (c) p, L^2 (d) σ_f, L^2

Fig. 7. Relative error in problem variables on progressively refined meshes for case 0917. The red and blue lines correspond to errors at ED and ES respectively.

Passive parameter estimates for a given set of ROUKF inputs were obtained on meshes 1, 2 and 3. The values were consistent at every ROUKF iteration, and the relative error in the parameters after 10 assimilation steps was < 5% between meshes 1 and 2, and < 2% between meshes 2 and 3.

Filter convergence was observed in all cases, both for the passive and active estimation procedures. At the same time, changes in ROUKF initial state and error covariance matrices in passive estimation resulted in a significant variation in the final estimates. Figure 8a illustrates how pressures computed using these estimates, $a^1 = (1.4, 0.9)$ kPa, $a^2 = (0.9, 2.6)$ kPa, $a^3 = (0.7, 3.4)$ kPa, compare to the data. The map of the errors in diastolic pressures $\|P - \lambda^l(a_1, a_2)\|$ over the passive parameter space (Figure 8b) shows that instead of a clear minimum there is a valley of parameter combinations that minimize the l^2-norm pressure functional. This indicates a coupling between the parameters, suggesting that the model requires additional data to achieve reliable passive parameter estimation. Finally, the estimated active tension curves are presented in Figure 8c. All cases exhibit fast growth post-activation, and sustained (sometimes increasing) tension through systole, with a tailing off in the deactivation stage.

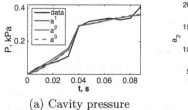
(a) Cavity pressure

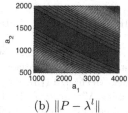
(b) $\|P - \lambda^l\|$

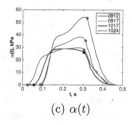
(c) $\alpha(t)$

Fig. 8. Estimation based on pressure data in diastole and systole: (a) matching of cavity pressure data P by the Lagrange multiplier λ^l in diastole using different parameter combinations, (b) map of distances between the vectors of simulated and observed cavity pressures over the passive parameter space (a_1, a_2), (c) estimates for the active tension over time

4 Discussion

The mechanics model incorporated cavity pressure-volume data to simulate deformation of the left ventricles for four canines through the whole cardiac cycle. Model personalisation was achieved through estimation of passive model parameters and time-dependent active tension scaling. A good fit for PV data was obtained, as well as reasonable physiological deformations, although total exclusion of the right ventricle from the model appears to produce higher errors in attachment areas. Simulation and estimation results were verified through a series of convergence tests.

In the setup presented there is limited potential for model personalisation based on bulk measures. Incorporating distances to surfaces at ED and ES could potentially result in a better fit, but was impractical to implement in a short time span and was only used for validation. An augmented set of data, *e.g.* time-resolved images of cardiac motion, could be included in the workflow to compute reliable estimates, allowing the use of parameters as biomarkers. In addition, assimilation of local displacements would enable better data fitting and stress computation, as well as studying the effects of tissue heterogeneity.

Acknowledgments. The authors would like to acknowledge funding from the BHF New Horizons program (NH/11/5/29058) and support from the Wellcome Trust-EPSRC Centre of Excellence in Medical Engineering (WT 088641/Z/09/Z) and the NIHR Biomedical Research Centre at Guy's and St. Thomas' NHS Foundation Trust and KCL. The views expressed are those of the authors and not necessarily those of the NHS, the NIHR, or the DoH. The authors would also like to thank Radomir Chabiniok for his input.

References

1. Augenstein, K., Cowan, B., LeGrice, I., Nielsen, P., Young, A.: Method and apparatus for soft tissue material parameter estimation using tissue tagged magnetic resonance imaging. J. Biomech. Eng. **127**(1), 148–157 (2005)

2. Bonet, J., Wood, R.: Nonlinear Continuum Mechanics for Finite Element Analysis. Cambridge University Press (2008)
3. Brezzi, F., Fortin, M.: Mixed and hybrid finite element methods. Springer, Heidelberg (1991)
4. Chabiniok, R., Moireau, P., Lesault, P.-F., Rahmouni, A., Deux, J.-F., Chapelle, D.: Estimation of tissue contractility from cardiac cine-MRI using a biomechanical heart model. Biomech. Model. Mechan. 11(5), 609–630 (2012)
5. Chapelle, D., Fragu, M., Mallet, V., Moireau, P.: Fundamental principles of data assimilation underlying the Verdandi library: applications to biophysical model personalization within euHeart. Med. Biol. Eng. Comput. 51(11), 1221–1233 (2013)
6. Hadjicharalambous, M., Lee, J., Smith, N., Nordsletten, D.: A displacement-based finite element formulation for incompressible and nearly-incompressible cardiac mechanics. Comput. Method. Appl. M. 274, 213–236 (2014)
7. Hadjicharalambous, M., Asner, L., Chabiniok, R., Sammut, E., Wong, J., Carr-White, G., Razavi, R., Nordsletten, D.: Analysis of cardiac constitutive laws for parameter estimation using 3D tagged MRI. Biomech. Model. Mechan (accepted for publication)
8. Holzapfel, G., Ogden, R.: Constitutive modelling of passive myocardium: a structurally based framework for material characterization. Philos. T. R. Soc. A 367, 3445–3475 (2009)
9. Kerckhoffs, R., Bovendeerd, P., Prinzen, F., Smits, K., Arts, T.: Intra- and inter-ventricular asynchrony of electromechanics in the ventricularly paced heart. J. Eng. Math. 47, 201–216 (2003)
10. Klotz, S., Hay, I., Dickstein, M., Yi, G., Wang, J., Maurer, M., Kass, D., Burkhoff, D.: Single-beat estimation of end-diastolic pressure-volume relationship: a novel method with potential for noninvasive application. Am. J. Physiol.-Heart C 291, H403–H412 (2006)
11. Marchesseau, S., Delingette, H., Sermesant, M., Ayache, N.: Fast parameter calibration of a cardiac electromechanical model from medical images based on the unscented transform. Biomech. Model. Mechan. 12(4), 815–831 (2013)
12. Moireau, P., Chapelle, D.: Reduced-order unscented Kalman filtering with application to parameter identification in large-dimensional systems. ESAIM Contr. Op. Ca. Va. 17(2), 380–405 (2011)
13. Nordsletten, D., Niederer, S., Nash, M., Hunter, P., Smith, N.: Coupling multi-physics models to cardiac mechanics. Prog. Biophys. Mol. Bio. 104, 77–88 (2011)
14. Wang, V., Lam, H., Ennis, D., Cowan, B., Young, A., Nash, M.: Modelling passive diastolic mechanics with quantitative MRI of cardiac structure and function. Med. Image Anal. 13(5), 773–784 (2009)
15. Xi, J., Lamata, P., Niederer, S., Land, S., Shi, W., Zhuang, X., Ourselin, S., Duckett, S., Shetty, A., Rinaldi, A., Rueckert, D., Razavi, R., Smith, N.: The estimation of patient-specific cardiac diastolic functions from clinical measurements. Med. Image Anal. 17(2), 133–146 (2013)

Identifying Myocardial Mechanical Properties from MRI Using an Orthotropic Constitutive Model

Zhinuo J. Wang[1]([✉]), Vicky Y. Wang[1], Sue-Mun Huang[1],
Justyna A. Niestrawska[2], Alistair A. Young[1,3], and Martyn P. Nash[1,4]

[1] Auckland Bioengineering Institute, University of Auckland,
Auckland, New Zealand
{zwan145,shua078}@aucklanduni.ac.nz,
{vicky.wang,a.young,martyn.nash}@auckland.ac.nz
[2] Institute of Biomechanics, Graz University of Technology, Graz, Austria
niestrawska@tugraz.at
[3] Department of Anatomy with Radiology, University of Auckland,
Auckland, New Zealand
[4] Department of Engineering Science, University of Auckland,
Auckland, New Zealand

Abstract. This paper presents a method to characterise the passive orthotropic and contractile properties of left ventricular (LV) myocardial tissue using MRI data of cardiac anatomy, structure and function. Personalised anatomical LV models were fitted to image data from four canine hearts. Diffusion tensor MRI data from the same hearts were parameterised using finite element fitting to provide fibre angle fields that represent longitudinal axes of the myocytes. Fitted fibre angle fields were combined with laminar-sheet orientation data extracted from the Auckland dog heart model and embedded into the customised LV anatomical models. A modified Holzapfel-Ogden orthotropic constitutive relation was parameterised using published data from *ex vivo* shear tests on myocardial tissue blocks. This parameterised constitutive model was scaled for each case in the present study by fitting the individualised LV models to end-diastolic image data. Contractile tension was then estimated by comparing LV model predictions to the end-systolic image data. Personalised models of this kind can be used to predict the 3D deformation and regional stress distributions throughout the LV wall during the entire cardiac cycle.

Keywords: Myocardial mechanical properties · Orthotropic constitutive model · Parameter estimation · Canine heart · Passive stiffness · Active contraction · Cardiac cycle

1 Introduction

The physiological function of the heart is determined by the mechanical properties of the myocardial tissue. Abnormalities in the mechanical function of the

© Springer International Publishing Switzerland 2015
O. Camara et al. (Eds.): STACOM 2014, LNCS 8896, pp. 135–144, 2015.
DOI: 10.1007/978-3-319-14678-2_14

heart affects its ability to pump blood through the circulatory system, which can lead to fatal consequences. Estimating the mechanical properties of the *in vivo* heart through the use of image-extracted geometries and biophysical modelling provides important information about the stresses and strains that occur during the cardiac cycle. This biomechanical analysis depends on the choice of constitutive model to describe the mechanical properties of myocardial tissue. Many studies have used transversely isotropic constitutive models, for which the fibre and cross-fibre directions can reproduce distinctly different mechanical responses [5]. However, experimental studies have reported that myocardial tissue is not only characterised by the myocardial fibre axis, but also by a distinct laminar organisation, where the tethering between the myocardial cells within a sheet is stiffer than that between adjacent sheets [5]. This motivates the use of orthotropic constitutive models to describe the three distinct axes of microstructural symmetry inherent within the myocardium.

This paper presents a modified version of the Holzapfel-Ogden orthotropic constitutive model [3] for modelling the passive mechanical response of the canine LV. The data used in this paper were provided as part of the MICCAI-STACOM 2014 LV mechanics challenge, which involved comparing model predicted LV displacements with those measured using tagged magnetic resonance imaging (MRI) techniques. The methods presented in this paper have the capability of predicting regional distribution of strain and stress of the LV at both the end-diastolic (ED) and end-systolic (ES) stages of the cardiac cycle.

2   Methods

2.1   LV Mechanics Modelling

Anatomical Model Customisation. Regular truncated prolate spheroid shaped 16 (4 x 4 x 1) element tricubic Hermite finite element (FE) models were fitted to the diastasis canine LV image-derived surface data of each of four cases. For each case, a generic model was first registered to the cardiac coordinate system of the experimental surface data, and then the endocardial and epicardial surfaces were fitted to the data using previously published methods [7].

In order to describe the orthotropic mechanical response of the myocardium, it was necessary to embed fibre and sheet angles into the LV model. Microstructural orientations were described using Euler angles with respect to the short-axis and epicardial tangent planes. Fibre angles were calculated as the helix angles between the projections of the supplied diffusion tensor imaging (DTI) vector data onto the wall tangent plane, and the circumferential axis. Imbrication angles were quantified as the transverse angles that the DTI vectors made with the wall tangent plane, and were found to be sufficiently small to be negligible in this study.

Subject-specific laminar sheet orientation data were not available for the canine hearts in this study, therefore sheet angle data from the Auckland dog heart (ADH) model [5] were incorporated into each of the models. Firstly, each canine LV model was transformed to match the geometry defined by the ADH model. Then fibre and sheet angle data, extracted directly from the ADH model, were fitted using tricubic Hermite interpolation into each transformed canine model. Since both sets of angles were defined with respect to the local FE material coordinates, the microstructural orientation fields could be directly mapped from the ADH geometry to the new canine models. The embedded sheet angles were adjusted to align the sheet-normal material axes between the DTI and ADH fields in order to produce the best match with the sheet planes described by the ADH model.

For comparative purposes, another set of models were generated based on ADH fibre and ADH sheet data. Predictions using these models were compared to those of the DTI fibre fitted models. The primary difference between the two sets of models was that the ADH data had a broader transmural distribution of fibre angles compared to the DTI-derived models as illustrated in Fig. 1 (see [8] for a detailed comparison).

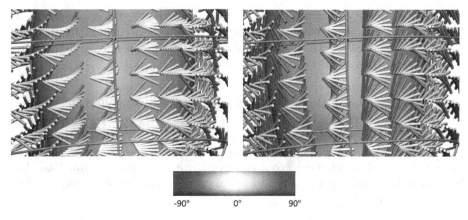

Fig. 1. Transmural variation in fibre angles for a mid-posterior portion of the LV model for case A. Left: DTI fitted fibre field. Right: ADH fitted fibre field.

Myocardial Mechanical Properties. The passive mechanical response of the myocardium was modelled using a modified version of the Holzapfel-Ogden orthotropic constitutive model [3]. The isotropic (first) term in the original formulation did not allow the mechanical response in each of the material directions to be independently controlled. To decouple the axial terms, the isotropic term was omitted from the original formulation and an additional exponential term describing the sheet-normal direction response was added [2]. The modified formulation is given by

$$W = \sum_{i=\mathrm{f,s,n}} \frac{a_i}{2b_i} \left(e^{b_i (I_{4i}-1)^2} - 1 \right) + \frac{a_{\mathrm{fs}}}{2b_{\mathrm{fs}}} \left(e^{b_{\mathrm{fs}} I_{8\mathrm{fs}}^2} - 1 \right) \tag{1}$$

where $I_{4f} = \mathbf{f}_0 \cdot (\mathbf{Cf}_0), I_{4s} = \mathbf{s}_0 \cdot (\mathbf{Cs}_0), I_{4n} = \mathbf{n}_0 \cdot (\mathbf{Cn}_0), I_{8fs} = \mathbf{f}_0 \cdot (\mathbf{Cs}_0)$ (2)

and $\mathbf{f}_0 = [1\,0\,0]^T, \mathbf{s}_0 = [0\,1\,0]^T, \mathbf{n}_0 = [0\,0\,1]^T$ (3)

where $\mathbf{C}$ is the right Cauchy-Green deformation tensor referred to the fibre (f), sheet (s) and sheet-normal (n) microstructural material axes, and $a_f, a_s, a_n, a_{fs}, b_f, b_s, b_n, b_{fs}$ are the constitutive parameters. In keeping with the original Holzapfel-Odgen model, the axial exponential terms only contribute to the strain energy function when their associated invariants I_{4f}, I_{4s} and I_{4n} are larger than 1.

The contractile mechanical response of the myocardium was modelled using the steady-state Hunter-McCulloch-ter Keurs active tension constitutive model [4], which is given by

$$T_a = T_{Ca} \times [1 + \beta(\sqrt{I_{4f}} - 1)]$$ (4)

where T_a is the active tension produced within the tissue, T_{Ca} is the contractile stress associated with calcium release from the sarcoplasmic reticulum at resting sarcomere length, β is the myocardial length-dependence parameter, and $\sqrt{I_{4f}}$ quantifies the fibre extension ratio.

LV Mechanics Simulations were performed for the diastolic slow filling phase (from diastasis to end-diastole) by applying the given LV cavity pressures on the endocardial surfaces of the LV models, while the LV base was constrained to match the motion of the basal epicardial surface data. Diastasis was assumed to be the stress-free reference geometry. Systolic contraction was simulated by increasing the active tension and endocardial pressure loads until the end-systolic values were reached.

2.2   Constitutive Parameter Estimation

Objective Function. Constitutive parameters were estimated by minimising the mean squared error (MSE) of the projections of the MRI-derived surface data points onto the endocardial and epicardial surfaces of the predicted model.

It was noted that there were discrepancies between the basal motion of the provided surface data and the supplied basal boundary constraints which had been derived from the tagging data. For the purposes of parameter estimation, which was designed to match the supplied surface data, the motion of the base of the LV models was constrained to match that of the surface data so as to exclude this discrepancy from the MSE calculation.

Even though the basal motion was taken from the surface data, following the FE simulations, it was observed that a rotational motion of the model gave a poor match to the surface data for the majority of the ventricle, apart from near the base. To address this problem, the LV models were rigidly aligned with the surface data prior to the computation of the surface projections at each stage in the parameter estimation process. This method allowed an unbiased comparison of the overall geometry between the model predictions and the surface data, which was independent of the questionable reliability of the prescribed basal motion.

Parameter Estimation. Passive parameters were estimated for each of the four cases. The parameters of the passive constitutive model have previously been fitted to simple shear experimental data [1] through a multivariate optimisation process for all six modes of shear. Details of this method can be found in [2]. The fitted values are listed in the Table 1.

Table 1. Orthotropic material parameters obtained by fitting to simple shear data [1]

a_f (kPa)	a_s (kPa)	a_n (kPa)	a_{fs} (kPa)	b_f	b_s	b_n	b_{fs}
24.84	6.94	6.35	0.37	11.32	7.07	0.22	11.67

For the purposes of the passive parameter estimation in this study, just two parameters were fitted due to the limited information provided by the diastolic deformation data. With reference to Eq. 5, one parameter (M_f) was used to scale the term associated with the stiffness in the fibre direction, while the second parameter (M) was used to scale the remaining terms in the constitutive equation. The rationale behind this model simplification lay in the fact that the LV surface data available for constitutive model parameterisation were only provided at two time points in the cardiac cycle (i.e. ED and ES), which would not contain sufficient kinematic information to estimate all eight passive parameters. Two scaling parameters were estimated instead of just one bulk scaling parameter because analyses showed that there was a substantial improvement in the fit to the ED surface data (data not shown).

$$W = M_f \left(\frac{a_f}{2b_f} \left(e^{b_f(I_{4f}-1)^2} - 1 \right) \right)$$
$$+ M \left(\sum_{i=s,n} \frac{a_i}{2b_i} \left(e^{b_i(I_{4i}-1)^2} - 1 \right) + \frac{a_{fs}}{2b_{fs}} \left(e^{b_{fs}I_{8fs}^2} - 1 \right) \right) \tag{5}$$

To estimate the contractile parameters for the four cases, the maximum activation level ($T_{Ca_{max}}$) was determined by matching model predictions to the supplied ES surface data. The length-dependency parameter (β) in the Hunter-McCulloch-ter Keurs model (Eq. 4) was set to 1.45 as previously reported in [4].

Simultaneous vs. Sequential Parameter Estimation Schemes. The framework was set up to estimate the passive and active parameters simultaneously by summing the errors in projecting the supplied ED and ES surface data onto the surfaces of the model predictions for those states. This approach worked well for the LV models embedded with the ADH fibre data, however the simultaneous estimation method failed for models based on the DTI fibre fields because these models predicted significant apex-to-base lengthening during systole (see Fig. 2 and a discussion of this effect in Section 3.2). Therefore, a sequential parameter estimation method was adopted instead for the models with DTI fibre fields.

2.3   Challenge Results

The 2014 LV mechanics challenge required the predictions of material point displacements and fibre stress distributions at ED and ES for each of the four canine hearts. The estimated constitutive parameters from Section 2.2 were used in conjunction with basal constraints that were provided as part of the challenge (these constraints had been derived from the MR tagging data). Regional fibre stress distributions were evaluated as part of the mechanical simulations. The displacements and fibre stresses were evaluated for the material point locations at which the DTI fibre field data were provided. Due to minor discrepancies between the geometric location of the DTI fibre field data and the MRI-derived surface data, some of the material points were found to be positioned outside of the fitted models. This was particularly evident near the base of the LV models. These external points (between 527 and 704 out of 9225 material points for each of the four cases) were excluded from the displacement and stress evaluations.

2.4   Computational Modelling Tools

The geometric, fibre and sheet orientation data were fitted using a combination of MATLAB and the computational back-end of the Continuum Mechanics, Image analysis, Signal processing and System identification (CMISS) software package (www.cmiss.org). The CellML open-standard (www.cellml.org) was used to describe the constitutive equation. All three-dimensional model visualisations were rendered using CMGUI (www.cmiss.org/cmgui).

3   Results

Parameter estimation results are presented for the sets of models fitted with the DTI and the ADH fibre fields.

3.1   Parameter Estimation Using the DTI Fibre Field

The models based on the DTI fibre fields predicted significant apex-to-base lengthening during systole, which yielded large MSEs of the projections at ES. This caused the simultaneous estimation method to fail, with the M and M_f parameters reaching the upper bound (10) because the ED projections were outweighed by the much larger ES projections. To address these issues, the passive and active parameters were estimated sequentially instead of simultaneously. This allowed the passive parameters to be estimated by fitting only the ED model predictions to the ED surface data, eliminating the issues associated with the apex-to-base lengthening of the ES model predictions. The active parameter ($T_{Ca_{max}}$) was subsequently estimated while fixing the passive parameters. The estimated passive and active parameters are presented in Tables 2(a) and 2(b), respectively.

For the contraction phase, the observed apex-to-base lengthening of the LV models led to unreliable projections of the surface data near the LV apex. In an attempt to overcome this problem, the projected locations of the surface data points on the model at DS were embedded and tracked throughout the cardiac cycle, so that a point-to-point vector could be constructed at ES from each surface data point to their corresponding tracked location on the model surface. The longitudinal components of these vectors were substituted for the longitudinal components of the untracked surface projections at ES to construct a mixed objective function for fitting these DTI-based models. This mixed objective function was designed to penalise apex-to-base model lengthening while remaining insensitive to model twisting in the short-axis plane. However, the lengthening problem was not eliminated even at the optimal value of $T_{Ca_{max}}$ (see Fig. 2), resulting in the large MSE values presented in Table 2(b).

Table 2. Passive (M_f and M) and active ($T_{Ca_{max}}$) parameters estimated for LV models embedded with the DTI fibre field data

Cases	M_f	M	ED MSE (mm^2)		Cases	$T_{Ca_{max}}$ (kPa)	ES MSE (mm^2)
A	0.98	1.18	0.38		A	53.8	43.9
B	0.60	1.09	0.45		B	46.8	18.7
C	0.70	1.23	0.37		C	31.9	26.5
D	4.93	3.51	0.15		D	30.1	23.8
(a)					(b)		

3.2 Parameter Estimation Using the ADH Fibre Field

The results of simultaneously estimating the passive and active constitutive parameters for the LV models based on the ADH fibre data are presented in Table 3. The use of ADH fibre data with optimal constitutive parameters gave rise to substantially smaller surface data projections at ES.

A comparison between the model predictions based on the DTI versus ADH fibre fields (Fig. 2) showed that the apex-to-base lengthening observed for the models based on the DTI fibre fields was reduced for the models based on the ADH fibre field in all four cases.

Table 3. Simultaneous estimation of the passive (M_{f} and M) and active ($T_{\mathrm{Ca_{max}}}$) parameters for LV models embedded with the ADH fibre field data

Cases	M_{f}	M	$T_{\mathrm{Ca_{max}}}$ (kPa)	ED MSE (mm^2)	ES MSE (mm^2)	Total MSE (mm^2)
A	2.30	1.77	125.1	0.46	1.31	0.89
B	0.56	0.94	60.3	0.47	0.99	0.73
C	0.86	1.25	46.1	0.40	1.42	0.91
D	3.07	4.48	50.4	0.13	2.62	1.38

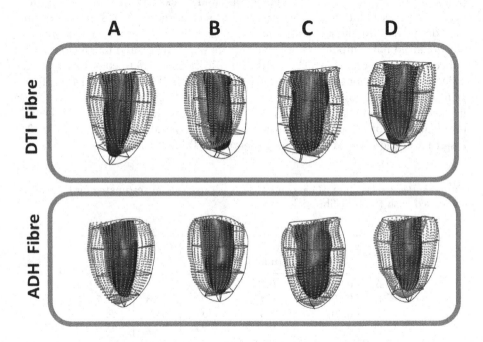

Fig. 2. Optimal end-systolic (ES) models for cases A, B, C and D, comparing deformation predictions for LV models based on the DTI fibre field (top panel) against those based on the ADH fibre field (bottom panel). The endocardium (brown surfaces) and epicardium (brown lines) of the predicted LV models are superimposed with the supplied surface data (green points) for the ES state.

3.3   Regional Strain and Stress Distributions

The individualised FE models were used to predict the strain and stress distributions throughout the ventricular walls during the cardiac cycle. An example of the stress distribution evaluated for case A is shown in Fig. 3.

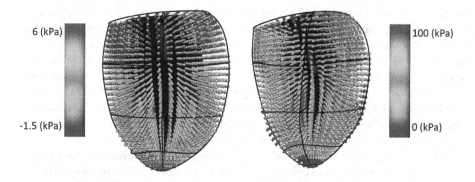

Fig. 3. Total Cauchy fibre stress distribution using the ADH fibre field at ED (left) and ES (right)

4   Discussion and Conclusions

In this study, an orthotropic passive constitutive model and an active tension model were parameterised using MRI-derived surface data. The objective function was the MSE of the projections from the MRI-derived data to the surfaces of the predicted LV models.

Sets of models were constructed using DTI-derived fibre fields, and the ADH fibre field. The major point of difference between the predictions for the two sets of models was that the LV long axis dimension of the ADH fibre field models did not lengthen as much as the DTI fibre field models during systolic contraction. The mechanism for this difference is most likely to be related to the differences in the transmural ranges of fibre orientations between the two sets of models, which have been quantified in [8].

Even though the constitutive model was orthotropic, just two passive parameters could be estimated due to insufficient information contained within the supplied surface data, which did not track myocardial material points, but instead simply characterised the LV surface shapes. The parameter estimation process was constrained such that the stiffness in the fibre direction was able to vary independently to the stiffness for the other components of the constitutive equation. It would be interesting to explore further the performance of a transversely isotropic constitutive model in biomechanical analysis and parameter estimation using these data.

A simultaneous passive and active parameter estimation method was performed for the models fitted with the ADH fibre field. The inclusion of ES error projections in the estimation of passive parameters allowed them to be tuned using a larger range of deformations. This was particularly important when the diastolic deformations were very small, as observed in case D in this study, which made it difficult to identify the optimal passive parameters using just the ED data. Simultaneous parameter estimation failed for the DTI fibre field fitted models because the predicted elongation caused the large ES projection errors to markedly outweigh the ED projection errors in the objective function. This sent the passive parameters to their upper bounds during the estimation process. When LV models based on the ADH fibre fields were used for parameter estimation, the objective function was more balanced in terms of the contributions of the ED and ES projection errors. In consequence, the parameter estimation procedure was much more stable compared to that of the DTI fibre models. A limitation of the simultaneous estimation method was that correlation was found between the M_f and M parameters as well as between the M and $T_{\mathrm{Ca}_{\max}}$ parameters. These correlations should be investigated further.

The model predicted regional distributions of fibre stress could provide insights into the mechanical behaviour of the myocardium that are not derivable from cardiac imaging techniques. These stress distributions could also be useful for investigating the myocardial work performed across different regions of the LV wall during the cardiac cycle.

References

1. Dokos, S., Smaill, B.H., Young, A.A., LeGrice, I.J.: Shear properties of passive ventricular myocardium. American Journal of Physiology **283**, H2650–H2659 (2002)
2. Niestrawska J.: A structure-based analysis of cardiac remodelling - a constitutive modelling approach. Masters Thesis, RWTH Aachen University of Technology, Germany (2013)
3. Holzapfel, G.A., Ogden, R.W.: Constitutive modelling of passive myocardium: a structurally based framework for material characterisation. Philosophical Transactions of the Royal Society A **367**(1902), 3445–3475 (2009)
4. Hunter, P.J., McCulloch, A.D., Ter Keurs, H.E.D.J.: Modelling the mechanical properties of cardiac muscle. Progress in Biophysics and Molecular Biology **69**(2–3), 289–331 (1998)
5. LeGrice, I.J., Hunter, P.J., Smaill, B.H.: Laminar structure of the heart: a mathematical model. American Journal of Physiology **272**, H2466–H2476 (1997)
6. Nielsen, P.M.F., LeGrice, I.J., Smaill, B.H., Hunter, P.J.: Mathematical model of geometry and fibrous structure of the heart. American Journal of Physiology **260**(4), H1365–H1378 (1991)
7. Wang, V.Y., Lam, H.I., Ennis, D.B., Cowan, B.R., Young, A.A., Nash, M.P.: Modelling passive diastolic mechanics with quantitative MRI of cardiac structure and function. Medical Image Analysis **13**(5), 773–784 (2009)
8. Wang, V.Y.: Modelling in vivo cardiac mechanics usng MRI and FEM. PhD Thesis, Auckland Bioengineering Institute, University of Auckland, New Zealand (2012)

Regular Papers

Evaluating Local Contractions from Large Deformations Using Affine Invariant Spectral Geometry

Dan Raviv[1]([⊠]), Jon Lessick[2], and Ramesh Raskar[1]

[1] Camera Culture Group, Media Lab, MIT, Cambridge, MA, USA
darav@mit.edu
[2] Rambam Medical Center, Haifa, Israel

Abstract. We propose a geometric tool for quantifying dense local contractions of the left ventricle given its three dimensional segmented computed tomography (CT). Our approach is based on metric invariants in spectral geometry coupled to a non-rigid alignment algorithm, and can be implemented on data obtained by any modality as only a segmented surface is used. We assume local affine movement of the tissue, and generate a global piecewise constant affine invariant model to regularize the alignment. In contrast to traditional methods which seek diffeomorphic deformation, we show that an isomorphic paradigm can enhance alignment results. We show the superiority of utilizing the proposed metric as part of known non-rigid alignment algorithms on synthesized examples. We further analyzed local contractions and provide statistics for 9 healthy patients and demonstrate abnormal local contractions in atrial fibrillation.

1 Introduction

The mechanical contraction of the heart is regulated by electric stimulus, as depolarization of the myocytes leads to an influx of calcium, which is responsible for the habitual contractions. Therefore, both the electrical signal and the mechanical movement are valuable for diagnosing abnormalities in the cardiac cycle. Methods for monitoring the mechanical and electrical signals have been studied for decades, where first attempts were done using mechanical recorders [1] and imaging techniques such as Kymograph [2]. Modern approaches for tracking soft tissues are based on tagged magnetic resonance imaging (MRI) [3,4], doppler tissue imaging (DTI) [5] and speckle tracking echocardiography (STE) [6]. Although these methods provide high spatial and temporal resolution, they track only a small number of points, and have major limitations in robustness. More details can be found in [5]. In order to evaluate movement of the heart for a dense set of points, a computational approach is added on top of the tagged data by tracking visible features and regulating in time and space for a smooth solution. For example, one can consider the popular *syngo* Velocity Vector Imaging system from SIEMENS, and the 3D strain assessment in ultrasound comparison paper [7].

© Springer International Publishing Switzerland 2015
O. Camara et al. (Eds.): STACOM 2014, LNCS 8896, pp. 147–157, 2015.
DOI: 10.1007/978-3-319-14678-2_15

Tracking soft tissues is one of the most challenging problems in compu
vision, since parameterization of the deformations is nontrivial. Traditionally, tracking has been done by aligning points according to the intensity values of the scanned data in sequential frames. However, ambiguity rises when neighbor pixels share similar values, and a regularization term must be added. Common approaches for aligning soft tissues are based on either surfaces or volumes. Although the latter can potentially provide higher accuracy [8,9] due to three dimensional information, acquiring high quality data might require unwanted prolonged radiation of the patient. For example, ultrasound involves no radiation, but the resulting data is inferior compared to CT or MRI. Adding regularization to the process can provide more accurate alignment such as in [10] or better statistical analysis as in [11]. On the other hand, when dealing with low quality imaging data, the surface boundary of the imaged organ can still be extracted, even if the volumetric data suffers from low signal to noise ratio. Several algorithms for non-rigid surface alignment have been proposed in the past, including non-rigid iterative closest points (ICP), [12,13], conformal mappings [14], mobius voting [15], spherical harmonics [16] and generalized multi-dimensional embedding [17].

In this work, we introduce global intrinsic distances measured from several anchor points as regularization terms. Those distances not only follow the intrinsic geometry, but also are affine invariant. We use a local affine metric, which was recently published in [18] as the building blocks for the intrinsic distances, and hence, those distances are locally affine. For example, even if only part of the surface contracts by unknown affine factors, then the global intrinsic distances remain the same. This approach can be adopted by various known algorithms and we specifically show how to apply it to a non-rigid ICP algorithm, and evaluate its superiority in a synthetic experiment with a known ground truth. Owing to the enhanced accuracy we were able to align segmented texture-less scans of the left ventricle in coarse temporal resolution and infer dense local contractions. We visualized the local contractions of the Left ventricle from apex to basal during the cardiac cycle, extract statistics, and detect abnormal behaviors in atrial fibrillation.

1.1 Main Contributions

- Design a dense non-rigid alignment algorithms for 2D surfaces with piecewise constant affine invariant regularization.
- Provide dense statistics of local contractions of the left ventricle in healthy patients and present local abnormal behavior for atrial fibrillation.

2   Methods

In this paper, we focus on alignment of segmented textureless surfaces based on geometric constraints. We present a novel non-rigid alignment algorithm where

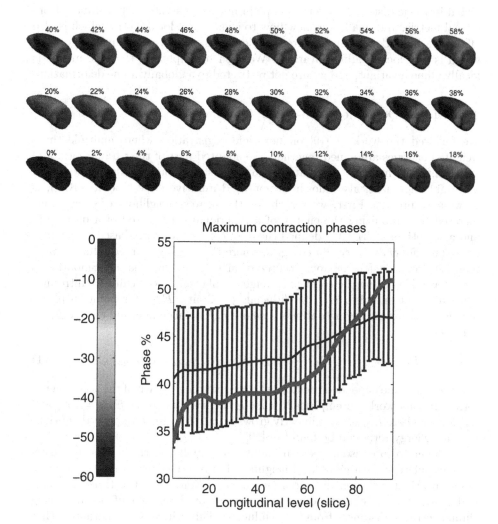

Fig. 1. Left: local contractions percent of the left ventricle during the systole cycle of a healthy individual. The data were up-sampled by a factor of 5. Right: the temporal phase of maximal contraction versus the longitudinal level (percentage of the long axis of the ventricle) for healthy subjects (blue, error bars represent one standard deviation). The results presented on the left are depicted in the red curve. An increasing curve represents a contraction from apex to base.

an affine invariant metric is used to compensate for large deviations between sequential images. Best algorithms today search for a smooth diffeomorphism between shapes, or isomorphisms based on Euclidean distances. Here we evaluate a smooth isomorphism which is also piecewise constant affine invariant.

In what follows, we elaborate on the three key ingredients of the proposed approach. We start by exploring a non-rigid alignment algorithm governed by global intrinsic distances. We then explain how to generate such distances from a local metric, and finally we show how to construct a local metric which is also affine invariant. Combining all three provides a global dense alignment algorithm which is also locally affine invariant. We wish to emphasize that the metric is locally affine invariant, and we are not restricted to a globally affine deformation.

2.1 Metric Depended Non-Rigid Alignment

We followed the work of [19] on non-rigid registration where multiple time-weighted energies are joined together. We adopted part of their framework, and added intrinsic metric constraints to gain robustness for large deformations. A non-rigid alignment, also known as non-rigid iterative closest points (ICP), is a two-step process. First, we search for the nearest neighbors of each point, followed by minimizing the energy of a functional constructed of a data term and a smoothness term. We defined the data consistency term based on *point to plane* and *fiducials proximity* energies, where three easily marked fiducials were manually selected (tip of apex, center of artery, and mid basal). Smoothness term was added using the cotangent weight Laplacian. Specifically, we introduce three different energies, E_{fid} for fiducials proximity, E_{p2pl} for point to plane, and E_{smooth} for forcing a continuous solution. The accumulating energy E_{total} becomes

$$E_{total} = \alpha_{fid}(t)E_{fit} + \alpha_{p2pl}(t)E_{p2pl} + \alpha_{smooth}(t)E_{smooth}, \tag{1}$$

where α_* are time depended coefficients corresponding to each of the three energy terms. In this work we empirically choose the weights to be $E_{fit} = 100$, and $E_{p2pl} = 1$, where $E_{smoothness}$ linearly grows from 100 to 1000. Explicit definitions for each energy term can be found in [19].

In order to force isometric constraints from global intrinsic measurements, we manipulate the search of local neighbors between the iterations. We evaluate affine invariant diffusion distances (see next section) from the three fiducials, and search for the closest points in space out of the subset of points having similar intrinsic distances from those fiducials. This critical step guarantees that the solution is not just smooth but also as isometric as possible with relation to the long intrinsic regularization. The system of equations converges following 10 iterations.

2.2 Spectral Geometry

In signal processing, operating in the Fourier domain is a classic that can be generalized to Riemannian manifolds. Differential geometry is widely used in computer vision for handling bendable shapes, as the local structure encapsulates needed quantities of length, angles and area. The eigenfunctions set of the Laplace Beltrami operator defined by the local Riemannian manifold, is a non-Euclidean analog to the Fourier basis that allows us to analyze information on manifolds.

We model a shape as a complete two dimensional Riemannian manifold X with a metric tensor g, noted by (X, g). As we assume X is embedded into $\mathbb{R}^3$ by a regular map $\mathbf{x} : U \subseteq \mathbb{R}^2 \to \mathbb{R}^3$, the metric tensor can be expressed in coordinates as the coefficients of the first fundamental form $g_{ij} = \left\langle \frac{\partial \mathbf{x}}{\partial u_i}, \frac{\partial \mathbf{x}}{\partial u_j} \right\rangle$, where u_i are the coordinates of U. Hence, the arc-length becomes $dp^2 = g_{11} du_1^2 + 2g_{12} du_1 du_2 + g_{22} du_2^2$.

Spectral geometry is based on the partial differential equation

$$\left(\frac{\partial}{\partial t} + \Delta_g \right) f(t, x) = 0, \tag{2}$$

which is called the *heat equation*. It describes heat propagation, where $f(t, x)$ is the heat distribution at a point x in time t , and Δ_g is the Laplace-Beltrami operator (LBO) which is evaluated from the local metric g. The fundamental solution of the heat equation is called the *heat kernel* and can be expressed using the spectral decomposition of Δ_g,

$$h_t(x, x') = \sum_{i \geq 0} e^{-\lambda_i t} \phi_i(x) \phi_i(x'), \tag{3}$$

where ϕ_i and λ_i are, respectively, the eigenfunctions and eigenvalues the Δ_g. Here we used finite elements framework (FEM) presented in [20] to compute the spectral decomposition of the Laplace-Beltrami operator. Out of the heat kernel we can construct a family of intrinsic metrics known as *diffusion metrics*,

$$d_t^2(x, x') = \int \left(h_t(x, \cdot) - h_t(x', \cdot) \right)^2 da = \sum_{i > 0} e^{-2\lambda_i t} (\phi_i(x) - \phi_i(x'))^2, \tag{4}$$

which measure the diffusion distance of the two points for a given time t. The parameter t can be considered as *scale*, and the family $\{d_t\}$ can be thought of as a scale-space of metrics.

2.3 Locally Affine Metric Invariants

The seminal work of Blaschke [21] and Su [22] showed that if scaling is known, an *equi-affine metric*, also known as special-affine, can be constructed on a two dimensional (surface) manifold. This research was a breakthrough later to be used in many numerical schemes such as curve evolution [23], flows [24] and shape analysis [25]. The equi-affine re-parametrization invariant metric [21,22] reads $q_{ij} = |r|^{-\frac{1}{4}} r_{ij}$, where $r_{ij} = \det \left(\frac{\partial \mathbf{x}}{\partial u_1}, \frac{\partial \mathbf{x}}{\partial u_2}, \frac{\partial^2 \mathbf{x}}{\partial u_1 \partial u_2} \right)$, and $r = \det(r_{ij}) = r_{11} r_{22} - r_{12}^2$.

A different approach for constructing local invariants was recently studied by [26] who built a locally *scale invariant metric*. Specifically, consider the surface (X, g), then the scale invariant metric takes the form $|K| g_{ij}$, where K is the Gaussian curvature.

Surprisingly, it is possible to combine the two results, equi-affine and scaling, in one framework and removing the annoying *equi* limitation. First shown in [18], one needs to replace the Gaussian curvature in the scale invariant metric definition with an equi-affine invariant curvature K^q, leading to $a_{ij} = |K^q| q_{ij}$, a locally affine invariant metric. Going back to the previous section, we need to replace g with a in order to evaluate affine invariant distances. More details on the numeric construction can be found in [18].

3   Results

The study population included nine patients with normal heart rhythm and normal left ventricular function, as well as three patients with heart disease. One had a dilated cardiomyopathy causing a global reduction in LV function, while the other two had atrial fibrillation (one also had abnormal apical contraction). The healthy population is composed of seven males and two females of the ages 46 to 88. We performed a gated cardiac CT angiography every 5% of the cardiac cycle, and automatically segmented the shapes as described in [27]. The spatial resolution was 2 mm with 1 mm overlap, which generated approximately 140 slices of 256 squared pixels each. We modeled the LV as a triangular shape, and evaluated the metric per triangle and distances in between vertices (see [25]) for more details).

3.1   Temporal Up-Sampling and Periodic Closed Loop

For high temporal (100 frames per cycle) we found that non-rigid ICP with local smooth regularization to be good enough (see Figure 3). Hence, we aligned the low temporal data (20 frames per cycle) using the proposed approach and quadratically resampled in time per matched point. This sampling is used to provide visually appealing results. In addition, in order to compensate for accumulating errors we performed two cycles of mappings. One from the first phase to the last, and another from the last phase to the first. We chose a weighted average of the two as the final alignment.

3.2   Local Contractions

Local isotropic contraction of a point $x \in X$ is the ratio between its local area $A^t(x)$ in time t divided by its local area at the first cycle ($t = 0$). We defined the local neighborhood for each point in every scale according to the one measured in $t = 0$, and averaged the value with a local kernel of 2% , which relates to 160 from 8000 model points. We projected a point and it's neighbors into the local tangential plane, and evaluated the standard deviation of their position, whose square root multiplication linearly grows with scaling. Thus, the ratio between time t and $t = 0$ provides an estimation of isotropic contraction. in Figure 2 we depict local contraction graphs of four levels (apical, sub-papillary, papillary and basal). In Figure 1 we show part of the systole contraction cycle of one healthy individual. Our alignment and up-sampling successfully captures the local contractions from apex to basal of a healthy cycle.

3.3   Abnormal Contractions

We can easily detect abnormality in the cardiac cycle, as seen in Figure 2, where we illustrate three abnormal cases (red curves). One patient (dotted curve) has a severe case of functional reduction, where the remaining two cases (dashed and solid curves) were diagnosed with atrial fibrillation. Such conditions result in irregular beating of the upper chambers of the heart. With our proposed method, we can observe local abnormal contractions.

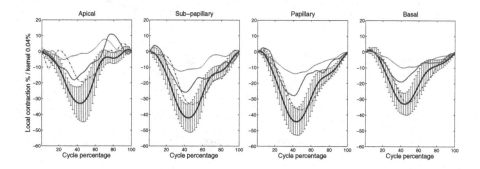

Fig. 2. Mean local contractions (in %) along the cardiac cycle on four levels (apical, sub-papillary, papillary and basal) of a healthy population. We aligned each scanning such that the first sampling has the maximum global area, and the contraction ratio was measured according to that. A kernel of 2 percentage was chosen, which relates to local averaging over 160 out of 8000 points. We depict in blue the mean and standard deviation of 9 individuals, and in red 3 abnormal cases.

3.4   Numeric Validation

In order to validate the superiority of metric regularization we generated a semi-synthetic experiment where the ground truth of every point is known (Figure 3). We used a model of the left ventricle and globally contracted it up to 70 percentages of the original long axis length. We aligned the surfaces using two algorithms, non-rigid ICP [19] and Generalized Multi-Dimensional Scaling (GMDS) [17] with and without affine invariant metric regularization. Non-rigid ICP is more robust to stretches and we witnessed the advantage of the new regularization above 25 percentage of contraction, while the GMDS is more sensitive to distances as it takes into account the long geodesics, hence we can see an improvement in all levels.

4   Discussion

Today's gold standard in alignment of medical data is based on diffeomorphisms, where a smooth regularization is enforced on the captured data. In this work, we

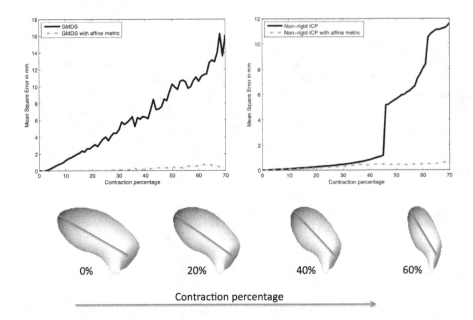

Fig. 3. We evaluated the mean square error (MSE) for two alignment algorithms; non-rigid ICP (top right) and Generalized Multi-Dimensional Scaling (top left), with and without the usage of affine invariant regularization. In each experiment we contracted the model according to the long axis (bottom row), and evaluated the alignment error with relation to the ground-truth. Non-rigid ICP is more robust to contractions and we witnessed the advantage of the new regularization above 25 percentage of contraction, while the GMDS is more sensitive to distances, hence we can see an improvement in all levels of contractions.

demonstrate that a stronger assumption on the deformation can be used and it can lead to better alignment results. Specifically, preserving global intrinsic distances between sampled points can be useful in alignment of deformable shapes. Until now, such regularizations could not have been used on structures that expand and stretch over time since the intrinsic distances (geodesics or diffusion) change during the deformations. Recent developments in metric invariants have allowed for considering global (long) normalization during the alignment process, since the long geodesics are constructed from local invariant measures.

While the term 'affine-invariant' has been used in literature in medical imaging, here we relate the affinity to the distances measured on the surface due to an affine deformation. We assume that the deformation is piecewise constant as the equations do not hold on the boundary in between parts. However, we do not need to know a priori where those segmented sub structures are. This fundamental observation is the main advantage of our approach. Usually, one must perform a two stage optimization switching between alignment and parcellation, while here the metric itself compensates for local stretching.

We believe our assumptions follow the natural behavior of soft tissues as internal forces generate a locally affine deformation. In practice, we witness continuous deformations rather than piecewise constant, which forces us to iterate until convergence. Compared to the diffeomorphisms paradigm, this approach better describes the process, and provides more accurate results in the provided experiments.

Two limitations must be taken into account. (1) A higher (second) derivative of the structure is required, and no solution exists for points with vanishing Gaussian curvature. In most biological tissues, the boundary is convex for which the solution is not degenerated, and encapsulating the metric with a random walk (PDE) approach provides a stable solution for second derivatives. (2) Affine invariant metric is known only for surfaces, hence we are forced to consider a segmented data as an input for our calculations. In some scenarios, consistently deriving the boundary over time is challenging and can affect the results. In addition, since the alignment is performed on the boundary we can not generate the conventional strain/stress statistics.

In summary, adding global metric constraints to current computational methods, turning a diffeomorphism into an isomorphism, can provide better alignment of biological tissues. Additional validation is required both for synthetic and captured datasets, and will be the subject of future research.

5 Conclusions

Local metric invariants can enhance alignment of non-rigid soft tissues, especially under large affine deformations. This approach is solely based on geometric assumptions on surfaces of segmented volumes, which can be extracted from any tomographic procedure. Moreover, it can complement numerous known tracking methods, including speckle echocardiography and MRI tagging, creating a multiple tracking technique. It can be used as an additional layer to current state-of-the-art approaches based on diffeomorphisms, providing stronger claims on the results. We demonstrated the added value of the local metric invariants in semi-synthetic experiments using non-rigid ICP and Generalized Multi-Dimensional Scaling algorithms, and quantified known medical phenomena on healthy and abnormal real cases.

References

1. Wiggers, C.: Studies of ventricular fibrillation caused by electric shock. American Heart Journal **5**, 351–365 (1930)
2. Scott, W., Moore, S.: Roentgen kymography in diseases of the heart. a realtively new and efficient aid in diagnosis. The Journal of the American Medical Association (JAMA) **107**, 1951–1954 (1936)
3. Zerhouni, E., Parish, D., Rogers, W., Yang, A., Shapiro, E.: Human heart: tagging with MR imaging - a method for noninvasive assessment of myocardial motion. Radiology **169**, 59–63 (1988)

4. Axel, L., Dougherty, L.: Heart wall motion: improved method of spatial modulation of magnetization for mr imaging. Radiology **127**, 349–350 (1989)
5. Bansal, M., Sengupta, P.P.: Longitudinal and circumferential strain in patients with regional LV dysfunction. Current Cardiology Reports **15**(339) (2013)
6. Hodt, A., Stugaard, M., Hisdal, J., Stranden, E., Atar, D., Steine, K.: Regional LV deformation in healthy individuals during isovolumetric contraction and ejection phases assessed by 2D speckle tracking echocardiography. Journal of Clinical Physiology and Functional Imaging **32**(5) (2012)
7. De Craene, M., Marchesseau, S., Heyde, B., Gao, H., Alessandrini, M., Bernard, O., Piella, G., Porras, A., Tautz, L., Hennemuth, A., Prakosa, A., Liebgott, H., Somphone, O., Allain, P., Makram Ebeid, S., Delingette, H., Sermesant, M., D'hooge, J., Saloux, E.: 3d strain assessment in ultrasound (straus): a synthetic comparison of five tracking methodologies. IEEE Transactions on Medical Imaging **32**(9) (2013)
8. Beg, F., Miller, M., Trouvé, A., Younges, L.: Computing Large Deformation Metric Mappings via Geodesic Flows of Diffeomorphisms. International Journal of Computer Vision (IJCV) **61**(2), 139–157 (2005)
9. Reuter, M., Rosas, H., Fischl, B.: Highly accurate inverse consistent registration: A robust approach. Neuroimage **53**(4), 1181–1196 (2010)
10. De Craene, M., Piella, G., Camara, O., Duchateau, N., Silva, E., Doltra, A., D'hooge, J., Brugada, J., Sitges, M., Frangi, A.F.: Temporal diffeomorphic free-form deformation: Application to motion and strain estimation from 3d echocardiography. Medical Image Analysis **16**(2), 427–450 (2012)
11. Durrleman, S., Pennex, X., Trouvé, A., Braga, A., Gerig, J., Ayache, N.: Toward a comprehensive framework for the spatiotemporal statistical analysis of longitudinal shape data. International Journal of Computer Vision (IJCV) **103**(1), 22–59 (2013)
12. Chen, Y., Medioni, G.: Object modeling by registration of multiple range images. In: Proc. Conf. Robotics and Automation (1991)
13. Besl, P.J., McKay, N.D.: A method for registration of 3D shapes. Trans. on Pattern Analysis and Machine Intelligence (PAMI) **14**(2), 239–256 (1992)
14. Wang, S., Wang, Y., Jin, M., Gu, X., Samaras, D.: Conformal geometry and its applications on 3D shape matching, recognition, and stitching. IEEE Transactions on Pattern Analysis and Machine Intelligence (PAMI) **29**(7), 1209–1220 (2007)
15. Lipman, Y., Funkhouser, T.: Mobius voting for surface correspondence. Proc. ACM Transactions on Graphics (SIGGRAPH) **28** (2009)
16. Huang, H., Shen, L., Zhang, R., Makedon, F.S., Hettleman, B., Pearlman, J.D.: Surface alignment of 3D spherical harmonic models: application to cardiac MRI analysis. In: Duncan, J.S., Gerig, G. (eds.) MICCAI 2005. LNCS, vol. 3749, pp. 67–74. Springer, Heidelberg (2005)
17. Bronstein, M.M., Bronstein, A.M., Kimmel, R., Yavneh, I.: Multigrid multidimensional scaling. Numerical Linear Algebra with Applications (NLAA) **13**, 149–171 (2006)
18. Raviv, D., Kimmel, R.: Affine invariant non-rigid shape analysis. CIS-2012-01, Technion. Israel Institute of Technology (2012)
19. Li, H., Sumner, R., Pauly, M.: Global correspondence optimization for non-rigid registration of depth scans. Computer Graphics Forum **27**(5) (2008)
20. Dziuk, G.: Finite elements for the beltrami operator on arbitrary surfaces. In: Partial Differential Equations and Calculus of Variations, pp. 142–155 (1988)
21. Blaschke, W.: Vorlesungen uber Differentialgeometrie und geometrische Grundlagen von Einsteins Relativitatstheorie, vol. 2. Springer (1923)

22. Su, B.: Affine differential geometry. Science Press, Beijing (1983)
23. Sapiro, G.: Affine Invariant Shape Evolutions. PhD thesis, Technion - IIT (1993)
24. Sochen, N.: Affine-invariant flows in the beltrami framework. Journal of Mathematical Imaging and Vision $20(1)$, 133–146 (2004)
25. Raviv, D., Bronstein, A.M., Bronstein, M.M., Waisman, D., Sochen, N., Kimmel, R.: Equi-affine invariant geometry for shape analysis. Journal of Mathematical Imaging and Vision (JMIV) (2013)
26. Aflalo, Y., Kimmel, R., Raviv, D.: Scale invariant geoemtry for non-rigid shapes. Journal of Imaging Science (SIAM) $6(3)$, 1579–1597 (2013)
27. Ecabert, O., Peters, J., Walker, M.J., Ivanc, T., Lorenz, C., von Berg, J., Lessick, J., Vembar, M., Weese, J.: Segmentation of the heart and great vessels in CT images using a model-based adaptation framework. Journal of Medical Image Analysis $15(6)$, 863–876 (2011)

Image-Based View-Angle Independent Cardiorespiratory Motion Gating for X-ray-Guided Interventional Electrophysiology Procedures

Maria Panayiotou[1]([✉]), Andrew P. King[1], R. James Housden[1], YingLiang Ma[1],
Michael Truong[1], Michael Cooklin[2], Mark O'Neill[2], Jaswinder Gill[2],
C. Aldo Rinaldi[2], and Kawal S. Rhode[1]

[1] Division of Imaging Sciences and Biomedical Engineering,
King's College London, London SE1 7EH, UK
maria.panayiotou@kcl.ac.uk
[2] Department of Cardiology,
Guy's and St. Thomas' Hospitals NHS Foundation Trust, London SE1 7EH, UK

Abstract. Cardiorespiratory phase determination has numerous applications during cardiac imaging. We propose a novel view-angle independent prospective cardiorespiratory motion gating technique for X-ray fluoroscopy images that are used to guide cardiac electrophysiology procedures. The method is based on learning coronary sinus catheter motion using principal component analysis and then applying the derived motion model to unseen images taken at arbitrary projections. We validated our technique on 7 sequential biplane sequences in normal and very low dose scenarios and on 5 rotational sequences in normal dose. For the normal dose images we established average systole, end-inspiration and end-expiration gating success rates of 100 %, 97.4 % and 95.2 %, respectively. For very low dose applications, the method was tested on images with added noise. Average gating success rates were 93.4 %, 90 % and 93.4 % even at the low SNR value of $\sqrt{5}$, representing a dose reduction of more than 10 times. This technique can extract clinically useful motion information whilst minimising exposure to ionising radiation.

Keywords: Principal components analysis · Cardiac electrophysiology · Motion gating · X-ray fluoroscopy · 3D rotational angiography

1 Introduction

Electrophysiology (EP) procedures are minimally invasive catheter procedures that are used to treat cardiac arrhythmias. They are performed under two-dimensional (2D) X-ray fluoroscopy to guide the insertion and movement of catheters. However, the guidance of such procedures is compromised by the inability of the X-ray images to effectively visualise soft tissues. To overcome this limitation, intra-procedure X-ray fluoroscopy images can be registered and overlaid with

© Springer International Publishing Switzerland 2015
O. Camara et al. (Eds.): STACOM 2014, LNCS 8896, pp. 158–167, 2015.
DOI: 10.1007/978-3-319-14678-2_16

previously acquired 3D anatomical models derived from other imaging modalities, such as magnetic resonance imaging (MRI) [1,2]. X-ray fluoroscopy images can also be registered and overlaid with 3D rotational X-ray angiography (3DRXA), which is particularly suited to clinical workflow [3]. However, the anatomical models will be static and will not update with the intra-procedural situation. Cardiorespiratory motion causes mis-registration of these models, compromising the guidance accuracy. This is important when performing catheter-based ablation treatment or electrical measurement. Accurate determination of treatment or measurement sites relative to an anatomical model using two or more synchronized oblique X-ray views can be used for procedure guidance and retrospective biophysical modelling [4]. Motion gating is crucial for achieving this accuracy. Cardiac gating can be achieved by synchronizing the fluoroscopic images with the electrocardiogram. Nevertheless, this is normally an optional extra when purchasing an X-ray system and requires extra hardware. Respiratory gating can be achieved using the breath-hold technique, commonly used during MRI [5], although this is not practical in the catheter laboratory. Alternatively, detecting the cardiorespiratory phase using the fluoroscopy images is more suited to the routine clinical workflow. Image-based methods can be divided into those that measure respiratory phase only, cardiac phase only and both. Methods of measuring the respiratory phase only include diaphragm [6], heart border [7] and EP catheter [8–10] tracking. Methods of measuring the cardiac phase only include weighted centroid tracking [11]. Measuring both types of motion simultaneously is an advantage and successful methods include the use of phase-correlation between successive X-ray images [12] and hierarchical manifold learning [13], a model-based approach.

We have previously proposed a technique for automated image-based cardiorespiratory motion gating in normal and very low dose X-ray fluoroscopy images [14]. The technique can gate previously unseen frames based on a statistical model formed from normal dose images during a calibration phase using principal component analysis (PCA) of the motion of the coronary sinus (CS) catheter, a particular catheter that is nearly always present in EP procedures. One major limitation of this and other model-based approaches is the requirement to build a separate model for each X-ray view. We significantly extend our previous approach in this manuscript to make it X-ray system view-angle independent and therefore much more clinically useful. Our proposed approach is based on forming a PCA-based model of the CS catheter in a first or *training* view and then using this to determine both the cardiac and the respiratory phases prospectively in any arbitrary second or *current* view. We carry out comprehensive validation of our technique on clinical and phantom X-ray sequences. In particular, we show how this novel approach can be used for motion gating of 3DRXA for which current methods are limited to breath-holding for respiration and either no gating for cardiac motion or arresting the heart using adenosine or rapid pacing [15].

2   Methods

2.1   Statistical Model Formation in the Training View

CS Catheter Detection. The CS catheter is composed of 10 electrodes, distributed in pairs along the catheter. The CS tracking technique [8] uses a fast multi-scale blob detection method [16] to detect all electrode-like objects in an X-ray image and a cost function to discriminate the CS catheter from other catheters. After application of the tracking algorithm for all frames in the training view, θ_1, the x and y positions of each of the 10 electrodes is concatenated into a single column vector for each time point. Hence, the data generated by the tracking process consists of:

$$\mathbf{s}_i = (z_{i,1,x}, z_{i,1,y}, \dots z_{i,10,x}, z_{i,10,y})^T, 1 \leq i \leq N \tag{1}$$

where $z_{i,e,x}$ and $z_{i,e,y}$ represent the x and y coordinates of the eth electrode in the ith frame. $e = 1$ corresponds to the distal electrode, and N is the number of frames.

Principal Component Analysis. PCA transforms a multivariate dataset of possibly correlated variables into a new dataset of a smaller number of uncorrelated variables called principal components (PCs), without any loss of information [17]. We first compute the mean vector, $\bar{\mathbf{s}}$, and the covariance matrix, $\mathbf{S}$ [14]. The eigenvectors $\mathbf{v}_m$, $1 \leq m \leq M$ of $\mathbf{S}$ represent the PCs and the corresponding eigenvalues $\mathbf{d}_m$, $1 \leq m \leq M$ represent the variance of the data along the direction of the eigenvectors. For our application $M = 20$ since the s_i are of length 20. The result of the PCA gives possible CS catheter electrode positions in θ_1. It was found that the 1st and 2nd modes of variation represented the cardiac and respiratory motions, respectively [14].

2.2   Application of Statistical Model on the Current View

The task is to gate previously unseen frames in any arbitrary second or *current* view based on a statistical model formed in a first or *training* view. The technique could be used for either retrospective or prospective gating in very low dose X-ray fluoroscopy images. Prospectively, the gating will be performed with a phase-lag of 1 frame interval. In this section we are demonstrating its use for retrospective gating.

Epipolar Line Reconstruction. Epipolar reconstruction allows loss of depth information to be recovered from a 2D projection image if another 2D image is taken of the same target from a different view, assuming we know the complete camera parameters of the X-ray fluoroscopy projective modality [18]. The camera parameters are obtained from the DICOM header of the X-ray images. Using epipolar geometry, each of the 2D electrode positions obtained when forming our statistical model in θ_1 is backward projected to form a 3D line, $\mathbf{l}_b$, which is then forward projected to generate a 2D epipolar line, $\mathbf{l}_e$, in the current view, θ_2, that contains the corresponding electrode position. Hence, we generate 10 epipolar lines in θ_2 for each frame in the current view.

Blob Detection and CS Catheter Position Estimation. We now determine the position of the CS catheter in θ_2 and simultaneously determine its state of cardiorespiratory motion. We do this by determining the cardiorespiratory state in the PCA model of θ_1 that produces epipolar lines that intersect the catheter electrodes in the new image in θ_2. The fast multi-scale blob detector is used to detect all possible electrode-like objects in a new image. The positions of all detected blobs are concatenated into a blob list, **BL**. Using the PCA model, an instance of the CS catheter, $\hat{s}$, can be generated in θ_1 according to

$$\hat{s} = \bar{s} + \sum_m w_m \mathbf{v_m} \tag{2}$$

where w_m are the weights for each eigenvector. If the first two eigenvectors are used then we can represent the instance by $\hat{s}_{w_1 w_2}$. We estimate the weights $\hat{w}_1$ and $\hat{w}_2$ that represent the cardiorespiratory phase of the image for θ_2 according to

$$\hat{w}_1, \hat{w}_2 = \underset{w_1 w_2}{\operatorname{argmin}}[D(\hat{s}_{w_1 w_2}, \mathbf{BL}) + A(\hat{s}_{w_1 w_2})] \tag{3}$$

where $D(\hat{s}_{w_1 w_2}, \mathbf{BL})$ is a function that computes the sum of the minimum Euclidean distances between the epipolar lines generated by $\hat{s}_{w_1 w_2}$ and their nearest corresponding blobs from **BL**. Its purpose is to position the epipolar lines so that they pass through the electrodes in the new view. $A(\hat{s}_{w_1 w_2}$ is a function that computes the sum of angles between line segments joining successive blobs. Motivated by the 2σ rule, that states that for a normal distribution, about 95.45% of the values lie within 2 standard deviations of the mean, our search space for the weights varies from $-2\sqrt{d_m}$ to $+2\sqrt{d_m}$, where d_m is the mth eigenvalue, and $1 \leq m \leq 2$. We minimized the function using a coarse-scale exhaustive search followed by an iterative optimization using Matlab's lsqnonlin function with the trust-region-reflective algorithm. For the application of our model on rotational sequences, where the CS catheter position deviation was larger, the first 3 PCs were used to solve our optimization. The resulting weights indicate the cardiorespiratory phases and the blobs from **BL** nearest to the epipolar lines give the catheter location in the new image.

2.3   Cardiorespiratory Gating of the Current View

$\hat{w}_1$ is used to detect systolic frames, Ω_{sys}, of the image sequences which are represented by the peaks of the variation of $\hat{w}_1$ with frame number. The peaks of the variation of $\hat{w}_2$ at each time frame represent end-inspiration (EI) respiratory frames, Ω_{EI}, while the troughs represent end-expiration (EX) respiratory frames, Ω_{EX}.

$$\Omega_{sys} = \{i \mid w_{1,i-1} < w_{1,i} > w_{1,i+1}\} \tag{4}$$

$$\Omega_{EI} = \{i \mid w_{2,i-1} < w_{2,i} > w_{2,i+1}\}, \Omega_{EX} = \{i \mid w_{2,i-1} > w_{2,i} < w_{2,i+1}\} \quad (5)$$

3   Experiments

3.1   Data Acquisition

All imaging was carried out using a monoplane 25cm flat panel cardiac X-ray system (Philips Allura Xper FD10, Philips Healthcare, Best, The Netherlands). Clinical images were acquired from 6 patients undergoing radiofrequency abla-tion procedures. Phantom images were acquired using a bespoke beating and breathing left ventricular phantom [19] with an inserted CS catheter. X-ray imaging was performed at between 3 and 30 frames per second with an image size of either 512^2 or 1024^2.

3.2   Application to Multiplane Sequence Pairs at Normal and Low Dose

We validated our technique on 3 sequential biplane clinical sequences (244 frames, 6 runs in total, running from a minimum of 8.0 to a maximum of 19.3 seconds, cov-ering at least 2 respiratory cycles) and 2 sequential multiplane (one biplane and one triplane) phantom sequences (1741 frames, 5 runs in total, running from a minimum of 9.8 to a maximum of 15.8 seconds). The PCA model was formed for each sequence individually and the method run on each possible combination of sequence pairs, giving a total of 6 clinical and 8 phantom experiments. A compar-ison of our existing single-view method [14] was included to show the effect of the extra step of changing view angle. Comparison to all single view methods was not our objective in this paper, as this has already been done in [14].

Validation. To validate our technique, gold standard cardiorespiratory signals were generated along with a gold standard for the electrode positions in each X-ray image. The latter was done by the use of the CS tracking technique [8]. Manual tracking was performed in cases where the technique failed to accurately detect electrodes. This was done by manually localizing the centre of any mis-detected electrode of the CS catheter. For the clinical data, manual gating of the cardiac cycle at systole was performed by an experienced observer and res-piratory gating was done using either diaphragm or heart border tracking [7]. The respiratory signal obtained was cardiac gated using the manually identi-fied systolic frames. For the phantom sequences, two different regions of interest moving independently with cardiac and respiratory motion were automatically tracked. The signals obtained using the gold standard methods were then com-pared to the signals obtained using the model-based method. Furthermore, for both cardiac and respiratory gating, the absolute frame difference was computed between our technique and the gold standard techniques. Specifically, systolic, end-inspiration and end-expiration frames were recorded from our automatic and gold standard methods and their corresponding absolute frame differences were computed. Faultless gating results are signified when the absolute frame difference is zero. Even though we do detect the whole cycle, for evaluation, we use only peaks and troughs, where the gold standard is well-defined.

Application of Noise. The effect of noise was investigated by adding Poisson noise to both the clinical and phantom test images, specified in terms of the median value of the Poisson mean [14], and then repeating the algorithm. We used SNR values of $\sqrt{50}$, $\sqrt{10}$, $\sqrt{8}$, $\sqrt{6}$ and $\sqrt{5}$, where the SNR value of $\sqrt{5}$, represents a dose reduction of more than 10 times.

Application to Rotational Sequences at Normal Dose. We validated our technique on 3 clinical rotational angiography sequences (341 frames) and 2 phantom rotational sequences (540 frames). For the patient sequences our statistical model was formed on a monoplane sequence acquired for each patient in the AP view. For the application of our technique on the phantom rotational sequences, the model was formed on monoplane sequences in AP and RAO30° views in turn. The validation was done in the same way as for the multiplane sequences.

4   Results

4.1   Application to Multiplane Sequence Pairs at Normal and Low Dose

Figure 1 illustrates the results of the CS catheter tracking technique on the 1st image of (a) an uncorrupted example X-ray sequence and (b), (c), (d), on the simulated noisy images, with SNR of $\sqrt{50}$, $\sqrt{10}$ and $\sqrt{5}$, respectively.

Quantitative Validation of Cardiorespiratory Motion Gating. Figure 2 illustrates the frame difference errors in histogram plots, i.e. the number of peaks or troughs with 0, 1 or 2 frames separation from the gold standard for (a) and (b) for the patient and phantom biplane sequences, respectively, for all gating tasks and noise levels. Percentage success rates for all gating tasks were also calculated and demonstrated in Figure 3. They were computed using the equation $\frac{100x}{x_{total}}$, where x corresponds to the number of perfectly matched gold standard and automatic gating frames and x_{total} corresponds to the total number of gold standard gating frames. To comparatively validate our technique to our previously published technique [14], where the statistical model was formed from normal dose images during a calibration phase and applied to low dose images acquired from the same view-angle, % success rates from both techniques for the same sequences are illustrated on the figure. No false positives or negatives (i.e. extra/fewer detected peaks/troughs) over the processed sequences were found. Outcomes show that our technique is robust and accurate in cardiorespiratory motion extraction even at the lowest SNR values of $\sqrt{5}$. Regarding the algorithm's performance on the different experiments, depending on the step size, the execution time was between 0.76 and 1.73 seconds/frame running in Matlab on Windows 7 with a 3.4 GHz Intel Core i7 CPU and 8 GB of RAM.

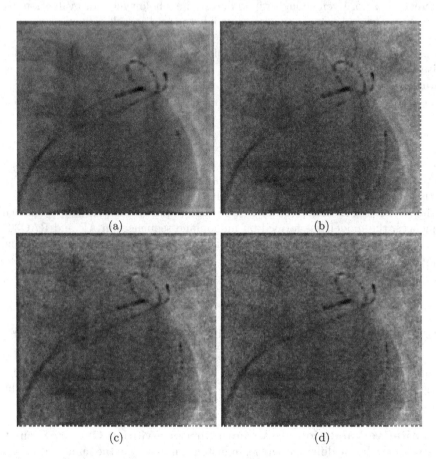

(a)

(b)

(c)

(d)

Fig. 1. (a) The PCA-view angle independent CS catheter tracking technique is illustrated in green crosses on an uncorrupted X-ray image during the ablation stage of a procedure to treat AF; (b), (c), (d), on the same X-ray image corrupted with different levels of Poisson noise. SNR values correspond to $\sqrt{50}$, $\sqrt{10}$ and $\sqrt{5}$, respectively.

4.2 Application to Rotational Sequences at Normal Dose

Quantitative Validation of Cardiorespiratory Motion Gating. For both cardiac and respiratory gating, the absolute frame difference was computed for the phantom procedures. For patient procedures the absolute frame difference was computed only for cardiac gating as patients were in breath-hold. Results of this experiment are that our proposed technique is doing a faultless job in extracting cardiorespiratory motion from any view-angle, over the range of

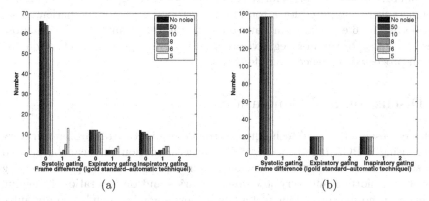

Fig. 2. Histograms of frame difference errors for cardiac, end-inspiration, and end-expiration gating for the uncorrupted and all noise corrupted X-ray sequences using our PCA-view-angle independent technique on (a) patient and (b) phantom sequences

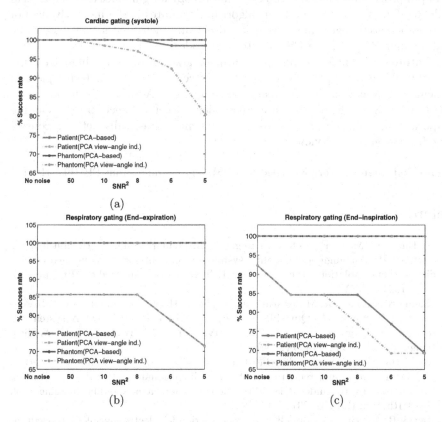

Fig. 3. % success rates for (a) cardiac, (b) end-expiration and (c) end-inspiration gating for the uncorrupted and all noise corrupted X-ray sequences computed for the application of our PCA view-angle independent and our PCA-based technique on patient and phantom sequences

180°, in normal dose scenarios for rotational acquisitions. Specifically, zero frame differences were computed for a total of 15 systolic frames for the patient cases and 26 systolic, 6 end-expiratory and 6 end-inspiratory frames for the phantom cases. No false positives or negatives (i.e. extra/fewer detected peaks/troughs) over all processed sequences were found.

5   Discussion and Conclusions

We have presented a novel technique for the determination of cardiorespiratory gating using a PCA-based model of CS catheter motion that can be applied to a secondary X-ray view. We validated our technique on 7 biplane imaging sequences in normal and very low dose scenarios and on 5 rotational imaging sequences in normal dose. Our technique is view-angle independent, fully automatic, requires no prior knowledge and can operate within a few seconds per image sequence. The method will be particularly useful for registration and overlay of pre-procedural images with X-ray fluoroscopy for guidance and biophysical modeling. The main reason for our algorithm's failures is the ineffectiveness of the blob detection algorithm in very low doses and view-angles that distort the solid circular shape of the CS catheter electrodes, resulting in their misdetection. Future work will focus on implementing a new more accurate blob detection algorithm in an attempt to increase the % success rates of our technique and reducing the execution time for real-time clinical use. Additionally, we are planning to investigate the effect of a more explicit catheter detection, by including temporal constraint, i.e. the electrode will not move drastically between consecutive frames on the 2nd view.

Acknowledgments. Work is funded by EPSRC programme grant EP/H046410/1.

References

1. De Buck, S., Maes, F., Ector, J., Bogaert, J., Dymarkowski, S., Heidbuchel, H., Suetens, P.: An augmented reality system for patient-specific guidance of cardiac catheter ablation procedures. IEEE Transactions on Medical Imaging **24**, 1512–1524 (2005)
2. Rhode, K., Sermesant, M., Brogan, D., Hegde, S., Hipwell, J., Lambiase, P., Rosenthal, E., Bucknall, C., Qureshi, S., Gill, J., Razavi, R., Hill, D.: A system for real-time XMR guided cardiovascular intervention. IEEE Transactions on Medical Imaging **24**(11), 1428–1440 (2005)
3. Li, J., Haim, M., Movassaghi, B., Mendel, J., Chaudhry, G., Haffajee, C., Orlov, M.: Segmentation and registration of three-dimensional rotational angiogram on live fluoroscopy to guide atrial fibrillation ablation: a new online imaging tool. Heart Rhythm (2), 231–237 (2009)
4. Kawal, R., Maxime, S.: Modeling and registration for electrophysiology procedures based on three-dimensional imaging. Current Cardiovascular Imaging Reports **4**(2), 116–126 (2011)

5. Paling, M., Brookeman, J.: Respiration artifacts in mr imaging: reduction by breath holding. Journal of Computer Assisted Tomography 10(6), 1080–1082 (1986)
6. Condurache, A., Aach, T., Eck, K., Bredno, J., Stehle, T.: Fast and robust diaphragm detection and tracking in cardiac X-ray projection images. In: Proceedings of SPIE Medical Imaging, vol. 5747, pp. 1766–1775 (2005)
7. Ma, Y., King, A., Gogin, N., Gijsbers, G., Rinaldi, C., Gill, J., Razavi, R., Rhode, K.: Clinical evaluation of respiratory motion compensation for anatomical roadmap guided cardiac electrophysiology procedures. IEEE Transactions on Biomedical Engineering 59(1), 122–131 (2012)
8. Ma, Y., King, A.P., Gogin, N., Rinaldi, C.A., Gill, J., Razavi, R., Rhode, K.S.: Real-time respiratory motion correction for cardiac electrophysiology procedures using image-based coronary sinus catheter tracking. In: Jiang, T., Navab, N., Pluim, J.P.W., Viergever, M.A. (eds.) MICCAI 2010, Part I. LNCS, vol. 6361, pp. 391–399. Springer, Heidelberg (2010)
9. Brost, A., Liao, R., Hornegger, J.: Respiratory motion compensation by model-based catheter tracking during EP procedures. Medical Image Analysis 14(5), 695–706 (2010)
10. Brost, A., Wimmer, A., Bourier, F., Koch, M., Liao, R., Kurzidim, K., Strobel, N., Hornegger, J.: Constrained registration for motion compensation in atrial fibrillation ablation procedures. IEEE Transactions on Medical Imaging 31(4), 870–881 (2012)
11. Lehmann, G., Holdsworth, D., Drangova, M.: Angle-independent measure of motion for image-based gating in 3d coronary angiography. Medical Physics 33(5), 1311–1320 (2006)
12. Sundar, H., Khamene, A., Yatziv, L., Xu, C.: Automatic image-based cardiac and respiratory cycle synchronization and gating of image sequences. In: Yang, G.-Z., Hawkes, D., Rueckert, D., Noble, A., Taylor, C. (eds.) MICCAI 2009, Part II. LNCS, vol. 5762, pp. 381–388. Springer, Heidelberg (2009)
13. Panayiotou, M., et al.: Extraction of cardiac and respiratory motion information from cardiac X-Ray fluoroscopy images using hierarchical manifold learning. In: Camara, O., Mansi, T., Pop, M., Rhode, K., Sermesant, M., Young, A. (eds.) STACOM 2013. LNCS, vol. 8330, pp. 126–134. Springer, Heidelberg (2014)
14. Panayiotou, M., King, A., Ma, Y., Rinaldi, C., Gill, J., Cooklin, M., O'Neill, M., Housden, R., Rhode, K.K.S.: A statistical model of catheter motion from interventional X-ray images: application to image-based gating. Physics in Medicine and Biology 58(21), 7543–7562 (2013)
15. Kriatselis, C., Nedios, S., Akrivakis, S., Tang, M., Roser, M., Gerds-Li, J.H., Fleck, E., Orlov, M.: Intraprocedural imaging of left atrium and pulmonary veins: a comparison study between rotational angiography and cardiac computed tomography. Pacing and Clinical Electrophysiology 34(3), 315–322 (2011)
16. Lindeberg, T.: Detecting salient blob-like image structures and their scales with a scale-space primal sketch: a method for focus-of-attention. International Journal of Computer Vision 11(3), 283–318 (1993)
17. Jolliffe, I.: Principal Component Analysis. Springer, New York (2002)
18. Hartley, R., Zisserman, A.: Multiple View Geometry in Computer Vision, 2nd edn. Cambridge University Press (2004) ISBN: 0521540518
19. Manzke, R., Lutz, A., Schenderlein, M., Bornstedt, A., Chan, R., Dietmeyer, K., Rasche, V.: A new pva-based dynamic cardiac phantom for evaluation of functional mr imaging methods at 3t. In: ISMRM Proceedings (2010)

Analysis of Mitral Valve Motion in 4D Transesophageal Echocardiography for Transcatheter Aortic Valve Implantation

Frank M. Weber[1]([✉]), Thomas Stehle[1], Irina Waechter-Stehle[1],
Michael Götz[1], Jochen Peters[1], Sabine Mollus[2], Jan Balzer[3],
Malte Kelm[3], and Juergen Weese[1]

[1] Philips Research Europe, Hamburg, Germany
frank.m.weber@philips.com
[2] Philips Research Europe, Aachen, Germany
[3] Klinik für Kardiologie, Pneumologie und Angiologie,
Universitätsklinikum Düsseldorf, Düsseldorf, Germany

Abstract. Transcatheter aortic valve implantation (TAVI) is used to treat aortic stenosis in high-risk patients that cannot undergo cardiac surgery. Because it is minimally-invasive, it could be beneficial to treat patients in better conditions as well. Because their expected lifetime is much longer, the long-term benefit of the TAVI implant must be ensured. If the TAVI stent is placed too far into the left ventricular outflow tract it can impair movement of the anterior mitral leaftlet. Case reports demonstrated endocarditis and leaflet damage due to such friction.

To predict possible complications, we identified mitral valve, aortic valve, and left ventricular outflow tract in 4D transesophageal echocardiography series using model-based segmentation. The segmentation model was a combined structure of the left heart with dynamic valves that was adapted as a whole. Valve dynamics were modeled using shape modes. In a leave-one-patient-out validation of 16 datasets, the respective mean segmentation error for mitral and aortic valve was 0.99 ± 1.16 mm and 1.27 ± 1.68 mm.

We further analyzed the overlap of the mitral leaflet trajectory with the target region for a possible TAVI implant in 18 patients. The overlap as a function of distance from the aortic annulus varied considerably with peak overlaps of 4.7 to 16.6 mm. Such information is potentially useful for procedure planning and device selection to avoid mitral valve impairment by TAVI.

Keywords: TAVI · Aortic Valve · Mitral Valve · 4D TEE

1 Introduction

Aortic valve (AV) stenosis is often treated by implanting an artificial AV via cardiac surgery. An alternative method for high-risk patients that cannot undergo open-heart surgery for aortic valve replacement is transcatheter AV implantation

© Springer International Publishing Switzerland 2015
O. Camara et al. (Eds.): STACOM 2014, LNCS 8896, pp. 168–176, 2015.
DOI: 10.1007/978-3-319-14678-2_17

(TAVI). In this technique, the compressed valve is introduced transfemorally or transapically using a catheter and then expanded in-place.

Although TAVI is less invasive, its long-term outcome is unclear [1]. A current discussion is therefore if TAVI is also beneficial for patients with only intermediate risk for valve replacement [2]. Because their expected lifetime is much longer, the long-term benefit of the TAVI implant must be ensured.

If the TAVI implant is placed too low, i.e. reaching too far into the left ventricular outflow tract (LVOT), it can impair movement of the anterior mitral leaflet. Case reports demonstrated that contact between the implant and the MV leaflet led to mitral endocarditis and leaflet aneurysms [3–5]. First, repetitive friction between the implant and the leaflet could damage the leaflet surface. Second, the implant could act as an endocarditis bridge that favours the spread of AV endocarditis to the mitral valve. Especially, the slow tissue degeneration caused by repetitive friction might become more relevant the longer the implant is present. Therefore, treatment planning should make sure to avoid such friction.

Imaging plays an important role in TAVI planning [6]. A powerful tool to evaluate these images is model-based segmentation of the valve apparatus. Segmentation of the AV has been demonstrated in CT using a combined model of heart and static AV [7]. Segmentation of the AV and MV in CT and transesophageal echocardiography (TEE) has been performed using a landmark-detection approach [8]. The MV alone without surrounding structures has been segmented using multi-atlas techniques [9]. AV segmentation results were also used to measure the aortic valve diameter to select the proper implant size [10,11].

We applied a model-based approach to segment aortic and mitral valve in 4D TEE recordings. We used a single model of the left heart and valves that incorporated the leaflet dynamics using artificial shape modes. The model was adapted as a whole without detecting individual landmarks or seed points.

The segmented dynamic valves over time defined the region that the mitral leaflets needed for free, friction-less movement. To assess implications of MV movement on TAVI placement, we defined the target region as prolongation of the elliptical LVOT cross-section towards the LV. Any implant that extends some distance into this target region might overlap with the MV leaflet region (see Fig. 1). We calculated the maximum overlap between the implant and MV leaflet region as a function of the implant depth. Then, we analyzed this overlap at typical implant depths, which are, e.g., around 12 mm for the Medtronic CoreValve [12]. This might help to identify patients with increased risk for friction between the anterior MV leaflet and a TAVI implant placed too low.

2   Dynamic Valve Model

2.1   Segmentation Framework

We use a method to segment cardiac structures in a multi-step approach. The model is represented as a triangular surface model with mean shape $\overline{m}$. Boundary detection for each triangle is trained as described in [13]. The adaptation process is described in detail in [14]. In summary: First, the heart position is located using

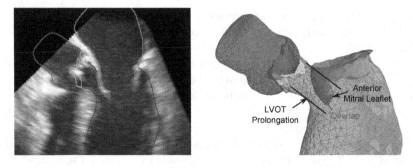

Fig. 1. Left: Example segmentation with left heart model. It consists of left ventricle (blue), left atrium (green), ascending aorta (red), mitral valve (orange), aortic valve (yellow). Right: 3D view of the model. We analyze the overlap between the anterior mitral leaflet and the prolongation of the left ventricular outflow tract. The more overlap, the more friction a TAVI implant is likely to cause if it is placed too low.

an adapted Generalized Hough Transform. The heart position and orientation are further refined using the available image information. For each triangle i of the N_T triangles, a target point x_i^{target} is detected based on the trained image feature. The deviation of the triangle centers c_i from their respective target points is described by the so-called external energy

$$E_{\text{ext}} = \sum_{i=1}^{N_T} w_i (\mathbf{n}_i \cdot (\mathbf{x}_i^{\text{target}} - \mathbf{c}_i))^2. \tag{1}$$

Weighting factors w_i may, for example, consider the reliability of the target point, and $\mathbf{n}_i$ are the triangle normals.

In a global adaptation step, heart position and orientation are iteratively refined by determining an affine transformation T that minimizes the external energy. The process of finding target points and minimizing the external energy is iterated, in this work up to 20 times.

Finally, we perform multiple iterations of a deformable adaptation. It is balanced between attraction to image boundaries and preservation of the mean shape. This shape preservation is mathematically described by the so-called internal energy

$$E_{\text{int}} = \sum_{i=1}^{V} \sum_{j \in N(i)} ((\mathbf{v}_i - \mathbf{v}_j) - (T[\overline{\mathbf{m}}_i] - T[\overline{\mathbf{m}}_j]))^2. \tag{2}$$

Here, V is the number of vertices in the model, $N(i)$ are the neighbors of the i-th vertex, $\mathbf{v}_{i/j}$ are the vertex positions in the deformed mesh, and $\overline{\mathbf{m}}_{i/j}$ are the vertex positions in the model. Internal energy increases when an edge $(\mathbf{v}_i, \mathbf{v}_j)$ deviates from the corresponding edge in the mean shape that was transformed with T. The total energy to be minimized is the weighted sum of E_{ext} and E_{int}

$$E_{\text{tot}} = E_{\text{ext}} + \alpha E_{\text{int}}. \tag{3}$$

It is iteratively minimized, in this work with up to 10 iterations. In each iteration, target points are searched starting at the current mesh location.

2.2 Problem-Specific Adaptations

We created a triangular surface model of the left heart from an annotated voxel bitmask. The model comprised endocardial surfaces of left ventricle, left atrium, and ascending aorta to model the anatomical context of the left heart valves. Furthermore, it contained detailed structures of aortic and mitral valve (MV). The model consisted of approximately 2700 vertices and 5700 triangles. A ring of triangles around the lower LVOT was marked with respective labels (see Fig. 2).

The mean shape $\overline{\mathbf{m}}$ contained the two valves in a half-open state. Because the valves undergo much stronger local deformations than other structures segmented in previous approaches, two linear modes $\mathbf{\Phi}_k$ were added to the model to describe valve dynamics. Here, $k = 1, 2$ corresponds to mitral and aortic valve, respectively:

$$\mathbf{m}(p_1, p_2) = \overline{\mathbf{m}} + p_1\mathbf{\Phi}_1 + p_2\mathbf{\Phi}_2. \tag{4}$$

This concept is similar to PCA modes, however, the valve modes were not calculated from PCA, but as linear interpolation between open and closed valve.

The coefficients p_k describe the current state of each valve. For all vertices outside the respective valves, the vector elements of $\mathbf{\Phi}_k$ were zero and did thus not influence the shape of the remaining model.

The model was adapted to the image as follows. After the Generalized Hough Transform, the mean model with half-open valves was used to estimate a global rigid transformation T. At this step, no valve dynamics were estimated. Then, the coefficients p_k were optimized during the deformable adaptation. The formulation of the shape constraining energy E_{int} was now given as

$$E_{\text{int}} = \sum_{i=1}^{V} \sum_{j \in N(i)} \left((\mathbf{v}_i - \mathbf{v}_j) - (T\left[\mathbf{m}_i(p_1, p_2)\right] - T\left[\mathbf{m}_j(p_1, p_2)\right]) \right)^2. \tag{5}$$

Thus, the mean shape used in equation 2 was replaced by the model containing the two linear valve modes. Furthermore, a penalty term was added to the total energy with weight β to avoid unphysiological mode coefficients p_k:

$$E_{\text{mode}} = \beta(p_1^2 + p_2^2). \tag{6}$$

2.3 Evaluation and Results

For eight patients, we generated ground truth for one cardiac phase with open MV and one with closed MV each, resulting in 16 meshes (all cardiac phases in between were not considered here). Images include pathological cases from patients suffering from aortic valve or mitral valve disease. For use in the model-based segmentation framework, boundary detectors were trained from the ground truth meshes. Because data in ultrasound acquisitions is only valid inside the acquisition cone, all image boundaries at the cone border between data and padding zeros were suppressed both during training and adaptation.

To assess segmentation accuracy, we performed a leave-one-patient-out analysis for training and segmentation. For every patient n, a mean shape and boundary detectors were trained from all other patients. With the resulting model, the two ground truth images of patient n were segmented and the resulting meshes were compared to the reference meshes. The mean surface-to-surface distance between segmentation and ground truth mesh was calculated for the MV and AV, both per dataset and over all datasets.

In the individual datasets of the leave-one-patient-out analysis, the mean segmentation error varied between 0.34 and 2.3 mm for the MV and between 0.47 and 2.5 mm (one outlier with 5.4 mm) for the AV. The mean segmentation error of all 16 datasets was 0.99±1.16 mm for the mitral valve and 1.27±1.68 mm for the aortic valve.

3   Motion Analysis

3.1   Methods

As input for the motion analysis we used 18 different 4D TEE acquisitions from patients considered for TAVI. These patients were not part of the training and validation process described in the previous section. Each acquisition comprised between 6 and 76 single cardiac phases covering at least one cardiac cycle.

All cardiac phases of each dataset were segmented using the model and framework described in the previous section. To this end, the first cardiac phase was segmented, and the result was used as initialization for the next cardiac phase. Only the deformable adaptation was then performed for the succeeding cardiac phases with the respective previous result as initialization.

To compensate for global movement or other displacements, we registered all meshes from one time series to the endsystolic mesh using the Kabsch algorithm [15]. In detail, we registered the AV annulus points onto each other to make all heart movement relative to the implant target region.

Furthermore, a local coordinate system was set up in the outflow tract to simplify the analysis. Origin and axes were determined from a reference ring around the outflow tract. An elliptical fit of the ring vertices determined center point and the three axes (major, minor, normal). In the local LVOT system, the x axis was aligned along the major axis, y along the minor axis, and z pointed along the normal towards LV/MV (Fig. 2). Finally, the origin was shifted along the z axis to the aortic valve plane. This way, all z distances were given with respect to the aortic annulus.

Next, the target region for an implant that extends into the LV was defined. To this end, the elliptical cross-section of the LVOT (as determined by the elliptical fit of the reference ring, Figure 2) was extended along the z axes.

The trajectory of each vertex in the anterior MV leaflet was determined from the registered meshes and transformed into the local LVOT system. Next,

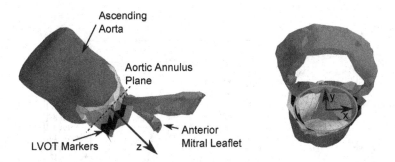

Fig. 2. Calculation of LVOT coordinate system. Left: A reference ring at the lower LVOT is marked with special labels in the model (shown black). The ellipse normal defines the z direction. The origin was shifted to the aortic annulus plane. Right: View along z from left ventricle with schematic elliptical fit in green. The major axis defines the x direction and the minor axis marks the y axis. The overlap between the mitral leaflet trajectories and the z-prolongation of the ellipse was analyzed as a measure for possible TAVI complications.

all points in all trajectories were combined into a point cloud. Points were binned according to their local z position (step size 2.5 mm). For every bin, we calculated the maximal overlap with the target region to receive an overlap curve $d_{max}(z)$.

3.2 Results and Discussion

The maximum overlap as function of implant depth is shown in Fig. 3. It can be clearly seen that the overlap was much stronger in some patients (e.g. Pat 7) than in others (e.g. Pat 1). The patient with the smallest overlap (Pat 1) had a maximum overlap of 4.7 mm, whereas the patient with largest overlap (Pat 11) had an overlap of 16.6 mm. Also, the overlap at a given implant depth varied considerably. At an implant depth of 12.5-15 mm (typical extension of clinically available implants) the overlap varied between around 2.6 and 13.4 mm. Figure 4 shows two examples of patients with low and high overlap.

The maximum overlap per patient was in the range of 4.7 to 16.6 mm and thus around five to ten times larger than the mean segmentation error. From this, we conclude that the segmentation error does not impair our analysis results.

A typical implant such as the Medtronic CoreValve [12] extends around 12 mm into the outflow tract. In this study, the overlap at a comparable implant depth of 12.5-15 mm varied between around 2.6 and 13.4 mm. If parts of the tissue are blocked by a an implant while others move freely, this could cause friction. It is plausible to assume that the deeper the mitral leaflet moves into the implant region before implantation, the more friction will occur after implantation. So the amount of overlap could allow to identify patients in which a deeper placed implant is likely to induce increased friction.

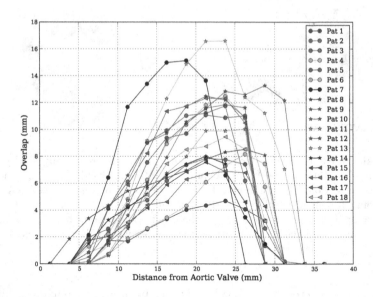

Fig. 3. Overlap $d_{\max}(z)$ between anterior mitral leaflet movement and LVOT prolongation as function of distance from AV. The maximum overlap varies considerably between patients and could be an indicator for risk of friction between MV and a TAVI implant. Also, the overlap in some patients increases closer to the AV than in other patients. This could allow to identify patient-individual zones at risk.

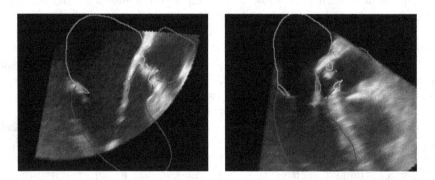

Fig. 4. Example segmentations at maximal MV opening. In Patient 6 (left), the overlap between the anterior MV leaflet and the LVOT prolongation was around 8 mm, the maximum overlap was located quite far from the AV. In Patient 7 (right), the maximum overlap was over 15 mm, and Fig. 3 shows that the maximum overlap was closer to the AV than in other patients.

The comparison with the CoreValve was exemplary and solely based on the typical length of one frequently used implant. Beside the CoreValve, there are other implants, such as the Edwards Sapien [16] or the Jena Valve [17]. We did not attempt to explicitly cover all available implants. We rather think that by analyzing the overlap as a function of implant depth, our approach is as general as possible.

A limitation of the current approach is that deformations caused by the actual implant are not considered. The implant in its initial shape is circular and will thus prolong the minor axis of the LVOT while shortening the major axis. Of course, a more complex analysis could incorporate such deformation into a biomechanical simulation to get an even more precise result. However, such an upward force onto the superior outflow tract or the anterior mitral leaflet is rather supposed to increase friction. Therefore, our analysis can be considered as best-case scenario to identify those patients with highest risk for friction.

4 Conclusions

In this paper, we demonstrated an automated dynamic segmentation of aortic valve, mitral valve and left ventricular outflow tract in 4D TEE images. To account for strong local valve deformations, we used linear interpolation modes to model valve opening and closing. We have validated the model using a leave-one-patient-out analysis on 16 datasets and demonstrated its feasibility. To our knowledge, this is the first combined model of LV and dynamic valves that is adapted as a whole, i.e. without detecting single landmarks, and that uses artificial dynamic shape modes.

From the segmentation results on 18 example 4D TEE datasets, we analyzed the overlap of anterior leaflet motion with the prolongation of the left ventricular outflow tract. The amount of overlap varied considerably between different patients. In the context of TAVI implants, this suggests that some patients are much more sensitive than others to implants that are placed further down in the LVOT.

This analysis shows that there can be large overlap between mitral leaflet motion and possible TAVI implant locations. The presented quantitative analysis could help in TAVI treatment planning, avoid leaflet friction, and thus increase success rates in patients that require long-term freedom from complications.

Acknowledgments. This work was supported by NRW, Germany and the European Union ("NRW Heart valve initiative", Med in.NRW 005-GW01-235C).

References

1. Vahanian, A., Himbert, D., Iung, B.: Transcatheter aortic valve implantation. Journal of the American College of Cardiology 58(20) (2011)
2. Vahanian, A., Alfieri, O., Andreotti, F., Antunes, M.J., et al.: Guidelines on the management of valvular heart disease (version 2012). Eur. Heart J. **33**(19), 2451–2496 (2012)
3. Wong, D., Boone, R., Thompson, C., Allard, M., Altwegg, L., Carere, R., Cheung, A., Ye, J., Lichtenstein, S., Ling, H., et al.: Mitral valve injury late after transcatheter aortic valve implantation. Journal of Thoracic and Cardiovascular Surgery **137**(6), 1547–1549 (2009)

4. Comoglio, C., Boffini, M., El Qarra, S., Sansone, F., D'amico, M., Marra, S., Rinaldi, M.: Aortic valve replacement and mitral valve repair as treatment of complications after percutaneous core valve implantation. Journal of Thoracic and Cardiovascular Surgery 138(4), 1025 (2009)
5. Piazza, N., Marra, S., Webb, J., D'Amico, M., Rinaldi, M., Boffini, M., Comoglio, C., Scacciatella, P., Kappetein, A., de Jaegere, P., et al.: Two cases of aneurysm of the anterior mitral valve leaflet associated with transcatheter aortic valve endocarditis: A mere coincidence? Journal of Thoracic and Cardiovascular Surgery 140(3), e36–e38 (2010)
6. Gessat, M., Frauenfelder, T., Altwegg, L., Grünenfelder, J., Falk, V.: Transcatheter aortic valve implantation. role of imaging. Aswan Heart Centre Science & Practice Series 2011(1) (2011)
7. Waechter, I., Kneser, R., Korosoglou, G., Peters, J., Bakker, N.H., Boomen, R., Weese, J.: Patient specific models for planning and guidance of minimally invasive aortic valve implantation. In: Jiang, T., Navab, N., Pluim, J.P.W., Viergever, M.A. (eds.) MICCAI 2010, Part I. LNCS, vol. 6361, pp. 526–533. Springer, Heidelberg (2010)
8. Ionasec, R.I., Voigt, I., Georgescu, B., Wang, Y., Houle, H., Vega-Higuera, F., Navab, N., Comaniciu, D.: Patient-specific modeling and quantification of the aortic and mitral valves from 4-d cardiac ct and tee. IEEE Transactions on Medical Imaging 29(9), 1636–1651 (2010)
9. Pouch, A.M., Wang, H., Takabe, M., Jackson, B.M., Gorman, J.H., Gorman, R.C., Yushkevich, P.A., Sehgal, C.M.: Fully automatic segmentation of the mitral leaflets in 3D transesophageal echocardiographic images using multi-atlas joint label fusion and deformable medial modeling. Med Image Anal 18(1), 118–129 (2014)
10. Korosoglou, G., Gitsioudis, G., Waechter-Stehle, I., Weese, J., Krumsdorf, U., Chorianopoulos, E., Hosch, W., Kauczor, H.U., Katus, H.A., Bekeredjian, R.: Objective quantification of aortic valvular structures by cardiac computed tomography angiography in patients considered for transcatheter aortic valve implantation. Catheterization and Cardiovascular Interventions 81(1), 148–159 (2013)
11. Kherada, N., Mehran, R.: Pursuit of perfection: three-dimensional ct angiographic objective quantification of aortic valve structures for transcatheter aortic valve implantation. Catheterization and Cardiovascular Interventions 81(1), 160–161 (2013)
12. Medtronic, Minneapolis, MN, USA
13. Peters, J., Ecabert, O., Meyer, C., Kneser, R., Weese, J., et al.: Optimizing boundary detection via simulated search with applications to multi-modal heart segmentation. Med. Image Anal. 14(1), 70–84 (2010)
14. Ecabert, O., Peters, J., Schramm, H., Lorenz, C., von Berg, J., Walker, M.J., Vembar, M., Olszewski, M.E., Subramanyan, K., Lavi, G., et al.: Automatic model-based segmentation of the heart in ct images. IEEE Trans. Med. Imag. 27(9), 1189–1201 (2008)
15. Kabsch, W.: A discussion of the solution for the best rotation to relate two sets of vectors. Acta Crystallographica Section A: Crystal Physics, Diffraction, Theoretical and General Crystallography 34(5), 827–828 (1978)
16. Edwards Lifesciences, Irvine, CA, USA
17. JenaValve Technology, Munich, Germany

Structural Abnormality Detection of ARVC Patients via Localised Distance-to-Average Mapping

Kristin McLeod[1,2,5]($\boxtimes$), Marcus Noack[1,5,6],
Jørg Saberniak[3,4,5], and Kristina Haugaa[3,4,5]

[1] Simula Research Laboratory, Oslo, Norway
kristin@simula.no
[2] INRIA Méditerranée, ASCLEPIOS Project, Sophia Antipolis, France
[3] Oslo University Hospital Rikshospitalet, Oslo, Norway
[4] University of Oslo, Oslo, Norway
[5] Centre for Cardiological Innovation, Lysaker, Norway
[6] Kalkulo AS, Oslo, Norway

Abstract. Many heart conditions result in irregular ventricular shape caused by, for example, increased ventricular pressure, regurgitated blood and poor electrical conduction, which affect the overall function of the heart. Structural abnormalities can be characteristic of a disease. Therefore, identifying structurally abnormal regions can give indicators for diagnosis and can provide useful information to guide long-term therapy planning. Given the difficulty in quantitatively measuring structural abnormalities in patients where the ventricular structure is significantly affected by the pathology, such as patients with arrhythmogenic right ventricular cardiomyopathy (ARVC), a method for computing the distance between a normal geometry and patient-specific geometries is presented. The proposed method involves computing distance maps that can visually emphasise regions with high variation from a normal geometry. A consistent parameterisation of the ventricular shape is imposed using an open-source implementation of the LDDMM algorithm on currents to deform patient-specific geometries to a mean surface, which is also computed using the LDDMM algorithm. The chosen shape parameterisation can be applied to meshes extracted from any segmentation algorithm, allowing a wide range of data to be analysed from different hospitals, different scanners and different imaging modalities. Given a consistent shape parameterisation of all meshes, distance maps can be generated by plotting the Euclidean distance point-wise on a triangulated mesh to visualise regions of high shape variability. The proposed method was applied to 10 ARVC patients to highlight patient-specific shape features.

1 Introduction: Clinical Context of ARVC

Arrhythmogenic right ventricular cardiomyopathy / dysplasia (ARVC) is a disease characterised by fibrofatty replacement of cardiac tissue, predominantly in the right ventricle of the heart. The disease affects between 1 in 2000 and 1

O. Camara et al. (Eds.): STACOM 2014, LNCS 8896, pp. 177–186, 2015.
DOI: 10.1007/978-3-319-14678-2_18

in 5000 people and can have devastating consequences due to the fact that the disease can affect anyone, including young people [1] and athletes [2]. In some cases, the first presentation of the disease is during fatal ventricular tachycardia or ventricular fibrillation events [3].

According to the latest diagnostic criteria for ARVC, the diagnosis relies on demonstrating structural, functional and electrophysiological abnormalities [4]. Detecting the structural abnormalities is generally focused on imaging via magnetic resonance imaging (MRI), echocardiography (ECHO) and in fewer cases using angiography of the right ventricle (RV). Previous structural analysis of ARVC patients was focused on the 'triangle of dysplasia' [5]. However, recent research indicates that these regions may not be discriminant identifiers for ARVC [6], and in fact RV apical involvement is generally only exhibited in severe cases as a part of global RV involvement.

Previous studies of structural abnormalities in ARVC patients have been focused on global measures such as volume, ejection fraction, ejection volume, as well as from 2D ECHO analysis [7]. However, given the poor image quality of ECHO, strain analysis is the primary analysis tool but is generally limited to the left ventricle (LV) due to the difficulty in visualising the RV with ECHO. Obtaining regional values in the RV is more difficult and thus less common. Recent studies have been conducted to include the right ventricle by measuring the longitudinal strain in six regions of the RV [8], indicating that the use of RV strain analysis for the diagnosis of ARVC may be promising. However, in general, obtaining ECHO images containing the RV is not straightforward, and strain analysis alone gives indicators towards the functional aspect of the disease, but less so towards the structural aspect. Given the better in-plane spatial resolution of MR images, the structure abnormalities can be better captured than in ECHO images. The structural abnormalities can be identified from visual inspection in severe cases, however, quantifying the severity of the structural abnormalities from visual inspection alone is a challenging tasks, and furthermore, qualitative analysis can be subject to user-bias. Automatic methods for structural abnormality detection can not only provide a more quantitative analysis of the abnormalities, but can also reduce the observer bias.

2   Background: Current Methods for Structural Analysis

Automatic methods for quantifying structural abnormalities have been proposed for other heart conditions and other organs using computational models. Registration-based methods have been widely used to quantify structural differences in two images by the deformation needed to deform one image to another. This methodology was used to study local brain atrophy in Alzheimer's patients [9] by comparing images acquired at different time points to quantify the longitudinal structural changes in the brain. This method is sufficient for quantifying the structural differences when there are small deformations between the two images (as is the case in single-subject analysis) as the registration algorithm is able to capture the deformations when they are sufficiently small. However, for inter-subject analysis, the deformations are generally greater due to the large structural variability observed from one subject to another, even for healthy subjects.

Cardiac surface analysis from deformations computed using the large deformation diffeomorphic metric mapping (LDDMM) on surfaces represented by currents (mathematical objects used to represent shapes non-parametrically) was applied to Tetralogy of Fallot patients to quantify the structural changes over time in [10]. In [10], the population-based shape variation was analysed from model order reduction applied to the deformations to extract the principal modes of shape variation around the mean shape (computed in the space of currents).

In contrast to the population-based shape analysis presented in [10], in the present work, we are rather focused on highlighting patient-specific shape variation. We propose a method to quantify patient-specific shape abnormalities by comparing the geometry extracted from a given subject to an average geometry generated from healthy subjects. The reference geometry is mapped to each patient-specific geometry to obtain a point-to-point correspondence between meshes. Previous methods for computing such correspondences were proposed for matching skull models using anatomical landmarks in [11], and more generalised for any shape in [12]. However, defining more than four anatomical landmarks on the heart consistently for a number of patients is challenging and thus a limitation of anatomical-based methods. Alternatively, the point correspondences could be defined in the segmentation step directly using, for example, level-set methods [13]. In the proposed work, a non-rigid registration algorithm is used to re-sample meshes to a common space with consistent point labelling. The chosen labelling can be applied to any segmented mesh acquired from any segmentation algorithm, which can allow a wider range of data-sets to be analysed and compared between groups that have access to different segmentation algorithms. Aside from potential errors in the original segmentation, the accuracy of the distance computation is dependent only on the LDDMM matching, which can be verified easily by comparing the original and warped meshes. Using the new labelling, distance maps between 10 ARVC patient meshes and an average healthy mesh computed from 15 healthy volunteers were computed to highlight localised patient-specific abnormalities.

3 Methods: Structural Abnormality Detection from a Registration-Based Perspective

Localising structural differences between a patient-specific geometry and an average geometry requires firstly the generation of an average geometry, followed by a way to parameterise all the geometries consistently, and finally a method to compute the distances between two geometries. By representing the geometries by surfaces, which can then be modelled by currents, the framework for computing an average geometry described in [14] can be applied. A brief introduction of the currents representation of surfaces is provided in Sec. 3.1, following the mean

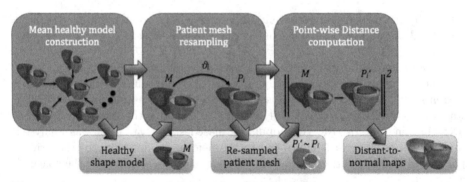

Fig. 1. The proposed method for patient-specific structural abnormality detection; beginning with the creation of a mean model of healthy biventricle shape, followed by a re-sampling of the patient-specific meshes to the parameterisation of the mean model, and finally a distance computation by taking point-wise Euclidean distances

surface computation of [14], which is described briefly in Sec. 4.3. The proposed method for defining a consistent parameterisation of all the surfaces in order to be able to compute distance maps is described in Sec. 3.3. The proposed pipeline is shown in Fig. 1.

3.1   Currents Representation of Surfaces

A key challenge in quantitatively comparing two geometries (such as two ventricles represented by surfaces), is determining where a given point in one geometry corresponds to in another geometry. Representing surfaces by currents rather than by triangulated meshes alleviates this issue by comparing sets of currents rather than points in a mesh. The key principle of currents is to characterise a surface by the flux integral of the surface through vector fields in a test space:

$$S(\omega) = \int_S \omega(x)^t n(x) d\lambda(x), \tag{1}$$

where ω is a square integrable 3D vector field, S is a set of piece-wise smooth surfaces, $n(x)$ is the unit normal of the surface at a point x, and $d\lambda$ is the Lebesque measure on the surface. A surface can then be characterised by the collection of all real numbers $S(\omega)$ calculated using this flux equation, for all possible vector fields in a test space W.

Essentially, each vector field characterises the surface from a different 'angle' or view, and given a sufficient number of vector fields, a complete characterisation of the surface is obtained. The key advantage of working in the space of currents is that it forms a vector space, meaning that standard statistical operations can be performed; currents can be added or subtracted from each other, and scalar multiplication of a current is possible. A sparse representation of currents was proposed in [14], which significantly reduces the size of the set of currents needed to represent the surface.

3.2   Iterative Computation of a Centred Mean

Given that the space of currents forms a vector space, the mean current can be computed for a given set of subjects, as described in [14]. Using this method, a forward strategy can be employed to model each subject as the deformation of the mean plus some residuals. Using this strategy, the mean current can be computed using an alternating iterative approach to minimise the deformations between the mean current and all the subjects, where the deformations are computed using the LDDMM registration of currents. The iterative approach is initialised by taking the mean current as a first approximation, which is then centred with respect to all the subjects. The mean is then updated, followed by a re-centring. This approach is continued until the mean is sufficiently well centred with respect to the population.

3.3   Patient-Specific Distance Mapping

By computing distance maps between a subject-specific geometry and an average geometry, regions of larger distance could highlight structural abnormalities with respect to the average geometry. Computing the distances between two meshes, however, is difficult due to the fact that the parameterisation is in general different from one mesh to another. Using the LDDMM approach, and given a mean surface mesh, the mean can be deformed to each individual, which essentially provides a close approximation of the original subject meshes, now with the same parameterisation as the mean surface mesh (see Fig. 2, right). Essentially, this results in a consistent parameterisation of all the meshes, which allows direct point-to-point distances to be computed between the meshes. From these distances, a colour-coded distance map can be computed for each subject characterising the degree of variation from the mean in each node by mapping the distances onto the patient meshes.

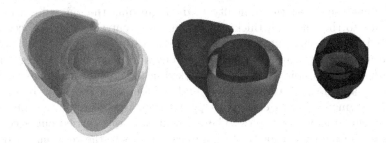

Fig. 2. Left: All the patient meshes shown together to visualise the shape variability in the population. Centre: The surface representation of the mean current used for the distance calculations. Right: The LV endocardium for one patient showing the original segmented mesh (in red) and the mesh computed by deforming the mean surface representation towards this mesh (black wire-frame) showing that the warped mesh used for the distance computation is close to the original mesh.

4   Experiments: Distance Map Generation of ARVC

In order to apply the proposed methodology, images covering both ventricles are required (see Sec. 4.1), from which the geometry can be extracted using image segmentation tools (see Sec. 4.2). The mean geometry can then be computed as a point of comparison and consistent mesh generation is required for the distance computations (see Sec. 4.3). Patient-specific structural abnormalities are highlighted using the distance maps computed between the ARVC patients and the mean normal model (see Sec. 4.4).

4.1   Subjects and Image Preparation

We illustrate these tools on 10 patients diagnosed with ARVC (5 male, mean age ± SD = 32 ± 12). SSFP MR images were acquired (one patient scanned with the Gyroscan NT Intera 1.5T System, Philips Medical Systems and nine with the SonataVision 1.5T System, Siemens) in the short axis view covering entirely both ventricles (10-14 slices; isotropic in-plane resolution:$1.25 \times 1.25mm^2$ to $1.64 \times 1.64mm^2$; slice thickness: $8 - 10mm$; 19-42 frames). In order to compare ARVC-specific shape features to healthy shape features, a control data-set of 15 healthy adult hearts from the STACOM 2011 motion tracking challenge was used [15]. Full details on the subject data and image acquisition can be found in [15].

4.2   Surface Mesh Preparation

The left ventricle endocardium and epicardium were segmented from the short axis cine-MR images at the end diastolic frame (chosen as the first frame of the cine loop, computed as the end diastolic frame from ECG gating). The right ventricle endocardium was also segmented, though the epicardium was excluded from the analysis given the difficulty in distinguishing the epicardium in MR images due to the thin wall thickness in the right ventricle. The surfaces were segmented using a semi-automatic tool provided within the Segment software[1]; freely available for research purposes [16]. The advantage of using Segment is that both basal and apical slices can be faked in to the analysis in cases where few basal / apical slices were acquired, and the long axis views can be used to guide the segmentation in cases with poor through-plane resolution and slice misalignment in short axis stack. The segmentation was carried out according to the guidelines for inclusion of the papillary muscles to the ventricular volume described in [17]. Once all images were segmented, manual rigid alignment of all meshes to a chosen reference was performed to globally align the bi-ventricle meshes (see Fig. 2 (left)).

---

[1] http://medviso.com/products/segment/

4.3   Mean ARVC Surface Model and Consistent Patient Meshing

Computation of the mean current was computed following the method of [14] as described in Sec. 3.2 using the ExoShape[2] toolbox. The two key parameters in the LDDMM registration that control the stiffness of the registration (λ_V) and the resolution of the currents controlling the level of detail to include in the model (λ_W) were set to $\lambda_V = 30, \lambda_W = 10$ according to the parameters used in previous work on similar meshes. Two iterations of the alternate minimisation was needed to reach convergence. Once the mean current was computed, a surface representation of this current was computed by warping the closest patient to the mean current. The mean surface representation is shown in Fig. 2 (centre).

4.4   Patient-Specific Structural Abnormality Analysis

Distance maps were computed for the 10 ARVC patients with colour maps to visualise the regions with greater distances. The distance maps were computed on the patient-specific meshes with and without scaling to analyse both global and local distances. The different level of analysis are exemplified in Fig. 3 on one patient. The mean distance of all patients before scaling is 9.1676 compared to the mean distance after scaling of 3.3307.

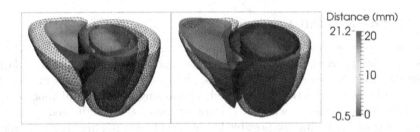

Fig. 3. Distance maps for one patient before (left) and after (right) re-scaling to show the different level of analysis either global (left) or local (right)

Since global shape differences are difficult to analyse and interpret given the range of ages of the patients used in this study, the local shape differences can give more insight into the pathology-specific shape features. The distance maps for the 10 patients after re-scaling are shown in Fig. 4. The patient with largest mean distance was the 7th patient with mean distance 4.95 (bottom row, second column in Fig. 4), which can be seen visually on the biventricle view of Fig. 4. Note that this patient had the highest ARVC diagnostic score, with five major criteria identified according to the diagnostic criteria defined in [4].

---

[2] http://www-sop.inria.fr/asclepios/projects/Health-e-Child/ShapeAnalysis/

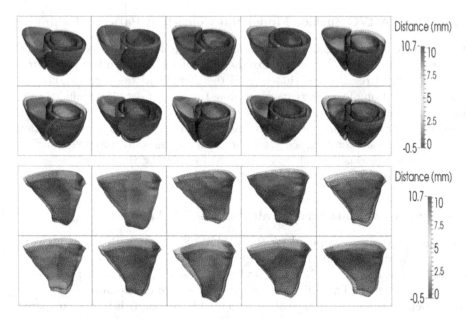

Fig. 4. Mean surface (left) and the 10 patient-specific distance maps after re-scaling shown for one biventricular view (top) and one view purely of the RV (bottom)

5   Discussion and Perspectives

The proposed methodology presents a simple method for detecting structural abnormalities by computing distance maps that highlight regions with large variability from a mean geometry. The application of the proposed method to ARVC patients suggests that the method is promising for structural abnormality detection. Some key issues with the current formulation are addressed in the following sections, including the possible bias caused by the required pre-processing steps, the discrepancy between the original meshes and the warped meshes used for the distance computation, and the difficulty in distinguishing pathological from non-pathological variability.

5.1   Segmentation and Rigid Registration

The proposed methodology relies on accurate segmentation and rigid pre-alignment (otherwise segmentation error and/or misalignment error are included in the distance maps). The rigid pre-alignment was performed manually in this work, though future work will be focussed on automating the pre-processing steps. Once the mesh-resampling step has been performed, the meshes can be rigidly aligned using the point-to-point correspondences in order to remove any bias in the distance maps.

5.2   Original Mesh vs. Warped Mesh

As mentioned briefly in Sec. 3.3, there are small differences between the original meshes and the warped meshes used for the distance computation. These differences can potentially introduce errors in the distance computation. For the present work, the order of these errors was considered to be low enough to not be significant for the analysis given that the errors are of the same order as the errors of the segmentation. The distances can be decreased by modifying the parameters of the LDDMM algorithm which control the stiffness of the regis- tration and the level of features included in the registration. These parameters were not optimised in the present work.

5.3 Pathological vs. Non-pathological Variability

Given the large shape variability observed between different individuals, both healthy and pathological, it may be difficult to distinguish between patholog- ical and non-pathological variability. In the present work, only the differences between pathological hearts and healthy hearts were analysed, however it is difficult to differentiate the distances from being related to pathological shape remodelling and normal remodelling due to age for instance. To address this, the distances between healthy subjects and a mean normal shape could be compared to the distances between diseased patients and a mean normal shape in order to define a measure for the limit of what is considered normal shape variability. Such analysis is limited in the present study due to the small size of the control data-set; more data is needed to create statistically significant cut offs for normal vs. abnormal.

6 Conclusion

A method for detecting structural abnormalities by computing distance maps from a mean geometry to patient-specific geometries was proposed and applied to ARVC patients. The proposed method relies on defining a consistent param- eterisation of the patient and mean meshes in order to be able to compute point-wise distances directly. The consistent parameterisation was defined using the LDDMM registration algorithm on currents which implicitly defines a point- to-point correspondence between the mean mesh and the patient meshes when deforming each patient mesh to the mean. Given the consistent mesh parame- terisation, distance maps were computed directly by computing the Euclidean distance between points. The method was applied to 15 healthy volunteers to compute the mean normal geometry, from which the patient-specific distance analysis was computed on 10 ARVC patients to visually highlight patient-specific deviations from the mean.

Acknowledgments. This project was carried out as a part of the Centre for Cardi- ological Innovation, Norway, funded by the Research Council of Norway.

References

1. Corrado, D., Basso, C., Rizzoli, G., Schiavon, M., Thiene, G.: Does sports activity enhance the risk of sudden death in adolescents and young adults? J. Am. Coll. Cardiology **42**(11), 1959–1963 (2003)

2. Firoozi, S., Sharma, S., Hamid, M.S., McKenna, W.J.: Sudden death in young athletes: Hcm or arvc? Cardiovascular Drugs and Therapy **16**(1), 11–17 (2002)
3. Corrado, D., Thiene, G.: Arrhythmogenic right ventricular cardiomyopathy / dysplasia: Clinical impact of molecular genetic studies. Circulation **113**(13) (2006)
4. Marcus, F.I., McKenna, W.J., Sherrill, D., et al.: Diagnosis of arrhythmogenic right ventricular cardiomyopathy / dysplasia: Proposed modification of the task force criteria. Euro. Heart J. **31**(7) (2010)
5. Anderson, E.L.: Arrhythmogenic right ventricular dysplasia. Am. Fam. Physician **73**(8) (2006)
6. Te Riele, A.S., James, C.A., Philips, B., et al.: Mutation-positive arrhythmogenic right ventricular dysplasia / cardiomyopathy: The triangle of dysplasia displaced. J. Car. Electro. **24**(12) (2013)
7. Tandri, H., Macedo, R., Calkins, H., et al.: Role of magnetic resonance imaging in arrhythmogenic right ventricular dysplasia: Insights from the north american arrhythmogenic right ventricular dysplasia (ARVD/C) study. Am. Heart J. **155**(1) (2008)
8. Healy-Brucker, A., Pousset, F., Almeida, S., Gandjbakhch, E., Duthoit, G., Hebert, J., Boubrit, L., Hammoudi, N., Isnard, R., Hidden-Lucet, F.: Usefulness of right ventricle 2D strain in arrythmogenic right ventricle dysplasia / cardiomyopathy. Euro. Heart J. **34** (2013)
9. Lorenzi, M., Ayache, N., Pennec, X.: Regional flux analysis of longitudinal atrophy in alzheimer's disease. In: Ayache, N., Delingette, H., Golland, P., Mori, K. (eds.) MICCAI 2012, Part I. LNCS, vol. 7510, pp. 739–746. Springer, Heidelberg (2012)
10. Mansi, T., Voigt, I., Leonardi, B., Pennec, X., Durrleman, S., Sermesant, M., Delingette, H., Taylor, A.M., Boudjemline, Y., Pongiglione, G., et al.: A statistical model for quantification and prediction of cardiac remodelling: Application to Tetralogy of Fallot. IEEE Trans. Med. Im. **30**(9) (2011)
11. Zhang, K., Cheng, Y., Leow, W.K.: Dense correspondence of skull models by automatic detection of anatomical landmarks. In: Wilson, R., Hancock, E., Bors, A., Smith, W. (eds.) CAIP 2013, Part I. LNCS, vol. 8047, pp. 229–236. Springer, Heidelberg (2013)
12. Praun, E., Sweldens, W., Schröder, P.: Consistent mesh parameterizations. In: Proc. Computer Graphics and Interactive Techniques, pp. 179–184. ACM (2001)
13. Angelini, E., Jin, Y., Laine, A.: State of the art of level set methods in segmentation and registration of medical imaging modalities. In: Handbook of Biomedical Image Analysis, pp. 47–101. Springer (2005)
14. Durrleman, S., Pennec, X., Trouvé, A., Ayache, N.: Statistical models of sets of curves and surfaces based on currents. Med. Im. Anal. **13**(5) (2009)
15. Tobon-Gomez, C., De Craene, M., Mcleod, K., Tautz, L., Shi, W., Hennemuth, A., et al.: Benchmarking framework for myocardial tracking and deformation algorithms: An open access database. Med. Im. Anal **17**(6), 632–648 (2013)
16. Heiberg, E., Sjögren, J., Ugander, M., Carlsson, M., Engblom, H., Arheden, H.: Design and validation of segment-freely available software for cardiovascular image analysis. BMC Med. Im.
17. Schulz-Menger, J., Bluemke, D.A., et al.: Standardized image interpretation and post processing in cardiovascular magnetic resonance: Society for cardiovascular magnetic resonance (SCMR) board of trustees task force on standardized post processing. J. of Cardio. Mag. Res. **15**, 35 (2013)

Joint Myocardial Motion and Contraction Phase Estimation from Cine MRI Using Variational Data Assimilation

Viateur Tuyisenge[1](✉), Laurent Sarry[1], Thomas Corpetti[3],
Elisabeth Innorta-Coupez[2], Lemlih Ouchchane[1], and Lucie Cassagnes[1,2]

[1] Clermont Université, Université d' Auvergne, ISIT UMR 6284 UdA-CNRS,
Clermont-ferrand, France
viateur.tuyisenge@udamail.fr
[2] Pôle de Radiologie et d' Imagerie Médicale, CHU Gabriel Montpied,
Clermont-ferrand, France
[3] COSTEL-LETG UMR 6554 CNRS-Université de Rennes 2, Rennes, France

Abstract. We present a cardiac motion estimation method with variational data assimilation that combines image observations and a dynamic evolution model. The novelty of the model is that it embeds new parameters modeling heart contraction and relaxation. It was applied to a synthetic dataset with known ground truth motion and to 10 cine-MRI sequences of patients with normal or dyskinetic myocardial zones. It was compared to the inTag tagging tracking software for computing the radial motion component, and to the diagnosis for dyskinesia. We found that the new dynamic model performed better than the standard transport model, and the contraction parameters are promising features for diagnosing dyskinesia.

1 Introduction

Non-invasive image-based analysis and quantification of cardiac motion provide important information on how pathology affects local and global deformation of the myocardium and its responses to a given therapy. The estimation of myocardial deformations helps to study and detect regions with an abnormal contraction in order to provide treatment for recovery. It includes a comprehensive study of the structural or architectural heart abnormalities, which provides an essential prognostic approach for therapeutic decisions, such as the implantation of defibrillators for infarction resynchronization, the adaptation of doses or treatments such as beta-blockers converting enzyme inhibitors.

Over the past few years, considerable efforts have been made to develop methods to track the myocardium in different available imaging modalities, such as ultrasound (US), magnetic resonance imaging (cine MRI or tagged MRI) or SPECT. However, accurate cardiac motion estimation is still a challenging and open problem due to low spatial and temporal resolutions and the complexity of the cardiac biomechanics [1]. Numerous categories of methods aim to

O. Camara et al. (Eds.): STACOM 2014, LNCS 8896, pp. 187–195, 2015.
DOI: 10.1007/978-3-319-14678-2_19

obtain cardiac contraction parameters and deformation fields from images and the underlying dynamics of the heart as reviewed in [2]. To improve the accuracy, knowledge about cardiac contraction can be used to constrain the solution in a data assimilation framework.

Initially, data assimilation has been used for meteorological image sequences [3]. To improve the diagnosis of cardiac diseases and therapy planning, different researchers have extended it to cardiac medical images to benefit from the robustness and accuracy of this estimation process. Sainte-Marie et al. [4] and Sermesant et al. [5] used data assimilation to estimate local cardiac contractility from cardiac synthetic data. Delingette et al. [6] and Sundar et al. [7] proposed methods to estimate the myocardial motion and contractility parameters of left and right ventricles using data assimilation and a full electromechanical model of the heart.

Although there is a significant work on the integration of imaging with cardiovascular mechanics, there is still a need to account for the active contraction/relaxation of the heart. To address this problem, we propose a novel method for myocardial motion and phase estimation in a variational data assimilation framework. To this end, a parameterized transport of velocity is used to accurately track the myocardium without imposing strong constraints over the motion field.

The novelty and contributions of our model with respect to previous works are two-fold. (1) It includes contraction parameters and makes displacement field estimation more accurate. In fact, the invariance assumption tends to smooth temporal variations in the transported values. It is adapted for uniformly accelerated movements, but not for cardiac dynamics. The sign function induces piecewise smoothing, independently for contraction and relaxation phases. (2) Flow fields and contraction parameters are simultaneously estimated and we show they are complementary features to diagnose cardiac dyskinesia. The method was applied to synthetic datasets and validated against a reference tagging MRI tracking software.

2   Method

We present a method for cardiac motion and contraction parameter estimation using variational data assimilation. Data assimilation was chosen because it incorporates a dynamical model that provides temporal coherency and makes results robust to poor quality and noisy images.

In this method, the standard transport equation used for meteo data is replaced by a parameterized transport equation of velocity thanks to cardiac dynamics. The mathematical derivation was simplified to keep it readable for wider audiences and obtained results are very encouraging. To the best of our knowledge so far, this kind of model has never been applied to cardiac imaging data.

Given the state vector $\mathcal{X}$ (variables to estimate), the observation vector $\mathcal{Y}$ (in our case, sequence of images), $\mathbb{H}$ an operator that links state variables to observations and the evolution model $\mathbb{M}$ of dynamic system, data assimilation aims to produce accurate estimates of the current (or the future) state variables of the dynamic system by solving the following system of three equations:

$$\begin{cases} \frac{\partial \mathcal{X}}{\partial t}(\mathbf{x}, t) + \mathbb{M}(\mathcal{X})(\mathbf{x}, t) = \nu_m(\mathbf{x}, t), \\ \mathbb{H}(\mathcal{X}, \mathcal{Y})(\mathbf{x}, t) = \nu_o(\mathbf{x}, t), \\ \mathcal{X}(\mathbf{x}, 0) = \mathcal{X}_b(\mathbf{x}) + \nu_b(\mathbf{x}, 0), \end{cases} \tag{1}$$

where $(\mathbf{x}, t)$ are the spatio-temporal variables, $\mathcal{X}_b$ is the background (*a priori* knowledge on state vector), and ν_m, ν_o and ν_b are the uncertainties of dynamic evolution, observation and background information respectively. Their respective covariance matrices are represented by Q, R and B.

2.1   Dynamic Evolution Model

The standard transport of velocity used in fluid dynamics [3] can overly smooth the estimated fields, especially when it is changing direction rapidly. To handle the case of cardiac dynamics, we propose to parameterize the transport equation. A sign function modeling myocardium contraction phase is embedded into the standard transport equation:

$$\mathbb{M}(\mathcal{X}) = sign\left(\sin\left(\omega(\mathbf{x})t + \varphi(\mathbf{x})\right) + a(\mathbf{x})\right) \boldsymbol{v}^T(\mathbf{x}, t) \nabla \mathcal{X}(\mathbf{x}, t), \tag{2}$$

where $sign$ is the sign function, $\mathcal{X} = (\boldsymbol{v}(\mathbf{x}, t), \varphi(\mathbf{x}), a(\mathbf{x}))^T$ is a state vector, $\boldsymbol{v}(\mathbf{x}, t) = (u(\mathbf{x}, t), v(\mathbf{x}, t))$ is the motion fields, $\omega = 2\pi/T$, with T the period of the cardiac cycle, $\varphi(\mathbf{x})$ and $a(\mathbf{x})$ are the phase angle and the temporal asymmetry (the ratio between systolic and diastolic time duration) respectively.

In fact, φ gives the phase of the contraction and a acts on the symmetry of the cardiac cycle. The assimilation process adjusts their values to synchronize the sign function with the cardiac cycle (positive and negative for contraction and relaxation respectively). In the following, the standard transport model without the *sign* function will be refered as DASS1 and our model (2) as DASS2.

2.2   Observation Terms

The observation operator on motion field relies on the optical flow equation combined with a nonlinear regulariser that acts as both quadratic and total variation smoothing [8] (OBS). In addition to the observation terms on the motion field, one can add observation terms to a and φ if *a priori* values are known. For example if $\varphi \in [\varphi_1, \varphi_2]$, then we can add a term of the form:

$$\begin{cases} \mathcal{Y}_\varphi(\mathbf{x}) = \mathbb{H}_\varphi(\varphi(\mathbf{x})) = 0, \\ \mathbb{H}_\varphi(\varphi(\mathbf{x})) = H(\varphi_1 - \varphi(\mathbf{x})) + H(\varphi(\mathbf{x}) - \varphi_2), \end{cases} \tag{3}$$

where H is the Heaviside function ($H(x) = 0$ if $x \leq 0$ and 1 elsewhere). The same kind of term can be applied to $a \in [a_1, a_2]$.

2.3 Cost Function and Minimization

The system (1) is solved by minimizing the following functional energy:

$$E(\boldsymbol{\mathcal{X}}) = \int_{\mathbf{x},t} \left(\frac{\partial \boldsymbol{\mathcal{X}}}{\partial t} + \mathbb{M}(\boldsymbol{\mathcal{X}}) \right)^T Q^{-1} \left(\frac{\partial \boldsymbol{\mathcal{X}}}{\partial t} + \mathbb{M}(\boldsymbol{\mathcal{X}}) \right) dxdt \qquad (4)$$

$$+ \int_{\mathbf{x},t} \mathbb{H}(\boldsymbol{\mathcal{X}}, \boldsymbol{\mathcal{Y}})^T R^{-1} \mathbb{H}(\boldsymbol{\mathcal{X}}, \boldsymbol{\mathcal{Y}}) dxdt + \int_{\mathbf{x}} (\boldsymbol{\mathcal{X}}_b - \boldsymbol{\mathcal{X}}_0)^T B^{-1} (\boldsymbol{\mathcal{X}}_b - \boldsymbol{\mathcal{X}}_0) dx.$$

Since it is minimized with respect to $\boldsymbol{\mathcal{X}}$, its differential is computed by determining the directional derivative and introducing an auxiliary variable known as the adjoint variable $\lambda(\mathbf{x},t) = \int_{\mathbf{x},t} Q^{-1} \left(\frac{\partial \boldsymbol{\mathcal{X}}}{\partial t} + \mathbb{M}(\boldsymbol{\mathcal{X}}) \right) dxdt$. As operators $\mathbb{M}$ and $\mathbb{H}$ are nonlinear, local linearization is applied and state vector becomes $\boldsymbol{\mathcal{X}} = \boldsymbol{\mathcal{X}}_b + \delta\boldsymbol{\mathcal{X}}$, with $\boldsymbol{\mathcal{X}}_b$ the background variable and $\delta\boldsymbol{\mathcal{X}}$ the incremental variable.

Differential and Adjoint Operators. We derive a linear tangent operator $\frac{\partial \mathbb{M}}{\partial \boldsymbol{\mathcal{X}}}(\delta\boldsymbol{\mathcal{X}})$ of operator $\mathbb{M}$ in the neighbourhood of $\boldsymbol{\mathcal{X}} + \delta\boldsymbol{\mathcal{X}}$. Using Gateau derivative $\left(\frac{\partial \mathbb{M}}{\partial \boldsymbol{\mathcal{X}}} \right) \delta\boldsymbol{\mathcal{X}} = \lim_{\beta \to 0} \frac{\mathbb{M}(\boldsymbol{\mathcal{X}} + \beta\delta\boldsymbol{\mathcal{X}}) - \mathbb{M}(\boldsymbol{\mathcal{X}})}{\beta}$, we have:

$$\frac{\partial \mathbb{M}}{\partial \boldsymbol{\mathcal{X}}}(\delta\boldsymbol{\mathcal{X}}) = \lim_{\beta \to 0} \left\{ \frac{[sign\,(\sin(\omega t + \varphi + \beta\delta\varphi) + a + \beta\delta a)]\,(v + \beta\delta v)^T \nabla(\boldsymbol{\mathcal{X}} + \beta\delta\boldsymbol{\mathcal{X}})}{\beta} \right.$$
$$\left. - \frac{[sign\,(\sin(\omega t + \varphi) + a)]\, v^T \nabla \boldsymbol{\mathcal{X}}}{\beta} \right\}. \qquad (5)$$

In practice, the function $sign(x)$ can be approximated by $\tanh(kx)$ with $k > 1$ in the continuous domain. After Taylor expansion $\tanh(k(x + \beta\delta x)) = \tanh(kx) + k\beta\delta x(1 - \tanh^2(kx))$ and $\sin(\omega t + \varphi + \beta\delta\varphi) = \sin(\omega t + \varphi) + \beta\delta\varphi \cos(\omega t + \varphi)$ and putting together terms in $\beta, \beta^2, ...$, the following equation is obtained:

$$\frac{\partial \mathbb{M}}{\partial \boldsymbol{\mathcal{X}}}(\delta\boldsymbol{\mathcal{X}}) = A_1(\delta v.\nabla v + v.\nabla\delta v) + A_k(v.\nabla\delta v)\delta\varphi + kA_2(v.\nabla\delta v)\delta a, \qquad (6)$$

with $A_1 = \tanh(k(\sin(\omega t + \varphi) + a))$, $A_2 = 1 - \tanh^2(k(\sin(\omega t + \varphi) + a))$ and $A_k = kA_2 \cos(\omega t + \varphi)$. The global linear tangent model is then: $\frac{\partial \delta\boldsymbol{\mathcal{X}}}{\partial t} + \frac{\partial \mathbb{M}}{\partial \boldsymbol{\mathcal{X}}}(\delta\boldsymbol{\mathcal{X}}) = \nu_m$. The adjoint model operator is given as follows (mathematical details are found in [3]):

$$\left(\frac{\partial \mathbb{M}}{\partial \boldsymbol{\mathcal{X}}} \right)^* = \begin{bmatrix} A_1(\nabla^T v - v^T\nabla + \nabla^T(\varphi + a)) \\ A_k(v.\nabla v - v^T\nabla + v^T\nabla\varphi) \\ kA_2(v.\nabla v - v^T\nabla + v^T\nabla a) \end{bmatrix}. \qquad (7)$$

Using the derivative definition from above, the linear tangent operator of $\mathbb{H}_\varphi(\varphi(\mathbf{x}))$ in the neighbourhood of $\varphi + \delta\varphi$ can be written as: $\left(\frac{\partial \mathbb{H}_\varphi}{\partial \boldsymbol{\mathcal{X}}} \right) \delta\varphi(\mathbf{x}) = [-\delta(\varphi_1 - \varphi(\mathbf{x})) + \delta(\varphi(\mathbf{x}) - \varphi_2)]\,\delta\varphi(\mathbf{x})$, where $\delta(x)$ is the Dirac function. In practice, we may use the continuous versions of the Heaviside and Dirac functions $H(x) = \frac{1}{2} + \frac{1}{2}\tanh(kx)$ and $\delta(x) = \frac{1}{2}(1 - \tanh^2(kx))$. The same can be done for the parameter a. The adjoint operator of $\left(\frac{\partial \mathbb{H}_\varphi}{\partial \boldsymbol{\mathcal{X}}} \right)$ is itself, $i.e.$,

$$\left(\frac{\partial \mathbb{H}_\varphi}{\partial \boldsymbol{\mathcal{X}}} \right)^* = \left(\frac{\partial \mathbb{H}_\varphi}{\partial \boldsymbol{\mathcal{X}}} \right).$$

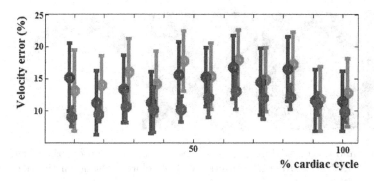

Fig. 1. Mean and standard velocity errors between ground truth and estimated velocities for the 3 methods on synthetic data: OBS (green), DASS1 (blue) and DASS2 (red)

Covariance Matrices. The appropriate covariance matrices R, Q, and B that represent errors in observation, evolution model and background have to be defined to avoid the influence of observation noise on the computed solution. To this end, we define the observation covariance matrix R as: $R(\mathbf{x}) = (1 - \exp^{-\frac{\|\nabla_3 I\|^2}{\sigma^2}})$, where $\nabla_3 I$ is spatio-temporal image gradient and σ standard deviation of intensity. The matrix B is chosen to be identity. In practice, covariance matrix Q can be learnt in a training process on real data by minimizing the error between the estimated velocities and a ground truth.

After defining the evolution and observations models, the adjoint operators and covariance matrices, we followed the procedure described in [3] to implement the algorithm.

3   Results and Discussion

3.1   Validation with Synthetic Data

The synthetic dataset was generated to evaluate the accuracy of the proposed method (DASS2). We simulated synthetic sequences using the transport equation from an initial image of a torus with a radial gray level ramp and a sinusoidal variable displacement identical to the one of (2). Parameters vary from $-\pi/6$ to $\pi/6$ all around the torus for φ and parameter a from 0.4 to 0.6 corresponding to a systolic time about twice as long as the diastolic time. Generated images were corrupted with a Gaussian noise (30 dB signal-to-noise ratio). Motion was estimated using the two assimilation methods DASS1 and DASS2 and the observation term alone (OBS). Fig. 1 shows the mean and standard error with respect to the simulated velocity field was smaller for DASS2 than for DASS1 and OBS.

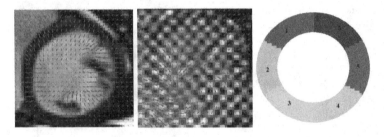

Fig. 2. Cine and tagged MRI in short axis view with surperimposed displacement field estimated by DASS2 and inTag respectively. The colored scheme on the right is the AHA sectorization.

3.2 Application to Clinical Data

We validated our method using cine MRI and tagged MRI image sequences for 10 patients: 6 were suffering from dyskinesia and 4 had normal kinetics. MRI was part of a post myocardial infarction protocol. MRI sequences were acquired with a *Siemens Avanto* 1.5T system: cine trufisp acquisitions in short axis view with and without a tagging pattern. The number of frames in both sequences varied from 17 to 33 with an image size of 208×256. As imaging parameters (x, y, z, resolutions, #slices, spacing etc.) were not the same for cine and tagged images, sequences were first spatially registered (two points manually selected in the middle of LV cavity and at junction to RV in order to center and reorientate images) and then temporally interpolated (only sequences qualitatively registered were selected for validation process).

Fig. 2 shows the recovered displacement field for one frame of one patient with DASS2 and inTag. Cardiac motion was estimated from cine MRI using the 3 methods DASS1, DASS2 and OBS, and retrieved from tagged MRI images using inTag software[1].

The covariance matrix Q was trained on the ground truth given by inTag for one of the patient data: minimum errors were obtained for variances of 10^2 and 0.1 for (u, v) and (a, φ) respectively. Comparable radial velocity variations were computed from cine MRI with the 3 methods DASS1, DASS2 and OBS and averaged over the 6 AHA divisions of the myocardium (Fig. 2, right) and then compared with the ones retrieved from tagged MRI by the inTag software (Fig. 3). Considering all the 10 patients, we recorded a slight trend for better results in terms of fitting to inTag gold standard for DASS2, but the p-value is far over 0.05.

Concerning the diagnosis of dyskinesia, discriminative power of each criterion depending on a and φ over the myocardial sectors was assessed using a generalized linear mixed model. The criterion was considered as response variable and expert diagnosis (agreement between a cardiologist and a radiologist) as binary explanatory variable, accounting for nested structure of the myocardial

---

[1] *inTag* is an open-source OsiriX plugin developed by the CREATIS laboratory (http://www.creatis.insa-lyon.fr/inTag/).

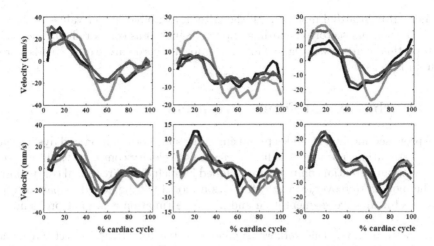

Fig. 3. Radial velocities estimated at 1 to 6 AHA sectors during one cardiac cycle with: inTag (black) from tagged MRI, DASS2 (red), DASS1 (blue) and OBS (green) from cine MRI

Table 1. Mean and standard errors of the 3 motion estimation methods with regard to inTag

Method	Mean±SE	p-value
DASS1	0.2879 ± 0.2006	
DASS2	0.2314 ± 0.1975	0.0954
OBS	0.3151 ± 0.2009	

Table 2. Mean and standard deviation of features and metric tests for significant discrimination of each continuous criterion regarding myocardial dyskinesia

Criterion	Expert diagnosis	mean±SD	p-value	AUROCC
$Max\,|\,a\,|$	Normal	0.0967 ± 0.0264	0.008	0.711
	Dyskinesia	0.2560 ± 0.0388		
$Max\,|\,\varphi\,|$	Normal	0.1276 ± 0.0276	0.477	0.666
	Dyskinesia	0.2398 ± 0.0405		
$\bar{a}$	Normal	0.0274 ± 0.0081	0.0648	0.635
	Dyskinesia	0.0574 ± 0.0118		
$\bar{\varphi}$	Normal	0.0297 ± 0.0078	0.0315	0.664
	Dyskinesia	0.0652 ± 0.0115		

sectors for each patient. A statistical inference was carried out seeking for significant difference between normal and dyskinetic myocardial sectors. The area under the ROC curve (AUROCC) was estimated for each criterion denoting the probability that two myocardial sectors range in the expected order (lower value for normal myocardial motion). All the criteria exhibited higher values in dyskinetic myocardial sectors (regarding expert diagnosis) as compared with normal sectors, this increase was significant except for $\bar{a}$ where only strong trends were found (Tab. 2).

4   Conclusion and Future Prospects

The proposed method provides promising results for both motion and dyskinesia index estimation. For now it is limited to radial velocity component, but extension to circumferential component is planned by including directional constraints to the model. Moreover, a wall deformation model will be added as part of the state vector to solve segmentation and motion estimation as a joint problem.

Acknowledgments. This work was supported by the 3DSTRAIN project through a grant from the French National Research Agency (ANR), programme "Technologies for health and autonomy", grant number ANR-11-TecSan-002.

References

1. Tobon-Gomez, C., De-Craene, M., McLeod, K., Lautz, T., Shi, W., Hennemuth, A., Prakosa, A., Wang, H., Carr-White, G., Kapetanakis, S., Lutz, A., Rasche, V., Schaeffter, T., Butakoff, C., Friman, O., Mansi, T., Sermesant, M., Zhuang, X., Ourselin, S., Peitgen, H., Pennec, X., Razavi, R., Reuckert, D., Frangi, A., Rhode, K.: Benchmarking framework for myocardial tracking and deformation algorithms: An open access database. Medical Image Analysis **17**, 632–648 (2013)
2. Wang, H., Amini, A.: Cardiac motion and deformation recovery from MRI: a review. IEEE Transactions on Medical Imaging **31** (2012)
3. Béréziat, D., Herlin, I.: Solving ill-posed image processing problems using data assimilation. Numerical Algorithms (2010)
4. Sainte-Marie, J., Chapelle, D., Sorine, M.: Data assimilation for an electromechanical model of the myocardium. In: Second M.I.T. Conference on Computational Fluid and Solid Mechanic, pp. 1801–1804 (2003)
5. Sermesant, M., Moireau, P., Camara, O., Sainte-Marie, J., Andriantsimiavona, R., Cimrman, R., Hill, D., Chapelle, D., Razavi, R.: Cardiac function estimation from MRI using heart model and data assimilation: Advances and difficulties. Medical Image Analysis **10**, 642–656 (2006)
6. Delingette, H., Billet, F., Wong, K.C.L., Sermesant, M., Rhode, K., Ginks, M., Rinaldi, C.A., Razavi, R., Ayache, N.: Personalization of cardiac motion and contractility from images using variational data assimilation. IEEE Transactions on Biomedical Engineering **10**, 20–24 (2012)
7. Sundar, H., Davatzikos, C., Biros, G.: Biomechanically-constrained 4D estimation of myocardial motion. In: Yang, G.-Z., Hawkes, D., Rueckert, D., Noble, A., Taylor, C. (eds.) MICCAI 2009, Part II. LNCS, vol. 5762, pp. 257–265. Springer, Heidelberg (2009)

8. Tuyisenge, V., Albouy-Kissi, A., Cassagnes, L., Coupez, E., Merlin, C., Windyga, P., Sarry, L.: Variational myocardial tracking from cine-MRI with non-linear regularization. In: Proc. of the 10th IEEE Int. Symposium on Biomedical Imaging (ISBI) (2013)
9. Tuyisenge, V., Albouy-Kissi, A., Sarry, L.: Variational myocardial tracking from cine-MRI with non-linear regularization: validation of radial displacements vs. tagged-MRI. In: Ourselin, S., Rueckert, D., Smith, N. (eds.) FIMH 2013. LNCS, vol. 7945, pp. 334–341. Springer, Heidelberg (2013)
10. Arts, T., Prinzen, F., Delhaas, T., Milles, J., Rossi, A., Clarysse, P.: Mapping displacement and deformation of the heart with local sine-wave modeling. IEEE Transactions on Medical Imaging **29**, 1114–1123 (2010)

Segmentation of the Aortic Valve Apparatus in 3D Echocardiographic Images: Deformable Modeling of a Branching Medial Structure

Alison M. Pouch[1([⊠])], Sijie Tian[2], Manabu Takabe[1], Hongzhi Wang[3], Jiefu Yuan[1], Albert T. Cheung[4], Benjamin M. Jackson[1,5], Joseph H. Gorman III[1,5], Robert C. Gorman[1,5], and Paul A. Yushkevich[3]

[1] Gorman Cardiovascular Research Group, University of Pennsylvania, Philadelphia, PA, USA
alison.pouch@gmail.com
[2] Department of Computer and Information Science,
University of Pennsylvania, Philadelphia, PA, USA
[3] IBM Almaden Research Center, San Jose, CA, USA
[4] Department of Anesthesiology, Perioperative, and Pain Medicine,
Stanford School of Medicine, Stanford, CA, USA
[5] Department of Surgery, University of Pennsylvania, Philadelphia, PA, USA

Abstract. 3D echocardiographic (3DE) imaging is a useful tool for assessing the complex geometry of the aortic valve apparatus. Segmentation of this structure in 3DE images is a challenging task that benefits from shape-guided deformable modeling methods, which enable inter-subject statistical shape comparison. Prior work demonstrates the efficacy of using continuous medial representation (cm-rep) as a shape descriptor for valve leaflets. However, its application to the entire aortic valve apparatus is limited since the structure has a branching medial geometry that cannot be explicitly parameterized in the original cm-rep framework. In this work, we show that the aortic valve apparatus can be accurately segmented using a new branching medial modeling paradigm. The segmentation method achieves a mean boundary displacement of 0.6 ± 0.1 mm (approximately one voxel) relative to manual segmentation on 11 3DE images of normal open aortic valves. This study demonstrates a promising approach for quantitative 3DE analysis of aortic valve morphology.

Keywords: Medial axis representation · Deformable modeling · Aortic valve · 3D echocardiography

1   Introduction

Echocardiography is the most commonly used imaging modality for heart valve assessment and has a prominent role in valve diagnostics and surgical planning. Heart valve segmentation in echocardiographic data, particularly 3D echocardiographic (3DE) images, is a means of extracting visual and quantitative information about valve morphology. However, image segmentation in this context is particularly challenging due to the signal dropouts and noise that are characteristic of this imaging modality, as well as the fact that many clinically relevant valve landmarks are defined geometrically rather than by distinctive image intensity characteristics. For example,

© Springer International Publishing Switzerland 2015
O. Camara et al. (Eds.): STACOM 2014, LNCS 8896, pp. 196–203, 2015.
DOI: 10.1007/978-3-319-14678-2_20

several components of the aortic valve complex, such as the sinotubular junction (STJ), the commissures, and the basal attachments of the aortic cusps, are identified anatomically rather than by characteristic image intensity patterns.

Deformable modeling methods are well suited for tasks like shape-guided heart valve segmentation in 3DE images. These methods capture the geometry of an image region by deforming parametric surfaces under the influence of external data-driven forces and internal regularization forces. Shape constraints imposed on the deformable model can fill in areas of intensity inhomogeneity or establish boundaries between anatomical components that are not demarcated by image gradients. Once a parametric model of the valve is obtained, it can be interactively visualized, quantitatively analyzed, and statistically compared to other valve geometries.

Several deformable modeling methods for heart valve segmentation in 3DE images have been proposed. Ionasec et al developed a fully automatic technique for segmenting the aortic and mitral valves in 3DE images [1]. Given a database of manually landmarked images, machine learning algorithms globally locate and track several valve landmarks throughout the cardiac cycle. A spline model fitted through these points with the aid of learned boundary detectors represents valve geometry. In other work [2,3], the mitral and aortic leaflets are represented with a deformable model known as a continuous medial representation (cm-rep), which explicitly parameterizes the leaflets' medial axis (or morphological skeleton) [4]. The latter representation is volumetric; it defines the structure as one with locally varying thickness. One advantage of employing a geometrical model that explicitly defines thickness is that leaflet thickness is an important tissue parameter in biomechanical valve simulation [5].

While cm-rep has been effectively used to describe mitral and aortic leaflet morphology in 3DE images, applying it to the entire aortic valve complex (including the sinuses of Valsava) is challenging. The heart valve leaflets themselves can be described in terms of a single non-branching medial manifold. However, the entire aortic valve complex has a branching medial representation, in which the basal attachments of the aortic cusps are seams that join the medial manifolds of the cusps and sinuses. The cm-rep methodology described in [4] has the limitation that medial axes are difficult to explicitly parameterize along curves at which medial surfaces meet. Attempts to do so have been relatively ad hoc [6,7] and do not strictly adhere to the medial axis definition originally proposed in [8].

To overcome the challenge of modeling structures with branching medial topologies, a new boundary-centric deformable medial modeling paradigm has been proposed [9]. Rather than explicitly parameterizing a structure's medial axis and determining its boundary algorithmically as in [4], the new paradigm explicitly describes the model's boundary and implicitly maintains medial axis topology by imposing geometric constraints on the boundary of the model as it deforms. Since these constraints are nearly identical at the interior of the medial axis and along branch curves, the framework supports medial modeling of structures with branching medial axes while adhering to the medial axis definition in [8]. To date, the feasibility of modeling branching structures with this boundary-centric paradigm has only been demonstrated with a toy example and has not yet been translated to any real-world applications. The contribution of the present work is to leverage this paradigm for visual, quantitative, and statistical shape analysis of the aortic valve in 3DE images. This work conceptually demonstrates that deformable medial modeling is not limited to anatomical structures with simple shape; it is potentially applicable to a wider range of clinical problems that involve anatomical structures with complex geometries.

2   Materials and Methods

2.1   Background on Medial Axis Representation

Medial axis representation, which describes an object's geometry in terms of its morphological skeleton [8], combines the attractive features of boundary and region-based shape representations by defining a continuous relationship between the structure's boundary and interior. Suppose an object represented by the set $S \subset \mathbb{R}^N$ has a smooth boundary ∂S. The medial axis transform (MAT) of S is a mapping between points on ∂S and points on the object's interior that are centers of the maximally inscribed balls (MIBs) of S. An MIB is defined as a ball B inscribed in S that satisfies the condition that there exists no other ball $B' \subset S$ such that $B \subset B'$. Note that in 3D the centers of the MIBs define a continuous surface, i.e. a medial manifold. Multiple medial manifolds join at seams, which are curves in 3D.

In the deformable medial modeling framework originally proposed in [4], a 3D cm-rep is a discretized model of an object's continuous medial axis comprising one or more medial manifolds. Object thickness is parametrically represented as a scalar field defined over the medial manifold(s). The deformable medial model is defined by tuples of values $\{\mathbf{m}, R\}$, where $\mathbf{m}$ refers to the 3D coordinates of points on the medial manifold(s) and R is the radial thickness associated with $\mathbf{m}$, or equivalently the distance between $\mathbf{m}$ and the closest point on ∂S. During model deformation, the values $\{\mathbf{m}, R\}$ are updated to capture the medial geometry of the target object, and the model's boundary is derived analytically by inverting the MAT. Model deformation is an optimization problem that maximizes the overlap of the cm-rep with an image region. Constraints that ensure valid medial geometry are enforced as soft penalties in the objective function.

Alternatively, in the constrained boundary-centric deformable medial modeling framework proposed in [9], ∂S is explicitly parameterized and the MAT of S is encoded by grouping tuples of points on ∂S using "medial links". For example, two boundary points $\mathbf{x}_1, \mathbf{x}_2 \in \partial S$ are defined as being medially linked if they are both members of the same MIB in S. Note that MIBs may be associated with one, two, or three medially linked boundary points depending on their position along the medial axis (Fig. 1a). *This boundary-centric approach to medial representation leverages the fact that transformations of S that preserve medial links also preserve the branching structure of the medial axis.* The following are the sufficient conditions for a transformation to preserve medial links. A ball with center $\mathbf{m} \in S$ and radius R is tangent to ∂S at a point $\mathbf{x}$ if and only if $\mathbf{m} = \mathbf{x} - R\mathbf{N}$, where $\mathbf{N}$ is the outward unit normal to ∂S at $\mathbf{x}$. Such a ball is an MIB in S if $\forall \mathbf{y} \in \partial S, ||\mathbf{y} - \mathbf{m}|| \geq R$. This observation leads to the condition that two points $\mathbf{x}_1, \mathbf{x}_2 \in \partial S$ are medially linked if and only if there exists $R > 0$ such that $\mathbf{x}_1 - R\mathbf{N}_1 = \mathbf{x}_2 - R\mathbf{N}_2$ and $||\mathbf{y} - (\mathbf{x}_1 - R\mathbf{N}_1)|| > R$ for all $\mathbf{y} \in \partial S$. In [9], constrained optimization is used to ensure that these conditions are satisfied during model deformation. Additional hard constraints are used to enforce geometric quality on the discretization of ∂S during deformation. Since the constraints are nearly the same on the interior of the medial axis as they are along branch curves, this latter approach to deformable medial modeling circumvents the challenge of explicitly parameterizing the medial axis at branch curves.

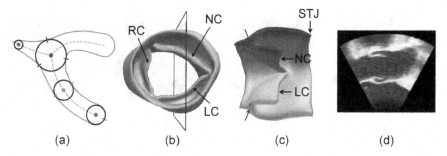

Fig. 1. (a) Diagram of 2D medial geometry showing an object's boundary (gray), medial axis (dashed green curves), and several MIBs (black circles). Centers of MIBs (red, pink, blue) are associated with one, two, or three linked boundary points (marked by colored lines) depending on their location along the medial axis. The blue point is a branch point in the medial axis. Note that this diagram is 2D for illustrative purposes only; model fitting is performed entirely in 3D. (b) Model of the aortic root and cusps viewed from the ascending aorta. (c) Deformable model of the aortic valve apparatus, clipped with respect to the red reference rectangle in (b). The model's medial manifolds are green and boundary is gray. Blue arrows point to branch points where the medial manifolds of the cusps and sinuses meet. (d) Slice of the original 3D image oriented with respect to the red reference rectangle in (b). (RC = right coronary cusp, LC = left coronary cusp, NC = non-coronary cusp).

2.2   Medial Modeling of the Aortic Valve Complex

The aortic valve apparatus is an anatomic structure with a branching medial axis, meaning that the medial axis consists of several surfaces that meet at curves, referred to as seams. Our delineation of the aortic valve extends from the outflow of the left ventricle to the STJ and includes the bulbous aortic sinuses and three cusps (Fig. 1b-c). The aortic root is modeled as a tubular shape to which three fin-like structures (the aortic cusps) are attached. The semilunar attachments of the cusps are seams in the medial axis. Free edges occur at the level of the left ventricular outflow and STJ, as well as the cusps' free margins.

Deformable modeling requires a pre-defined model, or template, of the anatomic structure of interest. Template generation involves manual interaction, but the deformable model is generated only once and thereafter is used to segment new instances of the target structure. To obtain a medial model of the aortic valve complex, the 3D Voronoi skeleton of a manually segmented valve is first generated (Fig. 2a-b). Then a triangulated mesh is created with an interactive tool that allows the user to select and triangulate points on the object's skeleton. The result is a coarse representation of the aortic valve's medial axis, shown in Fig. 2c. To obtain a boundary mesh from the skeleton, a duplicate of the medial mesh is created and the two copies of the mesh are "inflated" to give the aortic root walls and cusps finite thickness (Fig. 2d). Connectivity and vertex modifications are made to ensure proper medial linkage. Medial links are encoded on the boundary mesh by assigning each vertex i a medial link index $M_i \in \mathbb{N}$. Any two mesh vertices i, j that satisfy $M_i = M_j$ are considered medially linked, meaning that they are members of the same MIB. Boundary vertices may be medially linked to two, three, or no other boundary vertices depending on where the MIB is located on the medial axis (on the interior, along a seam, or on an edge).

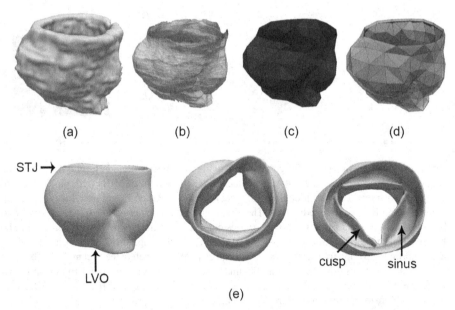

Fig. 2. The boundary template generation process. (a) Manual segmentation of the aortic valve complex viewed from the side. (b) Voronoi skeleton of the manual segmentation. (c) Triangulated mesh of the medial axis. (d) Boundary mesh (translucent) generated from the medial mesh (red). (e) Three views of the final template from a side (left), ventricular (center), and aortic (right) perspective. (LVO = left ventricular outflow).

Multi-atlas Segmentation. To guide model fitting to a target 3DE image, a preliminary segmentation of the aortic valve apparatus is obtained by multi-atlas label fusion. Briefly, a collection of atlases (3DE images and labels for the aortic valve components) is registered to a target image, first with a landmark-guided affine transformation and then diffeomorphic deformable registration. The candidate segmentations generated by each atlas are fused to create a consensus segmentation using the weighted voting method detailed in [10]. Five manually identified landmarks are used for registration initialization: three aortic commissures and two points marking the centers of the outflow tract at the level of left ventricle and the STJ. The reference atlas set is described in Section 2.3.

Model Fitting. In [9], the fitting of a medially constrained parametric boundary model to a target image is implemented as an iterative closest point (ICP) surface-matching problem. Since ICP is sensitive to initialization, deformable registration between the template in Fig. 2 and the multi-atlas segmentation of the target image is first performed to initialize the template prior to ICP surface matching. Then during ICP surface matching, the objective function of the constrained optimization function incorporates both the dissimilarity between the deforming model and target multi-atlas segmentation, as well as irregularity of the deforming mesh. The constraints include the inequalities described in Section 2.1 that preserve medial linkages, as well as mesh quality constraints. The variables in the optimization problem are the boundary vertex coordinates, as well as additional "helper" variables (such as the unit normal vector to each boundary vertex) introduced in order to make the constraints quadratic. Optimization is performed using the Ipopt method [11].

2.3   Dataset and Segmentation Evaluation

Automated segmentation of the aortic valve apparatus was evaluated in a leave-one-out cross-validation on a set of transesophageal 3DE images obtained from 11 human subjects with normal aortic valve morphology. These subjects underwent cardiac surgery for reasons unrelated to the aortic valve. The images were acquired pre-operatively with the iE33 platform (Philips Medical Systems, Andover, MA) using a 2 to 7 MHz matrix-array transducer. For each subject, a 3DE image of the aortic valve at mid systole was selected for analysis. The images were exported with an approximate size of 224 x 208 x 208 voxels with nearly isotropic resolution of 0.4 to 0.8 mm. To evaluate segmentation accuracy, each 3DE dataset was segmented using the other 10 datasets as reference atlases for multi-atlas segmentation. The automated and manual segmentations were compared based on symmetric mean boundary displacement.

3   Results

The original boundary mesh of the aortic valve complex had 433 vertices and 866 triangles. Fig. 3 illustrates a representative deformable model of the aortic valve (fitted to the results of multi-atlas segmentation) overlaid on the corresponding manual segmentation.

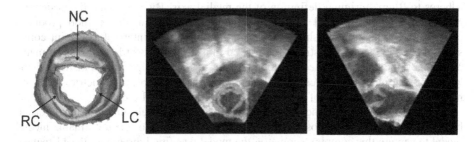

Fig. 3. (Left) Fitted model of the aortic valve complex (gray) overlaid on the manual segmentation (red) as viewed from the ascending aorta. (Right) Cross-sections of the 3DE image of the aortic valve with the manual segmentation in red and the model fitting in green. Overlap of the manual and automated segmentations is shown in blue. (RC = right coronary cusp, NC = noncoronary cusp, LC = left coronary cusp).

The mean boundary displacement (MBD) between the manual segmentations and the deformable model fitted to the results of multi-atlas segmentation was 0.6 ± 0.1 mm. The MBD and the mean difference in the radial thickness are shown in color on a mean model of the aortic valve in Fig. 4. For reference, the MBD between the manual segmentations and the deformable models fitted directly to the manual segmentations was 0.4 ± 0.03 mm, and the MBD between the manual and multi-atlas segmentations without any model fitting was 0.6 ± 0.1 mm.

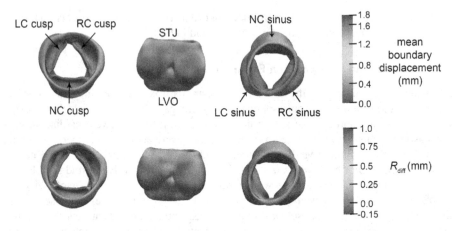

Fig. 4. Mean boundary displacement (top row) and mean difference in radial thickness (R_{diff}, bottom row) are displayed in color on a mean model of the aortic valve complex. The valve is shown from three viewpoints: aortic (left), side (center), and ventricular (right) perspectives. (LC = left coronary, NC = non-coronary, RC = right coronary, STJ = sinotubular junction, LVO = left ventricular outflow).

4   Discussion

This study is the first to demonstrate that deformable medial modeling can effectively represent an anatomical structure with a branching medial topology in a way that adheres to Blum's original definition of the medial axis. By preserving the branching configuration of the medial axis during model deformation, the method produces patient-specific anatomical shape representations that have inter-subject point correspondences and can be statistically compared in a straightforward manner. The method extends the utility of medial modeling for medical image and statistical shape analysis since many structures in the human body have complex geometries that cannot be represented in terms of a non-branching morphological skeleton.

The aortic valve has a branching medial geometry that is well suited for the deformable modeling paradigm proposed in [9]. To assess the ability of the deformable medial model to capture this complex geometry, the model was fitted directly to the 11 manual segmentations and the MBD was computed. The resulting MBD of 0.4 ± 0.03 mm demonstrates that the medial model can indeed capture the shape of the aortic valve apparatus. The MBD between the manual segmentation and the medial models fitted to the results of multi-atlas segmentation (0.6 ± 0.1 mm) was on the order of one voxel. The similarity of the multi-atlas and manual segmentations (without model fitting) was nearly identical, suggesting that improvements in multi-atlas segmentation could enhance the accuracy of deformable medial modeling. The advantage of a medial representation over the multi-atlas segmentation alone is that the model identifies landmarks and facilitates statistical comparison of shape features such as thickness.

The manual versus automatic segmentation comparison in this study is on par with one of few studies on automatic aortic valve segmentation in 3DE images, wherein the authors report an MBD of 1.54 ± 1.17 mm [1]. As shown in Fig. 4, the localized MBD is uniformly low across most of the sinus segments and cusps, with the largest error occurring at the STJ. This localized error is not surprising, since the STJ is an anatomical boundary rather than an intensity-based boundary in the 3DE image. While this study is a proof of concept of the branching medial modeling framework proposed in [9], future work will focus on the clinical application of medial modeling of the aortic valve apparatus, including image segmentation of pathological cases and of the valve at multiple time points in the cardiac cycle.

Acknowledgement. This work was supported by the National Institutes of Health: HL119010, HL103723, and EB014346.

References

1. Ionasec, R.I., Voigt, I., Georgescu, B., Wang, Y., Houle, H., Vega-Higuera, F., Navab, N., Comaniciu, D.: Patient-specific modeling and quantification of the aortic and mitral valves from 4-D cardiac CT and TEE. IEEE Trans. Med. Imaging **29**, 1636–1651 (2010)
2. Pouch, A.M., Wang, H., Takabe, M., Jackson, B.M., Gorman III, J.H., Gorman, R.C., Yushkevich, P.A., Sehgal, C.M.: Fully Automatic Segmentation of the Mitral Leaflets Using Multi-Atlas Label Fusion and Deformable Medial Modeling. Med. Image Anal. **18**(1), 118–129 (2014)
3. Pouch, A.M., Wang, H., Takabe, M., Jackson, B.M., Sehgal, C.M., Gorman III, J.H., Gorman, R.C., Yushkevich, P.A.: Automated segmentation and geometrical modeling of the tricuspid aortic valve in 3D echocardiographic images. In: Mori, K., Sakuma, I., Sato, Y., Barillot, C., Navab, N. (eds.) MICCAI 2013, Part I. LNCS, vol. 8149, pp. 485–492. Springer, Heidelberg (2013)
4. Yushkevich, P.A., Zhang, H., Gee, J.C.: Continuous Medial Representation for Anatomical Structures. IEEE Trans. Med. Imaging **25**(12), 1547–1564 (2006)
5. Rausch, M.K., Famaey, N., Shultz, T.O., Bothe, W., Miller, D.C., Kuhl, E.: Mechanics of the Mitral Valve: A Critical Review, An In Vivo Parameter Identification, and the Effect of Prestrain. Biomech Model Mechanobiol **12**(5), 1053–1071 (2013)
6. Pizer, S.M., Fritsch, D.S., Yushkevich, P.A., Johnson, V.E., Chaney, E.L.: Segmentation, Registration, and Measurement of Shape Variation via Image Object Shape. IEEE Trans. Med. Imaging **18**(1), 851–865 (1999)
7. Sun, H., Frangi, A.F., Wang, H., Sukno, F.M., Tobon-Gomez, C., Yushkevich, P.A.: Automatic cardiac MRI segmentation using a biventricular deformable medial model. In: Jiang, T., Navab, N., Pluim, J.P.W., Viergever, M.A. (eds.) MICCAI 2010, Part I. LNCS, vol. 6361, pp. 468–475. Springer, Heidelberg (2010)
8. Blum, H.: A transformation for extracting new descriptors of shape. In: Wathen-Dunn, W. (ed.) Models for the Perception of Speech and Visual Form, pp. 362–380. MIT Press, Cambridge (1967)
9. Yushkevich, P.A., Zhang, H.G.: Deformable modeling using a 3D boundary representation with quadratic constraints on the branching structure of the blum skeleton. In: Gee, J.C., Joshi, S., Pohl, K.M., Wells, W.M., Zöllei, L. (eds.) IPMI 2013. LNCS, vol. 7917, pp. 280–291. Springer, Heidelberg (2013)
10. Wang, H., Suh, J.W., Das, S., Pluta, J., Craige, C., Yushkevich, P.: Multi-Atlas Segmentation with Joint Label Fusion. IEEE Trans. Pattern Anal. Mach. Intell. **35**(3), 611–623 (2013)
11. Wächter, A., Biegler, L.T.: On the Implementation of an Interior-Point Filter Line-Search Algorithm for Large-Scale Nonlinear Programming. Mathematical Programming **106**, 25–57 (2006)

Estimation of Regional Electrical Properties of the Heart from 12-Lead ECG and Images

Philipp Seegerer[1,2], Tommaso Mansi[1(✉)], Marie-Pierre Jolly[1],
Dominik Neumann[1,2], Bogdan Georgescu[1], Ali Kamen[1], Elham Kayvanpour[3],
Ali Amr[3], Farbod Sedaghat-Hamedani[3], Jan Haas[3], Hugo Katus[3],
Benjamin Meder[3], and Dorin Comaniciu[1]

[1] Imaging and Computer Vision, Siemens Corporate Technology, Princeton, NJ, USA
Tommaso.mansi@siemens.com
[2] Pattern Recognition Lab, FAU Erlangen-Nürnberg, Erlangen, Germany
[3] Department of Internal Medicine III, University Hospital Heidelberg,
Heidelberg, Germany

Abstract. Computational models of cardiac electrophysiology are being investigated for improved patient selection and planning of therapies like cardiac resynchronization therapy (CRT). However, their clinical applicability is limited unless their parameters are fitted to the physiology of an individual patient. In this paper, a method that estimates spatially-varying electrical diffusivities from routine ECG data and dynamic cardiac images is presented. Contrary to current methods based on invasive electrophysiology studies or body surface potential mapping, our approach relies on widely available 12-lead ECG and motion information obtained from clinical images. First, a map of mechanical activation time is derived from a cardiac strain map. Then, regional electrical diffusivities are personalized such that the computed cardiac depolarization matches both the mechanical activation map and measured ECG features. The fit between measured and computed electrocardiography data after model personalization is evaluated on 14 dilated cardiomyopathy patients, exhibiting low mean errors in terms of the diagnostic ECG features QRS duration (0.1 ms) and electrical axis (10.6°). The proposed regional approach outperforms global personalization when 12-lead ECG is the only electrophysiology data available. Furthermore, promising results of a preliminary CRT study on one patient demonstrate the predictive power of the personalized model.

1 Introduction

Heart failure (HF) is a major cause of death in the western world (4-year survival rate of 50% [1]). Approximately 25% of HF patients are affected by a left bundle branch block, an obstruction in the cardiac conduction pathway, which decreases the speed of the electrical wave in the left ventricle [2]. Irregular mechanical activation of the myocardium is among its consequences. For patients with a prolonged QRS complex (QRS $\geq$ 120 ms) and low left ventricular ejection fraction, cardiac resynchronization therapy (CRT) is a well-established

© Springer International Publishing Switzerland 2015
O. Camara et al. (Eds.): STACOM 2014, LNCS 8896, pp. 204–212, 2015.
DOI: 10.1007/978-3-319-14678-2_21

treatment [3]. CRT consists in implanting electrodes into the heart to pace the myocardium artificially and "resynchronize" cardiac contraction. However, 25-30% of patients do not respond to CRT. Hence, more adequate patient selection and therapy planning is required [3]. Combining medical imaging with computational modeling of the heart could provide new tools towards this goal.

To that end, computational models of cardiac electrophysiology (EP) are being investigated. Recent developments enable fast EP computation when coupled with phenomenological models of the cardiac action potential [4,5]. However, model personalization, i. e. adjusting model parameters so that the model output fits clinical data of an individual patient, is a *sine qua non* for clinical applicability. Comprehensive and spatially-dense EP information can be gathered by invasive endocardial mapping or body surface potential mapping [6,7]. However, these measurements are often not available for diagnosis or disease monitoring purposes. Therefore, methods of personalizing EP models from routinely acquired 12-lead ECG have been proposed recently [8]. Due to the sparsity of the data, these approaches focus on the estimation of global parameters (one diffusion value per ventricle). As a consequence, complex pathologies like localized bundle branch blocks cannot be captured precisely.

Evidence is growing that irregularities in mechanical activation are related to abnormal electrical activation [9] and that indicators derived from such irregularities may be predictive for CRT outcome [10]. In order to measure mechanical activation, methods for quantifying myocardial strain from magnetic resonance images (MRI) have been developed [11]. The basic concept is to track the myocardium over time and compute the strain tensor from the estimated deformation field. This information can be used to estimate electrical activation patterns non-invasively [12].

In this paper, a method that estimates spatially-varying electrical diffusivity from ECG and strain maps is presented. While ECG provides global information of cardiac electrophysiology, strain maps are used to identify regional abnormalities. Mechanical myocardial activation is computed to identify the location of a block in the conduction system. Then, electrical diffusivity is estimated such that calculated ECG features match the measurements while the electrical depolarization pattern respects the block. The method is evaluated on 14 dilated cardiomyopathy patients, showing a significant improvement over global fitting in terms of goodness of fit between measured and simulated ECG features. Furthermore, the predictive power of the model is evaluated on one patient who underwent CRT, where better prediction accuracy is observed when using the proposed regional personalization compared to the global method.

2   Method

The workflow of our method is illustrated in Fig. 1. A mechanical activation map of the left ventricular myocardium is derived from Cine MRI, from which a line of block is localized (Sec. 2.1). The images are further used to create an anatomical heart model. Cardiac EP is calculated and the electrical potential propagated to

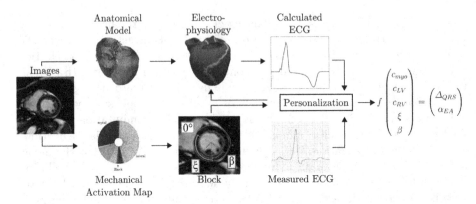

Fig. 1. Workflow of proposed cardiac electrophysiology personalization framework

the torso, where 12-lead ECG tracing is derived (Sec. 2.2). Eventually, the model parameters are personalized within a non-linear inverse optimization framework using clinically measured ECG data and the block information (Sec. 2.3).

2.1 Computation of Mechanical Activation Time

Mechanical activation time maps of the left ventricle (LV) are computed from short axis Cine MRI in four steps: *i)* left ventricular myocardium segmentation, *ii)* 2-D, slice-based myocardium tracking, *iii)* strain computation and *iv)* mechanical activation map calculation, as described below.

Myocardium Segmentation. The LV volume is automatically segmented on the 2-D slices using a 2-D+time algorithm [13]. First, the LV blood pool is automatically localized using temporal Fourier transform and isoperimetric clustering to find the most compact and circular bright moving object in the slices. Then, the myocardium boundaries are extracted using a shortest path algorithm in polar space. Temporal consistency is enforced by the backward and forward fields of an inverse consistent deformable registration. For each slice, all frames are registered to a reference frame at end-diastole. Contour sets are generated by successively segmenting each frame and propagating the contours to all the other frames. The best contour set is chosen as the final segmentation.

Myocardium Tracking. Deformable image registration is performed using an inverse consistent diffeomorphic algorithm [14]. The registration computes a dense deformation field between any two frames in a slice without having to register every possible pair of frames explicitly. To that end, the inverse consistency of the registration is exploited. The deformation field between frames f_j and f_k is obtained by compounding the deformation field between frame f_k and f_1 at end-diastole and the inverse deformation field between frames f_j and f_1. All frames f_i are registered to f_1 yielding the deformation fields Φ_i.

Strain Computation. The Lagrangian strain tensor E is derived from Φ_i according to $E = 1/2(\nabla\Phi_i + \nabla\Phi_i^T + \nabla\Phi_i\nabla\Phi_i^T)$. Computing the norm of the principal strain (eigenvectors of E) with the largest eigenvalue for every myocardium pixel in every frame yields a spatially and temporally resolved map of LV strain. Basal and apical slices are excluded from the subsequent analysis due to insufficient image quality.

Mechanical Activation Map. Afterwards, a polar map of mechanical activation is computed from the strain maps. More precisely, the LV is represented as a circle divided into 120 circumferential segments (Fig. 3, right panel). For each segment the strain is averaged across the myocardium. A polar strain map is computed for each time frame. Then, the time to peak of principal strain is identified per segment as the time of mechanical activation. Finally, median filtering is applied to remove outliers due to noise.

In a subject without block in the conduction system, the mechanical activation propagates uniformly from the septum to the lateral wall, i.e. the latest activated segment is at the lateral wall. However, if there is a block in the conduction system, the latest activated segment is shifted towards the septum, i.e. the myocardium does not contract uniformly. As shown in Fig. 1 ("Block"), the position of the line of block in the myocardium is described by an circumferential angle ξ (with respect to the long axis of the heart). The extent of the block is defined by an angle β. A voxel is considered to be inside the block if its circumferential angle is in a certain range Ω around ξ. In our experiments, we set $\Omega = [\xi - 0.5\beta; \xi + 0.5\beta]$.

2.2 Forward Model of Cardiac Electrophysiology

A fast cardiac electrophysiology model based on the lattice Boltzmann method is employed [4]. First, the heart is segmented automatically from MRI images by a data-guided machine learning algorithm [15]. A rule-based model of myocardial fiber architecture (fiber angles vary linearly from epi- to endocardium: from -40° to 65° [16]) is calculated in order to take anisotropy into account. This can be advanced without any modification by using fiber atlases (a sensitivity analysis is ongoing). Trans-membrane potentials are calculated according to the Mitchell-Schaeffer model [17], which is solved efficiently using the LBM-EP method [4].

The conduction velocity is governed by electrical diffusion parameters. Three domains with different diffusivities c are considered in the model, as pictured in Fig. 2: the slow-conducting myocardium (c_{myo}) and the fast-conducting left and right ventricular endocardia (c_{LV} and c_{RV}). Afterwards, the potentials are mapped to a torso atlas using the boundary element method [4], and the 12-lead ECG is calculated. Therefrom, important clinical ECG features, namely the duration of the QRS complex Δ_{QRS} and the electrical axis α_{EA}, are derived automatically.

Algorithm 1. Regional EP Personalization

Require: Initial diffusivity $c_{myo}^{init}, c_{LV}^{init}, c_{RV}^{init}$ and block parameters ξ^{init}, β^{init}

1: $\kappa^0 = \arg\min_\kappa d_{QRS}\left(\kappa \cdot (c_{myo}^{init}, c_{LV}^{init}, c_{RV}^{init})\right)$

2: $(c_{myo}^0, c_{LV}^0, c_{RV}^0) = \kappa^0 \cdot (c_{myo}^{init}, c_{LV}^{init}, c_{RV}^{init})$

3: **for** $i = 1$ **to** $i = N$ **do**

4:     $(c_{LV}^{i*}, c_{RV}^{i*}, \xi^i) = \arg\min_{c_{LV}, c_{RV}, \xi} (\lambda \cdot d_{QRS}(c_{LV}, c_{RV}, \xi) + d_{EA}(c_{LV}, c_{RV}, \xi))$

5:     $\beta^i = \arg\min_\beta (\lambda \cdot d_{QRS}(\beta) + d_{EA}(\beta))$

6:     $\kappa^i = \arg\min_\kappa d_{QRS}(c_{myo}^{i-1}, c_{LV}^{i*}, c_{RV}^{i*})$

7:     $(c_{myo}^i, c_{LV}^i, c_{RV}^i) = \kappa^i \cdot (c_{myo}^{i-1}, c_{LV}^{i-1}, c_{RV}^{i-1})$

8: **end for**

9: **return** Personalized EP parameters $c_{myo}^N, c_{LV}^N, c_{RV}^N, \xi^N, \beta^N$

2.3 Electrical Diffusivity Estimation

If the mechanical activation map shows an irregular pattern, i.e. the location of the latest contraction is significantly moved towards the septum, a block in the conduction system is considered and defined as a new domain in the EP model. Its position and extent are described by two angles ξ and β (Sec. 2.1). The diffusivity of the endocardial tissue inside the block region is set to the low myocardial diffusivity c_{myo} because the electrical wave propagates over the myocytes if the conduction pathways are obstructed.

The block region enables regional manipulation of the electrical wave propagation by targeted deceleration. The block position is estimated from the mechanical activation maps (Sec. 2.1). Then, the diffusivities c_{myo}, c_{LV} and c_{RV} and the block parameters ξ and β are personalized such that the calculated ECG features match the measurements $\Delta_{QRS,m}$ and $\alpha_{EA,m}$. This is achieved by nonlinear inverse optimization using BOBYQA, a robust gradient-free optimization technique [18]. First, a factor κ for the diffusivities c is optimized, as in [8]. Secondly, c_{LV}, c_{RV} and ξ are optimized. Thereby, ξ is refined inside a range of $\pm 45°$ around the position estimated from the mechanical activation maps to cope with inaccuracies in block localization. The diffusivity of the block region stays equal to c_{myo}. In the next steps, β and κ are optimized. These three steps are iterated (convergence typically after $N = 3$ iterations). The errors of the calculated ECG features are described by $d_{QRS}(\Psi) = (\Delta_{QRS,m} - \Delta_{QRS}(\Psi))^2$ and $d_{EA}(\Psi) = (\alpha_{EA,m} - \alpha_{EA}(\Psi))^2$, where Ψ denotes model input parameters. The weighting factor λ is chosen to cope with distinct units. All optimization steps (arg min) are initialized with the previously estimated parameters. The personalization workflow is sketched in Algorithm 1.

3 Experiment and Results

Experimental Setup. For experimentation, 14 dilated cardiomyopathy (DCM) patients who showed irregular contraction patterns in the estimated mechanical activation maps were selected. Tracked myocardium contours are presented in

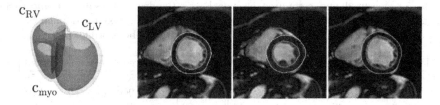

Fig. 2. *Left Panel:* Electrophysiology domains. *Right Panel:* Tracked endo- and epi-cardial contours (left ventricle) over time, showing good agreement to the image data.

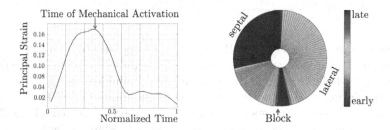

Fig. 3. *Left panel*: Principal strain of an example segment over time. The time of the peak is assumed to signify mechanical activation. *Right panel*: Polar map of mechanical activation (LV) with irregular contraction pattern and identified block location.

Fig. 2, right panel. The temporal changes in principal strain of an example sector of one patient are shown in Fig. 3, left panel. Fig. 3, right panel illustrates the mechanical activation map computed from the Cine MRI for a patient with block in the conduction system.

Personalization Performance. EP model personalization with the proposed regional approach was compared against a global state-of-the-art method that relies on 12-lead ECG only, similar as in [8]. The proposed approach differs from the global method only by the incorporation of the block (Algorithm 1, Lines 4 and 5). The output of the personalized models was compared to clinical measurements. Clinically plausible acceptance ranges were defined for both ECG features: $\varepsilon_{QRS} < 10$ ms and $\varepsilon_{EA} < 20°$. Both approaches captured Δ_{QRS} well with maximum errors of less than 1 ms. The average error of our method for α_{EA} was $10.6° \pm 20.0°$, which is well within the acceptance range. Using the global method, the average error was about twice as large: $21.9° \pm 33.8°$. In Tab. 1, the computed α_{EA} of both methods are compared to the measurements for each individual patient. According to the acceptance criteria defined above, α_{EA} was matched for 11 patients using our regional approach and only for 10 patients using the global approach. As a conclusion, the proposed regional approach can significantly improve EP model personalization over state-of-the-art global methods in terms of goodness of fit between measured and simulated ECG features.

Table 1. Measured and computed electrical axis (in degrees) using our approach ("Regional") and a state-of-the-art approach ("Global"), see text for details. Values that are outside of the acceptance ranges are highlighted in bold print.

Patient	Measured	Regional	Global	Patient	Measured	Regional	Global
1	-99	**-63**	-99	8	57	57	56
2	-3	-6	-3	9	90	89	**-172**
3	-40	-42	-40	10	-17	**22**	**24**
4	112	112	112	11	21	21	19
5	-15	-15	-15	12	45	45	26
6	32	**-31**	**-39**	13	60	60	**-9**
7	-12	-12	-12	14	-12	-16	-16

Predictive Power. After fitting the model to preoperative data using the proposed regional approach on the one hand, and the global approach on the other hand, CRT lead placement and programming were mimicked *in silico* for an LV and an RV pacing scenario on the employed model in order to evaluate its predictive power. The experiments were conducted on one CRT patient (Patient 14, Tab. 1), for whom pre- and postoperative ECG data were available. The outcome was compared to the postoperative measurements ($\Delta_{QRS,post}, \alpha_{EA,post}$): (149 ms, $-13°$) and (176 ms, $-40°$) for LV and RV pacing, respectively. Results show that while QRS prediction performs similarly well for both personalization methods and both pacing scenarios, for LV pacing the regional method (147 ms, $-25°$) predicted the change in electrical axis better, meeting the defined acceptance criteria, while the global method (149 ms, $-54°$) failed. RV pacing predictions were similar for both personalized models, as only the left ventricle is affected by the block estimation with little impact in RV pacing scenarios. The regional method predicted (177 ms, $-52°$) and the global method (175 ms, $-50°$), both well within the defined acceptance ranges. This preliminary CRT study suggests that our personalization framework could improve the ability of the model to predict CRT outcomes, which is an important result towards clinical applicability of computational cardiac models.

4   Discussion and Conclusion

This work presents a novel method to estimate regional electrical diffusivity from dynamic cardiac images and 12-lead ECG. The underlying assumption is that abnormalities in mechanical activation time are related to conduction system failure. Thus, we incorporated that knowledge in a gradient-free estimation framework. It can be used with any electrophysiology model or solver. Furthermore, our approach relies on data that is acquired non-invasively and is widely available, in contrast to other state-of-the-art methods. Results on 14 DCM patients showed that our approach achieves promising goodness of fit between measured and calculated ECG features. However, the personalization fails on 3 cases due to mismatched electrical axis. This could be caused by imprecise ECG lead positioning or the presence of complex pathologies which the model is not capable to capture. Hence, the next step will be to include further regionality in the personalization to allow the model to adapt to a larger variety of pathologies. Furthermore, the predictive power of the model will be evaluated more extensively in the future as soon as additional CRT cases are at our disposal. Moreover, fiber architecture can be modeled close to the real physiology once in vivo diffusion tensor imaging (DTI) data are available.

References

1. Dickstein, K., Cohen-Solal, A., Filippatos, G., McMurray, J.J., Ponikowski, P., Poole-Wilson, P.A., Strömberg, A., Veldhuisen, D.J., Atar, D., Hoes, A.W., et al.: Esc guidelines for the diagnosis and treatment of acute and chronic heart failure. European Journal of Heart Failure 10(10), 933–989 (2008)
2. Zannad, F., Huvelle, E., Dickstein, K., Veldhuisen, D.J., Stellbrink, C., Køber, L., Lechat, P.: Left bundle branch block as a risk factor for progression to heart failure. European Journal of Heart Failure (2007)
3. Kass, D.A.: Cardiac resynchronization therapy. Journal of Cardiovascular Electrophysiology 16(s1), 35–41 (2005)
4. Zettinig, O., Mansi, T., Neumann, D., Georgescu, B., Rapaka, S., Seegerer, P., Kayvanpour, E., Sedaghat-Hamedani, F., Amr, A., Haas, J., Steen, H., Katus, H., Meder, B., Navab, N., Kamen, A., Comaniciu, D.: Data-driven estimation of cardiac electrical diffusivity from 12-lead ECG signals. Medical Image Analysis (2014)
5. Talbot, H., Duriez, C., Courtecuisse, H., Relan, J., Sermesant, M., Cotin, S., Delingette, H.: Towards real-time computation of cardiac electrophysiology for training simulator. In: Camara, O., Mansi, T., Pop, M., Rhode, K., Sermesant, M., Young, A. (eds.) STACOM 2012. LNCS, vol. 7746, pp. 298–306. Springer, Heidelberg (2013)
6. Relan, J., Chinchapatnam, P., Sermesant, M., Rhode, K., Ginks, M., Delingette, H., Rinaldi, C.A., Razavi, R., Ayache, N.: Coupled personalization of cardiac electrophysiology models for prediction of ischaemic ventricular tachycardia. Interface Focus 1(3), 396–407 (2011)
7. Dössel, O., Krueger, M.W., Weber, F.M., Wilhelms, M., Seemann, G.: Computational modeling of the human atrial anatomy and electrophysiology. Medical & Biological Engineering & Computing 50(8), 773–799 (2012)
8. Neumann, D., Mansi, T., Grbic, S., Voigt, I., Georgescu, B., Kayvanpour, E., Amr, A., Sedaghat-Hamedani, F., Haas, J., Meder, B., Katus, H., Hornegger, J., Kamen, A., Comaniciu, D.: Automatic image-to-model framework for patient-specific electromechanical modeling of the heart. In: ISBI. IEEE (2014)
9. Risum, N., Strauss, D., Sogaard, P., Loring, Z., Hansen, T.F., Bruun, N.E., Wagner, G., Kisslo, J.: Left bundle-branch block: The relationship between electrocardiogram electrical activation and echocardiography mechanical contraction. American Heart Journal 166(2), 340–348 (2013)
10. Jackson, T., Sohal, M., Chen, Z., Child, N., Sammut, E., Behar, J., Claridge, S., Carr-White, G., Razavi, R., Rinaldi, C.A.: A u-shaped 'type ii' contraction pattern in patients with strict left bundle branch block predicts super-response to cardiac resynchronization therapy. Heart Rhythm (2014)

11. Oubel, E., De Craene, M., Hero, A.O., Pourmorteza, A., Huguet, M., Avegliano, G., Bijnens, B., Frangi, A.F.: Cardiac motion estimation by joint alignment of tagged mri sequences. Medical Image Analysis **16**(1), 339–350 (2012)
12. Prakosa, A., Sermesant, M., Allain, P., Villain, N., Rinaldi, C., Rhode, K., Razavi, R., Delingette, H., Ayache, N.: Cardiac electrophysiological activation pattern estimation from images using a patient-specific database of synthetic image sequences. IEEE Transactions on Biomedical Engineering **61**(2), 235–245 (2014)
13. Jolly, M.P., Guetter, C., Guehring, J.: Cardiac segmentation in mr cine data using inverse consistent deformable registration. In: ISBI, pp. 484–487. IEEE (2010)
14. Guetter, C., Xue, H., Chefd'Hotel, C., Guehring, J.: Efficient symmetric and inverse-consistent deformable registration through interleaved optimization. In: ISBI, pp. 590–593. IEEE (2011)
15. Zheng, Y., Barbu, A., Georgescu, B., Scheuering, M., Comaniciu, D.: Four-chamber heart modeling and automatic segmentation for 3-d cardiac ct volumes using marginal space learning and steerable features. IEEE T-MI **27**(11), 1668–1681 (2008)
16. Lombaert, H., Peyrat, J., Croisille, P., Rapacchi, S., Fanton, L., Cheriet, F., Clarysse, P., Magnin, I., Delingette, H., Ayache, N.: Human atlas of the cardiac fiber architecture: Study on a healthy population. IEEE T-MI **31**(7), 1436–1447 (2012)
17. Mitchell, C.C., Schaeffer, D.G.: A two-current model for the dynamics of cardiac membrane. Bulletin of Mathematical Biology **65**(5), 767–793 (2003)
18. Powell, M.J.: The bobyqa algorithm for bound constrained optimization without derivatives. Cambridge NA Report, University of Cambridge, Cambridge (2009)

Multi-source Motion Decoupling Ablation Catheter Guidance for Electrophysiology Procedures

Mihaela Constantinescu[1]([✉]), Su-Lin Lee[1], Sabine Ernst[2],
and Guang-Zhong Yang[1]

[1] The Hamlyn Centre for Robotic Surgery, Imperial College London, London, UK
mihaela.constantinescu12@imperial.ac.uk
[2] The Royal Brompton and Harefield Hospital, London, UK

Abstract. Accurate and stable positioning of the ablation catheter tip during the delivery of radiofrequency impulses in cardiac electrophysiology remains a challenge due to the endocardium motion from multiple sources (cardiac cycle and respiration) and inevitable slippage of the catheter tip. This paper presents a novel ablation catheter guidance framework during electrophysiology procedures. Catheter tip electrode position readings from intraoperative electroanatomical data are used to decouple tip motion from different motion sources as part of the pre-ablation mapping. The resulting information is then used to determine if there is relative slippage between the catheter tip and endocardial surface and is shown as a probability map for online decision support of the ablation process. The proposed decomposition method and the slippage assessment were performed on a retrospective cohort of 19 patients treated for ventricular tachycardia (13 cases) or atrial fibrillation (6 cases) and were also validated on artificially generated signals.

1 Introduction

Cardiac rhythm disorders are a major cause of sudden death worldwide, with atrial fibrillation and ventricular tachycardia being the most prevalent [1]. Globally, atrial fibrillation alone affects 33.5 million people and its related deaths doubled between 1990 and 2010 [2]; nevertheless, many patients are treated before the condition becomes critical.

One of the treatment options available is the ablation of the sources or paths for ectopic impulses under guidance from the CARTO system (Biosense Webster, Diamond Bar, CA, USA) which gives electroanatomical information from reference and mapping/ablation catheters, triggered at sparse points in the cardiac cycle. However, each patient still requires an average of 1.3 procedures with a 70 % success rate [3], among the causes being the lack of patient-specific dynamic guidance for both the scar development during ablation and the cardiac wall motion at the desired ablation point [4]. The motion of the cardiac wall, as well as the blood flow in the endocardium near the vessel wall, can cause

© Springer International Publishing Switzerland 2015
O. Camara et al. (Eds.): STACOM 2014, LNCS 8896, pp. 213–220, 2015.
DOI: 10.1007/978-3-319-14678-2_22

slippage of the ablation catheter tip which can be over 12 mm in 2.5 s (Fig. 1a), as measured from electroanatomical data used in this work. Such slippage may result in ablation lesions not originally planned by the interventional cardiologist and in repeated procedures for the patient. Although there are certain procedures where sliding along the endocardium is desired during ablation, the present study assumes focused ablation of an endocardial point.

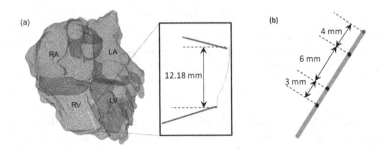

Fig. 1. (a) The cardiac chambers (RA – right atrium, RV – right ventricle, LA – left atrium, LV – left ventricle) with the catheter placed in the RV. Absolute catheter tip motion can be as high as 12 mm. The red catheter shapes indicate the motion range and the green curve is the trajectory of the ablation catheter tip. (b) Spatial distribution of the mapping and ablation (MA) catheter sensor and electrodes.

Several approaches have been investigated to estimate the motion of the catheter tip intraoperatively. Principal Component Analysis (PCA) has been applied on the reference catheter shape vectors extracted from fluoroscopy images [5]. Other image-based approaches proposed include 2D tracking of the interventional reference catheters [6], which was also extended to 3D under epipolar constraints [7]. While these methods are able to track the motion, they depend on X-ray fluoroscopy, whose use is avoided due to radiation exposure.

The respiratory and cardiac motions have also been estimated from 3D electroanatomical mapping datasets. Roujol *et al.* [8] simplified the motion model by removing the two signals from fixed frequency bands after analysing the catheter tip position in the Fourier domain. Another recent approach fitted a model of motion to the catheter tip by instantiating a bilinear atlas of patient-specific shapes and deformations [9]. These methods, however, need a good spread of the recorded points on the endocardium in order for the instantiation to have a small error.

This paper proposes a method for online assessment of ablation catheter tip contact with the endocardium based on recordings of catheter tip position. A probabilistic slippage map of the catheter tip with respect to the endocardium is provided for online guidance of the ablation catheter, allowing the operator to adjust the catheter, should slippage occur. Validation of the proposed method was performed on 19 data sets from patients treated for ventricular tachycardia and atrial fibrillation, as well as on artificially generated mixed signals.

2   Methods

2.1   Data Acquisition

Simulated Data with Known Ground Truth. Artificial data sets of 3D signals with their first order derivatives were generated in order to simulate 29 respiratory frequencies, $(12...40)\,\text{min}^{-1}$, and 96 different starting points of the recording relative to the respiratory cycle length, i.e. 96 different phase shifts, $(0...95)\,\%$. It was assumed that the cardiac and respiratory components follow phase-shifted sine waves with amplitudes of 5 and 20 mm, respectively. A linear drift of 2 mm/s, accounting for a slip of 5 mm in 2.5 s, was added to the 3D signal. No noise was added, as the real signals were smoothed with an average filter in the preprocessing step of the decomposition method.

Patient Studies. For the patient studies, data from a Navistar MA catheter were used (Fig. 1b). The sensor at the tip records the electrocardiogram (ECG) as well as the 3D position. Additionally, the 3D positions of the other four electrodes on the MA catheter and the first order derivatives of all signals were used for motion decoupling. All signals were linearly interpolated to generate 2500 time stamps. The intraoperative data comprised 19 studies from 13 ventricular tachycardia and 6 atrial fibrillation patients, each with a different number of mapping points. The ECG recordings were used to remove the mapping points acquired during arrhythmic episodes, i.e. cardiac period under 600 ms, as it was assumed that the ablation will be performed during episodes of normal heart beat so that the contact with the wall is more easily maintained. The number of normal sinus mapping points per study ranged from 10 to 63.

2.2   Motion Decoupling

Multivariate empirical mode decomposition (MEMD) [11] was used to decouple the three-dimensional position signals of the MA catheter sensor and electrodes. The method sorts the zero-mean components, called intrinsic mode functions (IMF), in descending order of their number of local extrema, which in the case of periodic events, such as cardiac and respiratory displacement, is equivalent to sorting them by the signal frequency (amplitude and frequency modulation of the mixed input signal).

In the original empirical mode decomposition (EMD) [10], the IMFs have a physical meaning in the original mixed EEG signal. Analogously, the component with the least number of local extrema showing the general trend in the signal must have a physical correspondence in the relative slippage. The next in periodicity was identified as the respiration, followed by the cardiac motion. Eq. (1) shows the composition of the mixed signal assumed by the MEMD algorithm, with $\mathbf{x}$, $\mathbf{y}$, and $\mathbf{z}$ being the original signals from the sensor and the four electrodes over 2.5 s, M the number of decomposed IMFs, $\mathbf{a}_{m,k}$ the amplitude value which modulates the oscillation vector $\boldsymbol{\Psi}_m$ of the m-th IMF at time stamp k, and $\mathbf{r}$ the residual trend vector for each channel.

$$\begin{bmatrix} \mathbf{x}_k \\ \mathbf{y}_k \\ \mathbf{z}_k \end{bmatrix} = \sum_{m=1}^{M} \mathbf{a}_{m,k} \boldsymbol{\Psi}_{m,k} + \mathbf{r}_k, \qquad\qquad k = 1..2500 \qquad\qquad (1)$$

The simultaneous decomposition with MEMD as compared to the single-channel EMD ensures not only the same number M of independent IMFs in all channels, but also their alignment in the frequency domain. EMD, the single-channel decomposition method, for a variable x can be summarised in the following steps [10, 12]:

1. Find the local extrema of x.
2. Perform spline interpolation between the local minima and local maxima, respectively, thus generating two envelope signals.
3. Calculate the mean $m(t)$ of the two envelopes.
4. Subtract $m(t)$ from $x(t)$ to obtain a candidate for IMF. $d(t) = x(t) - m(t)$ is an IMF if it has a zero mean and the number of zero crossings and extrema are equal or differ by one.
5. If $d(t)$ does not satisfy these two criteria, $x(t) = d(t)$ and reinitialise the algorithm.
6. If $d(t)$ is a valid IMF, $x(t) = x(t) - d(t)$ and restart the algorithm.
7. Run the algorithm until $x(t)$ (the residual) becomes a monotonic function.

The multivariate extension computes the mean in the multidimensional space by first generating a Hammersley sequence for projecting the 30-dimensional sequence (one sensor and four electrodes, each with three dimensions and their derivatives) onto certain directions. The means are calculated for the projection signals and then subtracted as in the one-dimensional algorithm [11].

2.3   Probabilistic Model

A Dynamic Bayesian Network was used to model the conditional dependency of the ablation catheter tip (Tip) on the cardiac motion (C), respiration (R), and slippage (S), in a probabilistic framework (Fig. 2). In a single step, Tip was the observed variable as measured by the electromagnetic position sensors, while the other variables were extracted using MEMD. $\mathbf{P}$ (S|Tip,C,R) in an intercausal reasoning approach and the interstate dependencies $\mathbf{P}$ (R'|S,R) and $\mathbf{P}$ (C'|S,C) were computed from a Gaussian Mixture Model trained on the slippage and the MA catheter tip position.

3   Results

Simulated Data with Known Ground Truth. Results from the artificial data sets are shown in Fig. 3. Both amplitude and frequency can be recovered in the respiratory signal with an error of under 10 % in the case of a respiratory rate between 12 and 30 min^{-1}, which is the normal respiratory rate in adults. The starting point of the recording interval relative to the respiratory cycle does not influence the recovery. The cardiac signal extraction for these cases yielded a mean amplitude error of 9.33 % and a mean frequency error of 11.73 %.

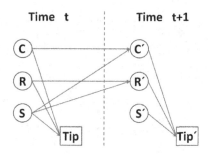

Fig. 2. Conditional dependency of the ablation catheter tip (Tip) on the cardiac motion (C), the respiration (R), and the slippage (S). Squared variables are observed, circled variables are unknowns. $\mathbf{P}$ (S|Tip,C,R) is sought.

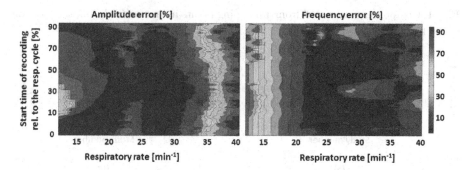

Fig. 3. MEMD respiration recovery using simulated data with known ground truth. The jagged contours indicate that there are some combinations of phase shift and respiratory rate for which the decomposition is either slightly better or worse than the trend.

Patient Studies. MEMD was applied to each sinus mapping point of the 19 studies. Fig. 4 shows the original catheter tip position recording, followed by the relative slippage and the respiratory and cardiac components for each axis and for four different points around a mapped right ventricle. The slippage accounted for the biggest motion of the catheter tip, exhibiting as a constant drift in the least periodic IMF. The second component was the respiratory motion, identified as the IMF next in frequency. Finally, the third factor was classified as the cardiac component due to its periodicity compared to the ECG. The relative error in the estimated heart rate (HR) was assessed (Fig. 5).

A Gaussian Mixture Model was trained on each set of mapping points, giving the conditional dependency $\mathbf{P}$ (S|Tip,C,R) as a normal distribution. Fig. 5 gives an overview of several study-specific values, including the maximum absolute slip in mm and the probability of this maximal relative slip. The heart rate error was higher for faster ECGs, at the arrhythmic border of the 600 ms period. In addition, two other probabilities were computed from the conditional dynamic network, estimating the recovery of the cardiac and respiratory motion after a

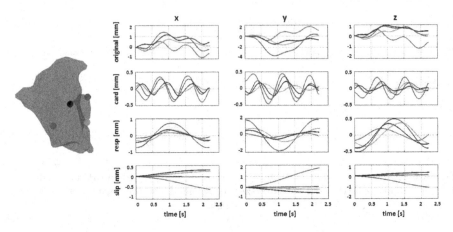

Fig. 4. Components extracted from 4 mapping points in one ventricle and the location of the points within the anatomy

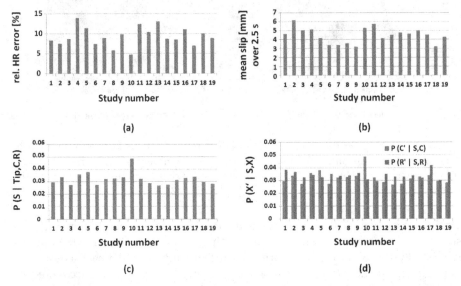

Fig. 5. (a) Relative heart rate error of the recovered cardiac motion compared to ECG, (b) Mean relative tip motion with respect to the endocardium, (c) Probability of slippage given the tip position, the cardiac motion and the respiration, (d) Probabilities of recovering the cardiac and respiratory components after slippage from the old endocardium point with a C-R motion to a new endocardium point C'-R'

slip of the catheter tip to a new endocardial point moving on different cardiac (C') and respiratory (R') waves.

Finally, Fig. 6 shows a visual indication of the probability of slippage at the mapping points in contact with the catheter tip when the electrode position and the cardiac and respiratory components are known. Additionally, the maximal expected slippage is shown. This combined information is able to provide the

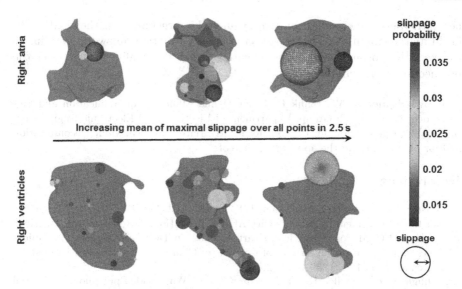

Fig. 6. Example of probabilistic maps of slippage with the radius of the sphere showing the maximum slippage computed over 2.5 s. The sphere is a real-size expectancy of relative slippage which may occur with the probability coded in the colour.

operator with online decision support of the ablation process and may influence the adjustment of the ablation point, force, or the use of robotic catheter stabilisation.

4   Discussion and Conclusion

MEMD provides an initial solution to the source decomposition problem in a simplified scenario of intracardial motion due to its suitability to decouple periodic signals from monotonic drifting trends. However, because of the short acquisition time of 2.5 s for each mapping point, the MEMD algorithm failed to decompose the signal into three clear physiological components when the respiratory sequence was a monotonic function. In this case, the method added the respiratory motion in the observed time interval to the monotonic relative slippage. Out of 517 sinus mapping points analysed with the decomposition method, in 183 cases the respiration could not be decoupled from the relative slippage. The outcome can be potentially improved with respiratory gating or by adding a full-period respiratory sequence as an additional channel to the algorithm.

Nevertheless, the source separation provided a good starting point for the novel probabilistic guidance. With an average of 27 mapping points per study, the trained Gaussian Mixture Model computed a reliable distribution of conditional dependencies. Significant information could be gained from the intercausal inference based on the known cardiac motion and respiration, i.e. $\mathbf{P}\,(S|\text{Tip},C,R)$.

In conclusion, a new method for the assessment of intracardiac ablation catheter motion by incorporating probabilistic estimation of the relative slippage from the moving endocardium was proposed. The method also provides a new intraoperative visualisation tool to guide the surgeon during the ablation, to facilitate the stabilisation of the catheter tip in a robotic framework, and finally to select the optimal ablation point with a lower probability of drift over the planned ablation period.

Acknowledgments. We thank Professor Danilo Mandic, Communication and Signal Processing Research Group, Department of Electrical and Electronic Engineering, Imperial College London, for the code for Multivariate Empirical Mode Decomposition and for his guidance in the application thereof.

References

1. Fuster, V., Ryden, L.E., Cannom, D.S., et al.: ACC/AHA/ESC 2006 Guidelines for the Management of Patients with Atrial Fibrillation: A Report of the American College of Cardiology/American Heart Association Task Force on Practice Guidelines and the European Society of Cardiology Committee for Practice Guidelines. Circulation **114**(7), e257–e354 (2006)
2. Chugh, S., Havmoeller, R., Narayanan, K., et al.: Worldwide Epidemiology of Atrial Fibrillation: A Global Burden of Disease 2010 Study. Circulation **129**, 837–847 (2014)
3. Cappato, R., Calkins, H., Chen, S.A., et al.: Updated worldwide survey on the methods, efficacy, and safety of catheter ablation for human atrial fibrillation. Circulation **3**, 32–38 (2010)
4. Klemm, H., Steven, D., Johnsen, C., et al.: Catheter motion during atrial ablation due to the beating heart and respiration: impact on accuracy and spatial referencing in three-dimensional mapping. Heart Rhythm **4**(5), 587–592 (2007)
5. Panayiotou, M., King, A.P., Ma, Y., et al.: Statistical model of catheter motion from interventional x-ray images: application to image-based gating. Phys. Med. Biol. **58**, 7543–7562 (2013)
6. Brost, A., Liao, R., Hornegger, J., Strobel, N.: Model-based registration for motion compensation during EP ablation procedures. In: Fischer, B., Dawant, B.M., Lorenz, C. (eds.) WBIR 2010. LNCS, vol. 6204, pp. 234–245. Springer, Heidelberg (2010)
7. Ma, Y., Gao, G., Gijsbers, G., Rinaldi, C.A., Gill, J., Razavi, R., Rhode, K.S.: Image-based automatic ablation point tagging system with motion correction for cardiac ablation procedures. In: Taylor, R.H., Yang, G.-Z. (eds.) IPCAI 2011. LNCS, vol. 6689, pp. 145–155. Springer, Heidelberg (2011)
8. Roujol, S., Anter, E., Josephson, M., Nezafat, R.: Characterization of respiratory and cardiac motion from electro-anatomical mapping data for improved fusion of MRI to left ventricular electrograms. PLoS ONE **8**(11), e78852 (2013)
9. Porras, A.R., Piella, G., Berruezo, A., et al.: Interventional endocardial motion estimation from electroanatomical mapping data: application to scar characterization. Transactions on Biomedical Engineering **60**(5), 1217–1224 (2013)
10. Huang, N., Shen, Z., Long, S., et al.: The empirical mode decomposition and the Hilbert spectrum for nonlinear and non-stationary time series analysis. Proc. R. Soc. Lond. **454**, 903–995 (1998)
11. Rehman, N., Mandic, D.P.: Multivariate empirical mode decomposition. Proc. R. Soc. **466**, 1291–1302 (2010)
12. Mandic, D.P., Rehman, N., Wu, Z., Huang, N.: Multivariate empirical mode decomposition. IEEE Signal Processing Magazine, 74–86, November 2013

Statistical Model of Paroxysmal Atrial Fibrillation Catheter Ablation Targets for Pulmonary Vein Isolation

Ahmad Al-Agamy[1], Rashed Karim[2], Aruna Arujuna[2], James L. Harrison[2], Steven E. Williams[2], Kawal S. Rhode[2], and Hans C. van Assen[1(✉)]

[1] Signal Processing Systems, Department of Electrical Engineering, Eindhoven University of Technology, Eindhoven, Netherlands
h.c.v.assen@tue.nl
[2] Division of Imaging Sciences and Biomedical Engineering, King's College London, London, UK

Abstract. Atrial fibrillation (AF) is the most common cardiac arrhythmia. Pulmonary vein isolation (PVI) by catheter ablation is a cornerstone treatment of paroxysmal AF. Low success rates are mainly due to reconnecting tissue. Local myocardial wall-thickness (WT) information is missing; lesion transmurality is impossible to estimate. WT information can be obtained from pencil beam high-resolution MRI, a time-consuming protocol. To reduce scan time, automatic selection of regions of interest is proposed. We developed a left atrial target probability model for paroxysmal AF ablation, based on intraprocedural ablation targeting data of fifteen patients, to support the selection of these regions. A common mesh serves as a reference for registration of the electroanatomical meshes and ablation targets using landmark registration and the Iterative Closest Points algorithm. This is followed by projection of the ablation targets onto the mean mesh model, closure of isolated ablation voids on the surface and Gaussian smoothing of the probability distribution.

The final probability distribution clearly shows PVI contours as suggested in the consensus statement by European associations. The right inferior pulmonary vein (RIPV) shows a lower ablation probability, which may be due to limited maneuverability of the ablation catheter and the proximity of the RIPV ostium and the transseptal puncture, where the catheter enters the left atrium.

Keywords: Atrial fibrillation · Left atrium · Catheter ablation · Pulmonary vein isolation · Statistical modeling

1 Introduction

Atrial fibrillation (AF) is the most common cardiac arrhythmia causing chaotic contraction of the atrium. AF becomes more prevalent with age [1], is frequently associated with atrial remodeling and fibrosis, and causes loss of atrial muscle mass, the severity of which reflects the duration of preexisting AF [2].

© Springer International Publishing Switzerland 2015
O. Camara et al. (Eds.): STACOM 2014, LNCS 8896, pp. 221–230, 2015.
DOI: 10.1007/978-3-319-14678-2_23

AF is classified based on the presentation and duration. Five types can be distinguished [3]. First diagnosed AF refers to patients who are first diagnosed with AF, irrespective of the duration. Paroxysmal AF is self-terminating, usually within 48 hours. Persistent and longstanding persistent AF refer to AF which lasts longer than 7 days and a year respectively. Finally, permanent AF refers to AF the patient has accepted and without pursued rhythm control interventions.

Catheter ablation is considered an established therapeutic alternative to antiarrhythmic medications for paroxysmal and persistent AF patients. Ablation of isolated points or small regions with fractionated potentials has been shown to be effective in both paroxysmal and chronic AF [4]. Since no single ablation technique is optimal for any AF mechanism, many elements of all techniques are often incorporated ad-hoc. However, depending on the type of AF, different lesion sets are devised; paroxysmal AF is commonly treated by pulmonary vein isolation (PVI), the creation of circumferential lesions around the PV ostia [5]. Clinical success rate of PVI at 5-year follow-up as low as 46% for single procedure intervention has been reported, which increases to 79% after at most three interventions [6]. Recovered PV conduction was found in 66 – 94%.

The success rate of PVI is dependent on accurate lesion placement, knowledge about the substrate and local wall-thickness. Intervention guidance systems include atrial anatomical information to improve lesion placement accuracy [7], while knowledge about the substrate can be obtained from fibrosis mapping [8]. Local atrial wall-thickness information is still missing. Therefore, it is impossible to know whether a placed lesion is transmural and electrically contiguous other than by continuing ablation until electrical blockage has been achieved. Whether this blockage is permanent or temporary is hard to tell immediately. Despite efforts to create contiguous transmural lesions, gaps are common [9]. Tissue recovering from *temporal* electrical block causes recurrences. Transient circumferential PVI may be caused by edema and inflammation induced by ablation, *temporarily* closing dormant conduction gaps [6]. Recurrences generally occur due to reconnecting tissue at PV ostia [10].

Motivations for creating an ablation probability model for paroxysmal AF are:

- for use in biophysical modeling of AF to predict likelihood of reconnection and to predict successful ablation strategies;
- to support region of interest (ROI) selection in pencil beam wall thickness imaging with MRI [11];
- to separate fibrotic lesions due to ablation from those due to AF;
- to support patient-specific ablation strategy planning and annotation;
- to study variations in ablation patterns between different centers;
- to drive robot-based ablation [12].

For biophysical modeling of AF knowledge of the local wall-thickness is crucial.

To assess atrial wall-thickness, segmentation of both endo- and epicardial walls are required. Pfeifer et al. proposed a combination of an AAM for blood pool segmentation and a morphological thresholding operation for the epicardium, based on MRI data [13]. Alternatively, an active contour approach was presented based on zoomed CT reconstruction [14]. However, the intrinsic contrast between muscle and fat tissue – which characterizes the epicardial atrial border for a large part – is very weak in CT. Since MRI is known for its superior soft-tissue contrast and the atrial wall thickness may vary between 1 and 4 mm [15,16], a high resolution MRI sequence has been developed recently [11]. Due to pencil beam imaging, this is a time-consuming protocol; therefore only a few smaller regions of interest (ROIs) can be imaged. To support the selection of these ROIs, we propose to build an ablation targeting atlas. Such an atrial surface model indicates where ablation is performed most, based on a database of PVI cases. The most ablated regions indicate the best ROIs to be imaged at high resolution. Furthermore, this model can help in separating fibrotic lesions due to ablation from those due to AF. Finally, strategy planning can benefit from statistical knowledge regarding ablation of similar types of AF.

The rest of this paper is organized as follows. Section 2 introduces the proposed method and implementation details. Section 3 presents the obtained results. The discussion and conclusions are presented in Section 4 together with a brief description of expected future work.

2 Method

The presented model is based only on patients with paroxysmal atrial fibrillation. We used an LA mean model mesh as a common reference for mapping and projecting ablation targets from all study cases. This was achieved using landmark registration (LM) and Iterative Closest Point (ICP) affine transformation [17]. The projected ablation targets were used to calculate target density. Hence, an ablation target probability density function is deduced to model PVI lesion sets, visualized on the LA mean mesh as a color encoded ablation map.

2.1 Left Atrial Mean Model

The left atrial mean model was obtained from an updated version of the whole heart segmentation framework by Peters et al. [18]. This framework includes an anatomical mesh model of the heart, including the four chambers and the trunks of the aorta, pulmonary artery and pulmonary veins. The original segmentation framework comprises a mean mesh and a number of deformation constraints and rules to localize myocardial borders in MRI images. From this whole heart mean mesh the left atrium was extracted to use in our ablation target probability model. The atrial mean mesh consisted of 5265 vertices combined in 10422 triangles. Attached to the atrial mesh are the PV antra, which are approximately

14 mm in length and 12 mm in diameter. It also includes the LA appendage, the length of which is approximately 15 mm from the LA body.

2.2   Landmark Registration and ICP Affine Transformation

The patient-specific LA mesh (originating from an electrical mapping suite) was registered to the mean LA mesh in two stages. In the first stage, landmark registration was employed to obtain an approximate registration. To achieve this, corresponding landmarks were manually selected for the ostium of each pulmonary vein and for the appendage, both on the patient mesh and on the mean LA model. A rigid-body registration was computed minimizing errors between corresponding landmarks in a least squares sense. In the second stage, an Iterative Closest Point (ICP) algorithm [17] was used to match individual vertices of the patient-specific LA shapes and the mean model. In this algorithm, each vertex on one surface is matched to the closest surface point on the other mesh (in a least squares sense) and an affine transformation is applied. This is iterated to get optimal convergence of the two surfaces. Using point correspondences established from landmark and ICP registrations, the ablation targets are then mapped to the LA mesh as follows.

2.3   Ablation Targets Probability Density Function

Mapping Ablation Targets to Patient-Specific and Mean Model Mesh.
In the electroanatomical 3D space, individual ablation targets are transferred to the patient-specific mesh by mapping them to the nearest vertex on this electroanatomical mesh. After landmark registration and ICP, the individual ablation targets defined in the 3D electroanatomical space have been transformed to the LA mean segmentation mesh space. In this stage, each ablation target is mapped to the closest mean mesh vertex, establishing point correspondence between the different patient-specific ablation target sets. After mapping of the ablation targets, those which are displaced by more than 10 mm (twice the ablation catheter tip width) in both mapping stages together have been discarded.

Estimation of Ablation Probability Density. After mapping the ablation target points to the mean mesh, certain vertices have received "votes" from the mapped ablation targets. Due to the inherent uncertainty in the target location both before and after mapping, every vote is copied to each of the neighbors – up the 4th level – of the vote-receiving vertex. The average distance between a vertex in the mean model mesh and its 4th level neighbor is comparable to twice the width of the ablation catheter tip (approx. 10 mm). Subsequently, the number of votes n_i each vertex i has received is converted to a probability p_i by normalizing with the total number of votes.

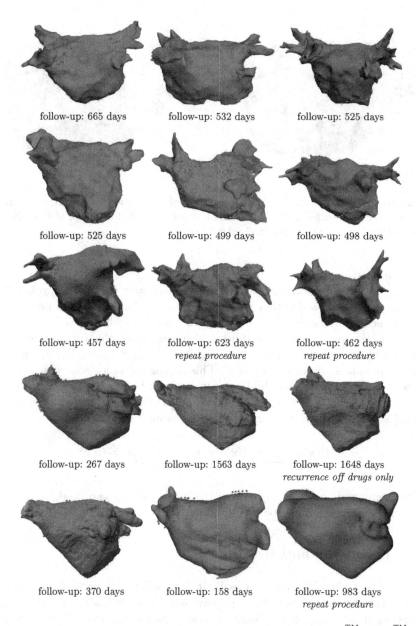

follow-up: 665 days   follow-up: 532 days   follow-up: 525 days

follow-up: 525 days   follow-up: 499 days   follow-up: 498 days

follow-up: 457 days   follow-up: 623 days   follow-up: 462 days
                                   repeat procedure   *repeat procedure*

follow-up: 267 days   follow-up: 1563 days   follow-up: 1648 days
                                                                      recurrence off drugs only

follow-up: 370 days   follow-up: 158 days   follow-up: 983 days
                                                                      repeat procedure

Fig. 1. All 15 cases in the dataset, either originating from the EnSite™ NavX™ (top three rows) or from the Carto® (Biosense Webster) (bottom two rows) electroanatomical mapping systems. Red dots indicate the locations targeted by ablation. Green dots show the mitral valve annulus and the location of the transseptal puncture where the catheter goes from the right to the left atrium. Three cases on rows 3 & 5 had a repeat ablation procedure. The last case on row 4 showed a recurrence when this patient came off medication only, the others were considered cured or AF was suppressed using antiarrhythmic drugs.

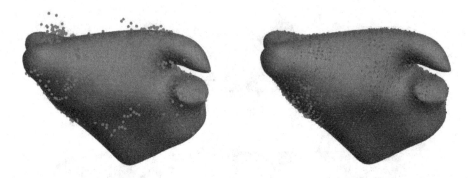

Fig. 2. (left) Ablation targets before mapping. (right) Ablation targets after mapping to the mean model surface. The size of the red dots is an indication of the number of votes that particular vertex has received.

In the resulting probability density map, gaps may exist. Gaps are vertices with zero probability surrounded only by vertices with a nonzero probability. These are post-processed with a 2D median filter, replacing the zero probability with the median probability value of all its 1st level neighbors.

Finally, the probability distribution resulting from the previous steps is smoothed by convolution with a Gaussian kernel. Each vertex is considered a signal point source, described by $\delta(\mathbf{x})$. This means the point source at vertex i at position $\mathbf{x}_i$ and with probability p_i can be described as $p_i\,\delta(\mathbf{x} - \mathbf{x}_i)$. Consequently, a global probability density function $P(\mathbf{x})$ can be generated by summing all local smooth probability density functions around the mesh

$$P(\mathbf{x}) = \sum_i p_i\,\delta(\mathbf{x} - \mathbf{x}_i) * \frac{1}{(\sigma\sqrt{2\pi})^3}e^{-\frac{\mathbf{x}^2}{2\sigma^2}}.$$

By sampling $P(\mathbf{x})$ at all vertices of the mean model mesh, a global smooth probability distribution can be projected onto this very mesh.

3   Experiments and Results

Our ablation probability model was built from electroanatomical models and ablation target points from fifteen paroxysmal atrial fibrillation patients; nine originating from an EnSite^{TM} NavX^{TM} system and six additional cases from a Carto® mapping system. Of these fifteen patients, three (20%) had a repeat procedure, one (6.7%) showed a recurrence when (s)he came off medication only; the other eleven (73.3%) did not show recurrences, meaning they were cured or AF was suppressed using antiarrhythmic drugs. Median follow-up period was

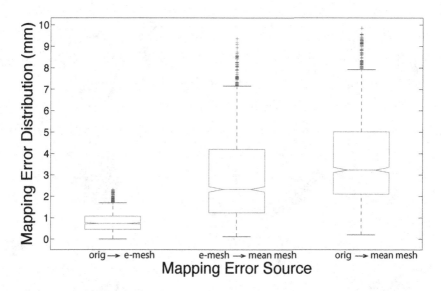

Fig. 3. Mapping error distributions. Mapping ablation targets from their original position to the electroanatomical mesh (left), from the electroanatomical mesh to the mean LA model mesh (middle) and the cumulative error (right). All points that showed a cumulative error above 10 mm have been discarded for probability distribution calculations, and from the error distribution calculations.

1.44 years (interquartile range was 1.26 – 1.76 years; total range was 0.43 – 4.51 years). For more details on all the training data, see fig. 1.

Both mapping operations, first mapping the ablation targets from their original positions to the respective electroanatomical meshes (NavX^{TM} and Carto$^{\circledR}$) (see fig. 1), and second, mapping electroanatomical mesh vertices to the mean LA model mesh by ICP (see fig. 2) introduce errors. Both error sources have been analyzed separately and combined. The resulting error distributions are shown in fig. 3. All points showing a cumulative error >10 mm have been discarded during probability distribution calculations, and in the error distribution calculations.

The probability distributions resulting from calculating a mapping density only are shown in fig. 4, top row. Furthermore, the distribution resulting from filling gaps – characterized by a zero mapping density surrounded by only nonzero mapping density mesh vertices – with the median value of the first level mesh neighbors can been seen in fig. 4, second row. The probability distribution resulting from propagation of the probability after the filling step along the surface with a Gaussian kernel with $\sigma = 0.5$ mm is shown in the bottom row of fig. 4.

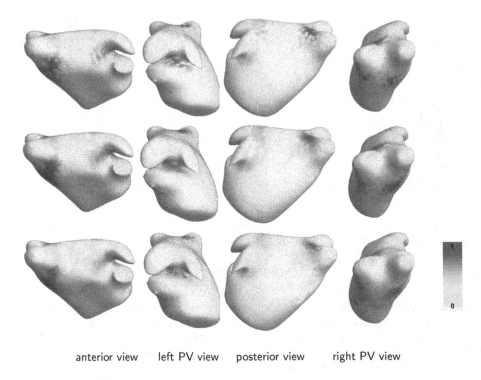

anterior view   left PV view   posterior view   right PV view

Fig. 4. Probability distributions projected on the LA mean model mesh. Resulting from ablation target mapping density only (top row); resulting from filling gaps in the projected mapping by means of the median value of their neighbors (middle row); resulting from propagation of the probability in the middle row along the surface with a Gaussian kernel with $\sigma = 0.5$ mm.

4   Discussion and Conclusion

We have presented an ablation probability density model for the cardiac left atrium built from the ablative treatment data from paroxysmal atrial fibrillation patients. Ablation target data were collected from Carto® (Biosense Webster) and EnSite™ NavX™ (St. Jude Medical) electroanatomical mapping suites.

The resulting probability distribution clearly shows PVI contours as suggested for paroxysmal AF treatment [5]. The right inferior pulmonary vein (RIPV) shows a lower overall ablation probability than the other PVs. This may be due to the fact that the RIPV is harder to reach with the ablation catheter, which enters the LA through a transseptal puncture right below the RIPV. To maximize maneuverability of the catheter in the LA in the context of robot-based ablation, Jayender et al. [19] investigated optimal transseptal puncture placement. In the future this model may also be used to drive robot-based ablation.

The ablation probability model can be of additional value in biophysical modeling of AF to predict likelihood of reconnection and to predict successful ablation strategies, to study variations in ablation patterns between different medical centers, and to support ROI selection in pencil beam MRI wall thickness imaging. Furthermore, during post-operative assessment of lesion formation, fibrotic lesions due to ablation can be separated from those due to AF.

In future work, more patient data should be obtained to make the model more representative of paroxysmal atrial fibrillation treatment strategies. Thus different ablation patterns may emerge for different medical centres reflecting their different strategies. Moreover, novel additional ablation lesion sets may be identified, and different lesion sets may be compared by their clinical outcome. Finally, nonrigid registration of the ablation target sets may reduce mapping errors as shown in fig. 3, and yield even sharper ablation patterns.

References

1. Feinberg, W.M., Blackshear, J.L., Laupacis, A., Kronmal, R., Hart, R.G.: Prevalence, age distribution, and gender of patients with atrial fibrillation. analysis and implications. Arch. Intern. Med. **155**(5), 469–473 (1995)
2. Allessie, M., Ausma, J., Schotten, U.: Electrical, contractile and structural remodeling during atrial fibrillation. Cardiovasc. Res. **54**(2), 230–246 (2002)
3. European Heart Rhythm Association, European Association for Cardio-Thoracic Surgery, Camm, A.J., Kirchhof, P., Lip, G.Y.H., Schotten, U., Savelieva, I., Ernst, S., Van Gelder, I.C., Al-Attar, N., Hindricks, G., Prendergast, B., Heidbuchel, H., Alfieri, O., Angelini, A., Atar, D., Colonna, P., De Caterina, R., De Sutter, J., Goette, A., Gorenek, B., Heldal, M., Hohloser, S.H., Kolh, P., Le Heuzey, J.Y., Ponikowski, P., Rutten, F.H.: Guidelines for the management of atrial fibrillation: the task force for the management of atrial fibrillation of the european society of cardiology (ESC). Eur. Heart J. **31**(19), 2369–2429 (2010)
4. Nademanee, K., McKenzie, J., Kosar, E., Schwab, M., Sunsaneewitayakul, B., Vasavakul, T., Khunnawat, C., Ngarmukos, T.: A new approach for catheter ablation of atrial fibrillation: mapping of the electrophysiologic substrate. J. Am. Coll. Cardiol. **43**(11), 2044–2053 (2004)
5. Calkins, H., Cappato, R., Brugada, J., et al.: 2012 HRS/EHRA/ECAS expert consensus statement on catheter and surgical ablation of atrial fibrillation. Heart Rhythm **9**(4), 632–696 (2012)
6. Ouyang, F., Tilz, R., Chun, J., Schmidt, B., Wissner, E., Zerm, T., Neven, K., Köktürk, B., Konstantinidou, M., Metzner, A., Fuernkranz, A., Kuck, K.H.: Long-term results of catheter ablation in paroxysmal atrial fibrillation: Lessons from a 5-year follow-up. Circulation **122**(23), 2368–2377 (2010)
7. Stevenhagen, J., Van Der Voort, P.H., Dekker, L.R.C., Bullens, R.W.M., Van Den Bosch, H., Meijer, A.: Three-dimensional ct overlay in comparison to cartomerge for pulmonary vein antrum isolation. J. Cardiovasc. Electrophysiol. **21**(6), 634–639 (2010)
8. Akoum, N., Daccarett, M., McGann, C., Segerson, N., Vergara, G., Kuppahally, S., Badger, T., Burgon, N., Haslam, T., Kholmovski, E., Macleod, R., Marrouche, N.: Atrial fibrosis helps select the appropriate patient and strategy in catheter ablation of atrial fibrillation: a de-mri guided approach. J. Cardiovasc. Electrophysiol. **22**(1), 16–22 (2011)

9. Jumrussirikul, P., Atiga, W.L., Lardo, A.C., Berger, R.D., Halperin, H., Hutchins, G.M., Calkins, H.: Prospective comparison of lesions created using a multipolar microcatheter ablation system with those created using a pullback approach with standard radiofrequency ablation in the canine atrium. Pacing. Clin. Electrophysiol. **23**(2), 203–213 (2000)

10. Ouyang, F., Antz, M., Ernst, S., Hachiya, H., Mavrakis, H., Deger, F.T., Schaumann, A., Chun, J., Falk, P., Hennig, D., Liu, X., Bänsch, D., Kuck, K.H.: Recovered pulmonary vein conduction as a dominant factor for recurrent atrial tachyarrhythmias after complete circular isolation of the pulmonary veins: lessons from double lasso technique. Circulation **111**(2), 127–135 (2005)

11. Koken, P., Holthuizen, R., Krueger, S., Heese, H.S., Weiss, S., Smink, J., Razavi, R., Schaeffter, T.: Atrial thickness mapping for ep ablation using black-blood restricted field of view mri. In: Proceedings 19th ISMRM Scientific Meeting, Montréal, Canada (2011)

12. Pappone, C., Vicedomini, G., Manguso, F., Gugliotta, F., Mazzone, P., Gulletta, S., Sora, N., Sala, S., Marzi, A., Augello, G., Livolsi, L., Santagostino, A., Santinelli, V.: Robotic magnetic navigation for atrial fibrillation ablation. J. Am. Coll. Cardiol. **47**(7), 1390–1400 (2006)

13. Pfeifer, B., Hanser, F., Trieb, T., Hintermüller, C., Seger, M., Fischer, G., Modre, R., Tilg, B.: Combining active appearance models and morphological operators using a pipeline for automatic myocardium extraction. In: Frangi, A.F., Radeva, P., Santos, A., Hernandez, M. (eds.) FIMH 2005. LNCS, vol. 3504, pp. 44–53. Springer, Heidelberg (2005)

14. Koppert, M.M.J., Rongen, P.M.J., Prokop, M., ter Haar Romeny, B.M., van Assen, H.C.: Cardiac left atrium CT image segmentation for ablation guidance. In: IEEE International Symposium on Biomedical Imaging: From Nano to Macro, ISBI 2010, pp. 480–483, April 2010

15. Sanchez-Quintana, D., Cabrera, J., Climent, V., Farre, J., Mendonca, M., Ho, S.: Anatomic relations between the esophagus and left atrium and relevance for ablation of atrial fibrillation. Circulation **112**(10), 1400–1405 (2005)

16. Hall, B., Jeevanantham, V., Simon, R., Filippone, J., Vorobiof, G., Daubert, J.: Variation in left atrial transmural wall thickness at sites commonly targeted for ablation of atrial fibrillation. J. Interv. Card. Electr. **17**(2), 127–132 (2006)

17. Zhang, Z.: Iterative point matching for registration of free-form curves and surfaces. International Journal of Computer Vision **13**(2), 119–152 (1994)

18. Peters, J., Ecabert, O., Meyer, C., Schramm, H., Kneser, R., Groth, A., Weese, J.: Automatic whole heart segmentation in static magnetic resonance image volumes. Med. Image. Comput. Comput. Assist. Interv. **10**(Pt 2), 402–410 (2007)

19. Jayender, J., Patel, R.V., Michaud, G.F., Hata, N.: Optimal transseptal puncture location for robot-assisted left atrial catheter ablation. In: Yang, G.-Z., Hawkes, D., Rueckert, D., Noble, A., Taylor, C. (eds.) MICCAI 2009, Part I. LNCS, vol. 5761, pp. 1–8. Springer, Heidelberg (2009)

Factors Affecting Optical Flow Performance in Tagging Magnetic Resonance Imaging

Patricia Márquez-Valle[1]([✉]), Hanne Kause[2], Andrea Fuster[3,4],
Aura Hernàndez-Sabaté[1], Luc Florack[3,4], Debora Gil[1], and Hans C. van Assen[2]

[1] Computer Vision Center, Autonomous University of Barcelona, Barcelona, Spain
pmarquez@cvc.uab.es
[2] Department of Electrical Engineering, Eindhoven University of Technology,
Eindhoven, The Netherlands
[3] Department of Biomedical Engineering, Eindhoven University of Technology,
Eindhoven, The Netherlands
[4] Department of Mathematics and Computer Science,
Eindhoven University of Technology, Eindhoven, The Netherlands

Abstract. Changes in cardiac deformation patterns are correlated with cardiac pathologies. Deformation can be extracted from tagging Magnetic Resonance Imaging (tMRI) using Optical Flow (OF) techniques. For applications of OF in a clinical setting it is important to assess to what extent the performance of a particular OF method is stable across different clinical acquisition artifacts. This paper presents a statistical validation framework, based on ANOVA, to assess the motion and appearance factors that have the largest influence on OF accuracy drop. In order to validate this framework, we created a database of simulated tMRI data including the most common artifacts of MRI and test three different OF methods, including HARP.

Keywords: Optical flow · Performance evaluation · Synthetic database · ANOVA · Tagging magnetic resonance imaging

1 Introduction

Tagging MRI (tMRI) is an important imaging technique that enables detailed motion analysis of the cardiac left ventricle (LV) [1]. Tagging MR images can be obtained by spatially modulating the MR magnetization field [2] so that images have a characteristic stripe or grid pattern that deforms along with cardiac tissue. This makes it possible to track information about motion and deformation over time, alterations of which are known to correlate with pathology [3–5].

A well-known technique to obtain motion information from image sequences is optical flow (OF), which results in a dense motion field by minimizing an energy functional that combines a data and a smoothness term [6]. OF techniques have two main types of error sources: model assumptions and numerics. Model assumption errors arise when images do not meet the expected appearance or motion patterns, such as the brightness constancy violated by signal decay, or

© Springer International Publishing Switzerland 2015
O. Camara et al. (Eds.): STACOM 2014, LNCS 8896, pp. 231–238, 2015.
DOI: 10.1007/978-3-319-14678-2_24

flow field irregularity. Numerical errors arise from the propagation of errors in the input data to errors in the output, e.g. signal decay or noise. Although it is impossible to avoid these errors, as they are inherent to any real world problem, some model assumptions, such as brightness constancy, can be modelled in the case of tMRI by using the harmonic phase of the original signal, which is constant over time [7–12]. Variable brightness OF has been studied in [13], where the signal decay was modelled by including decay terms in the OF equations. Still, resulting flow vectors can not be made error free.

Much work has been done on OF for tMRI [14–16]. However, signal decay and noise (among others) will always influence its accuracy [17]. In order to correctly interpret results it is, therefore, important to provide a quantitative estimate of the impact of the most influencing factors in OF accuracy. A qualitative comparison of four different algorithms for automatic motion analysis of the heart was carried out in [17]. The performance was assessed by a visual comparison of the box-plots as a function of SNR. From that paper, one can discern that the most stable method is the one working in the frequency domain. Still, it is worth noting that the extent to which the methods are stable in the presence of artifacts needs to be quantified.

In order to do so, as well as to be able to infer the OF accuracy range in the absence of ground truth (real images), we present in this paper a validation framework using Analysis of Variance (ANOVA [18]). This tool usually detects differences in performance, and evaluates the impact of different factors or assumptions across methodologies used for new diagnostic scores [19]. In this paper we do a step forward in the use of this statistical tool. We assess the performance of different algorithms against several factors using a 2-way ANOVA. In particular, we use ANOVA to evaluate the impact of clinical acquisition conditions (noise, signal decay, tagging acquisition), motion patterns and the influence on the results of the regularization built into some OF methods. The performance has been evaluated on three OF algorithms, two Harmonic Phase Flow (HPF) [11] implementations and HARP [7]. Our framework, presented in Section 2, is applied to a database of synthetic tagged MR images (subsection 2.1). This database contains realistic tagging images, which are either line tagged or grid tagged and with several motion patterns based on a cardiac motion simulator by Arts et al. [20]. Section 3 presents the experiments and section 4 the conclusions.

2   ANOVA Assessment of Influential Factors

The OF method best suited for a clinical application should be the one presenting the most stable performance across the artifacts arising in that particular clinical setting. In the context of cardiac deformation tracking, clinical settings prone to affect OF performance include, among others, variability in image acquisition conditions, radiological noise distorting image appearance and distorted motion patterns due to cardiac pathologies.

We propose to use Analysis of Variance (ANOVA) to compare the performance of multiple OF methods and explore the impact of specific clinical conditions. ANOVA's [18] are powerful statistical tools for detecting differences in performance across methodologies, as well as the impact of different factors or assumptions. We can apply ANOVA in case our data consists of one or several categorical explanatory variables (called factors) and a quantitative response of the variable. The variability analysis is defined as soon as the ANOVA quantitative score, different factors and methods are determined. The quantitative score taken from a sampling (individuals) of the clinical data is grouped according to such factors and differences among a quantitative response group mean are computed. ANOVA provides a statistical way to assess if such differences are significant with a given confidence level α.

In order to assess the impact of a given clinical setting on the performance of several OF methods, we propose to use a 2-way ANOVA with factors given by the OF method (denoted OF) and the clinical source of error (denoted CSE) whose influence on OF we want to assess. The ANOVA individuals should be defined as a random sampling of consecutive frames taken from a representative set of sequences. The quantitative ANOVA variable should be a measure of OF performance computed for each of the sampled frames. Such a measure could be the pixel-based OF error summarized for the whole frame or the error in a clinical functional score calculated from OF motion (such as strain or rotation).

The desired result of the 2-ANOVA test would be a significance in the methods factor, possibly a significance across CSE and, most important, no significant interaction. In case of significant interaction ($p-val < \alpha$), a 1-way ANOVA with the combined OF-CSE factor should be used to detect the sources of bias. Otherwise, the significance of each ANOVA factor can be correctly interpreted using its associated p-value. In case of significant differences ($p - val < \alpha$), we can compare group factors using a multiple comparison test with Tukey correction [21] to detect those groups that are significantly worse. In this paper we have considered 3 different types of CSE:

- **CSE1: Acquisition impact**. The typical tMRI acquisition can produce either two sequences with complementary stripes or a single sequence combining both magnetic fields into a single grid pattern. The two patterns define the CSE groups.
- **CSE2: Radiological noise impact**. The influence of the radiological noise should be assessed by considering sequences with decreasing SNR. The different SNR_S define the ANOVA groups of the CSE factor.
- **CSE3: Motion impact**. Finally, several kinds of pathologies should be considered in order to assess if OF methods are biased due to regularity assumptions or a priori models of motion. The different motion patterns define CSE factor groups.

As a first step towards a full validation of CSE influence using clinical data, we have simulated the above conditions using the model of cardiac deformation and SPAMM acquisition described in what follows:

L1 - F1   L2 - F2   L2 - F5   L2 - F12   G - F1   G - F5   G - F12

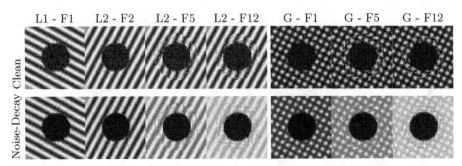

Fig. 1. Line (L1 and L2) and grid (G) tagging images (frames 1, 5 and 12) from the 3rd slice of the set with 2D cardiac motion. Clean data is shown above and data with noise and decay below. Arrows illustrate a sample of the ground truth.

2.1 Synthetic Image Database Construction

To test the framework described above, it is necessary to have images with a ground truth motion field. For this purpose we defined a database of synthetic MR images (Fig. 1), by making use of the cardiac motion simulator by Arts and Waks [20,22]. The heart motion was modelled using their 13-parameter model which includes radially-dependent compression, torsion, ellipticallization, shear, rotation and translation.

The initial shape of the left ventricle was modelled as a prolate sphere. A total number of 6.300 material points was sampled on the model and the deformation of the initial shape is computed using a time-dependent parametric model. We adapted the full 3D model by eliminating longitudinal motion to prevent out-of-plane motion. Different image datasets were created restricting motion to either rotation around the z-axis or radially-dependent contraction.

Although the model allows for slices with any orientation, we created datasets consisting of five short axis slices sampled across the prolate sphere. Every slice had 50×50 isotropic pixels and started with the longitudinal axis in the center of the image. For construction of the images from a set of points of transformed material coordinates with intensities, a linear interpolation approach was used. The cardiac cycle was split into 16 frames, but this can be further sub-sampled to account for low temporal resolution.

The datasets contained three sinusoidal SPAMM (spatial modulation of magnetization) [2] tagging sequences, two stripe tagging sequences (horizontal and vertical) and a grid sequence, that were modelled with signal decay according to [22].

The spatial period of the tagging patterns was set to 6.6 pixels. Rician noise was added with a constant SNR of 25 over time, defined as SNR $= \frac{\mu}{\sigma}$ with μ the mean signal and σ the standard deviation of the noise [23]. Two data variants have been generated: images with noise and decay and clean data without noise and decay.

3   Experiments

In this study, we choose motion estimation errors given by OF End-point-Error[1] (EE) [24] to define the ANOVA variable. Given that EE is computed for each pixel, the ANOVA variable is the EE average: $\mu(EE) := \frac{1}{N} \sum EE_i$, with EE_i the error for each pixel and N the number of pixels. In order to account for non-normality in the data, $\mu(EE)$ was transformed to the logarithmic scale [18]. ANOVA tests were performed at a significance level $\alpha = 0.05$.

Concerning ANOVA individuals and groups, we defined them using the dataset described in section 2.1. The CSE factor groups are given as:

- **CSE1.** We used the sequences without noise and decay (SNR_{100}) and with the full 2D motion grouped according to their tag pattern, which denoted as *grid* and *striped*. The ANOVA individuals were taken from a random sampling of 7 frames of sequences at basal, mid and apical levels. This ANOVA should assess the impact of the grid pattern under the best possible setting and it selects the pattern for the remaining experiments.
- **CSE2.** The impact of radiological noise was assessed by taking sequences without noise and without decay, denoted by SNR_{100}, and with decay and the constant Rician noise added, denoted by $\text{SNR}_{25} - D$. As before, the full 2D motion sequences with grid pattern at basal, mid and apical levels randomly sampled define the ANOVA individuals.
- **CSE3.** Finally, the impact of motion bias in OF assumptions is checked by considering 2D motion, noted by $2DF$, and its decoupling into rotation, denoted R, and contraction, denoted C, as CSE groups. Sequences were considered with Rician noise and decay to account for conditions as realistic as possible. This ANOVA should detect the impact of regularity assumptions in OF computation.

The OF factor groups are three methods working on the frequency domain and with different regularity assumptions for a fair assessment of CSE3:

- **Full HPF** (*HPF*). Implementation of the algorithm described by Garcia et al. in [11]. The data term is computed using the phase images of each tagging pattern and is combined with the smoothness term using variable weights given by the amplitudes of the Gabor filter responses.
- **Constant HPF** (*HPF_C*). Adaptation of [11] with constant weights set to 0.5.
- **HARP** (*HARP*). In-house implementation of the algorithm described by Osman et al. in [7].

In order to avoid introducing a bias in the results, we computed harmonic phase images for all of the input images, as described in [7]. These images were then used as input for all OF methods.

---

[1] $EE := \sqrt{(U - u)^2 + (V - v)^2}$ for (U, V) the ground truth flow field, and (u, v) the flow field computed using a given OF to be tested.

Table 1. ANOVA results

CSE1			CSE2			CSE3		
$p-OF$	$p-CSE$	$p-int$	$p-OF$	$p-CSE$	$p-int$	$p-OF$	$p-CSE$	$p-int$
$\ll 10^{-16}$	0.239	0.657	$\ll 10^{-16}$	0.058	0.251	$\ll 10^{-16}$	0.852	0.874

Table 1 reports the 2-ANOVA p-values for the CSE experiments: p-OF for the OF factors, p-CSE for CSE factors, and p-int for interaction. For all experiments, there is no evidence of significant interaction ($p - int > 0.05$), but there are significant differences in OF performance ($p - OF \ll 10^{-16}$). It follows that, OF performance ranking is independent of the considered CSE conditions and the most suitable OF method can be selected. Concerning the CSE factor there are no significant differences ($p - CSE > 0.05$), so that all OF methods are robust against the clinical settings considered. However, it is worth noticing that the presence of noise causes p-values to drop so a further decrease in SNR could affect OF performance.

In order to further explore group differences and, in the particular case of OF significant differences, discard the worse methods, we have applied the pairwise comparison with Tukey correction shown in Figure 2. For each factor, Figure 2 shows group mean differences represented as horizontal lines centred at the mean (in logarithmic scale) and vertically distributed according to the factor group. Group differences being in logarithmic scale, the more negative mean values are, the smaller the OF error is. We observe that, for all CSE conditions, the best OF method is HPF and the worst one $HARP$. Regarding the impact of CSE conditions, although there is not enough evidence of differences, plots reveal

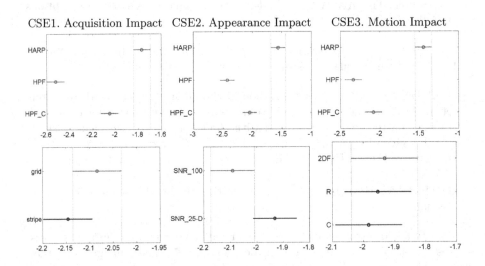

Fig. 2. Pairwise comparison with Tukey correction. Results on the EE group mean shown in logarithmic scale in the horizontal axis.

some interesting tendencies. First, we observed that considering two sequences with stripe lines has smaller error in OF computations. Second, OF methods performance is better without noise and decay, as expected. Finally, there is no difference across different motions, so that OF motion assumptions do not bias computations.

4   Conclusions

We presented a validation framework that uses ANOVA to detect significant differences in OF performance according to different clinical factors prone to have a large influence in OF accuracy. Our framework has been applied to quantitatively test the performance of three OF methods working on the frequency domain ($HARP$, HPF and HPF_C).

On the one hand, the presented experiments show that a method (HPF) that applies the regularity term only at areas where phase is not reliable performs better than the one using a global regularity constraint (HPF_C). Experiments also show the need for the regularity term to reduce $HARP$ sensitivity to noise.

On the other hand, experiments show that there is no bias due to CSE. First of all, using as input image stripes or a grid pattern does not affect OF performance significantly. Regarding the $SNR_{25} - D$ versus SNR_{100} sequences, although there are no significant differences, we observe that OF performance is better for clean sequences. Finally, motion assumptions do not bias computations. Summarizing, the chosen OF methods are robust against CSE artifacts.

This preliminary study encourages the use of the presented framework to explore OF performance in new settings. In the future we aim to apply it to the clinical sequences that were made available in the 2011 STACOM motion tracking challenge to assess the impact of tMRI features on the computation of scores of potential diagnostic value. This will also enable the comparison with other methods previously tested on this dataset. Although the framework was applied on two dimensional sequences in this study, it should be noted that the framework can be applied to three dimensional data as well.

Acknowledgments. Work supported by Spanish project TIN2012-33116. First author supported by FPI-MICINN BES-2010-031102 program. Second author is supported by the Dutch Technology Foundation STW, which is part of the Netherlands Organisation for Scientific Research (NWO), and which is partly funded by the Ministry of Economic Affairs. The authors would like to thank Marijke Dermois for support with the artificial tagging MR images.

References

1. Zerhouni, E., Parish, D., Rogers, W., et al.: Human heart: Tagging with MR imaging-a method for noninvasive assessment of myocardial motion. Radiology **169**(1), 59–63 (1988)
2. Axel, L., Dougherty, L.: MR imaging of motion with spatial modulation of magnetization. Radiology **171**(3), 841–845 (1989)

3. Mirsky, I., Pfeffer, J., Pfeffer, M., Braunwald, E.: The contractile state as the major determinant in the evolution of left ventricular dysfunction in the spontaneously hypertensive rat **53**, 767–778 (1983)
4. Götte, M., van Rossum, A., Twisk, J., et al.: Quantification of regional contractile function after infarction: Strain analysis superior to wall thickening analysis in discriminating infarct from remote myocardium. JACC **37**, 808–817 (2001)
5. Delhaas, T., Kotte, J., van der Toorn, A., et al.: Increase in left ventricular torsion-to-shortening ratio in children with valvular aorta stenosis **51**, 135–139 (2004)
6. Horn, B., Schunck, B.: Determining optical flow. AI **17**, 185–203 (1981)
7. Osman, N., Kerwin, W., McVeigh, E., Prince, J.: Cardiac motion tracking using CINE HARP magnetic resonance imaging **42**(6), 1048–1060 (1999)
8. Prince, J., McVeigh, E.: Motion estimation from tagged MR image sequences **11**(2), 238–249 (1992)
9. Florack, L., van Assen, H.: A new methodology for multiscale myocardial deformation and strain analysis based on tagging MRI (2010)
10. Xavier, M., Lalande, A., Walker, P., et al.: An adapted optical flow algorithm for robust quantification of cardiac wall motion from standard cine-MR examinations. Inf. Tech. in Biomed. **16**(5), 859–868 (2012)
11. Garcia-Barnes, J., Gil, D., Pujades, S., Carreras, F.: Variational framework for assessment of the left ventricle motion. Math. Mod. of Nat. Phen. **3**(6), 76–100 (2008)
12. Becciu, A., van Assen, H., Florack, L., et al.: A multi-scale feature based optic flow method for 3D cardiac motion estimation. In: SSVM, pp. 588–599 (2009)
13. Gupta, S., Prince, J.: On variable brightness optical flow for tagged MRI, pp. 323–334 (1995)
14. Carranza-Herrezuelo, N., Bajo, A., Sroubek, F., et al.: Motion estimation of tagged cardiac magnetic resonance images using variational techniques. Comp. Med. Im. and Graph. **34**(6), 514–522 (2010)
15. Alessandrini, M., Basarab, A., Liebgott, H., Bernard, O.: Myocardial motion estimation from medical images using the monogenic signal. IEEE Transactions on Image Processing **22**(3), 1084–1095 (2013)
16. Arts, T., Prinzen, F., Delhaas, T., et al.: Mapping displacement and deformation of the heart with local sine-wave modeling **29**(5) (2010)
17. Smal, I., Carranza-Herrezuelo, N., Klein, S., et al.: Reversible jump MCMC methods for fully automatic motion analysis in tagged MRI. Medical Image Analysis **16**(1), 301–324 (2012)
18. Arnold, S.: The theory of linear models and multivariate observations. Wiley (1997)
19. Jap, B., Lal, S., Fischer, P., Bekiaris, E.: Using eeg spectral components to assess algorithms for detecting fatigue. Expert Systems with Applications **36**(2), 2352–2359 (2009)
20. Arts, T., Hunter, W., Douglas, A., et al.: Description of the deformation of the left ventricle by a kinematic model. Journal Biomechanics **25**(10), 1119–1127 (1992)
21. Tukey, L.: Comparing individual means in the analysis of variance. Biometrics **5**, 99–114 (1949)
22. Waks, E., Prince, J., Douglas, A.: Cardiac motion simulator for tagged MRI. In: MMBIA-Workshops, pp. 182–191 (1996)
23. Gutberlet, M., Schwinge, K., Freyhardt, P., et al.: Influence of high magnetic field strengths and parallel acquisition strategies on image quality in cardiac 2D CINE magnetic resonance imaging. Eur. Radiol. **15**(8), 1586–1597 (2005)
24. Baker, S., Scharstein, D., Lewis, J., et al.: A database and evaluation methodology for optical flow. IJCV **92**(1), 1–31 (2011)

Multi-modal Validation Framework of Mitral Valve Geometry and Functional Computational Models

Sasa Grbic[1]([✉]), Thomas F. Easley[2], Tommaso Mansi[1],
Charles H. Bloodworth[2], Eric L. Pierce[2], Ingmar Voigt[1], Dominik Neumann[1],
Julian Krebs[1], David D. Yuh[3], Morten O. Jensen[2],
Dorin Comaniciu[1], and Ajit P. Yoganathan[2]

[1] Imaging and Computer Vision, Siemens Corporate Technology, Princeton, NJ, USA
Sasa.grbic@siemens.com
[2] The Wallace H. Coulter Department of Biomedical Engineering,
Georgia Institute of Technology and Emory University, Atlanta, GA, USA
[3] Section of Cardiac Surgery, Department of Surgery,
Yale University School of Medicine, New Haven, CT, USA

Abstract. Computational models of the mitral valve (MV) exhibit significant potential for patient-specific surgical planning. Recently, these models have been advanced by incorporating MV tissue structure, nonlinear material properties, and more realistic chordae tendineae architecture. Despite advances, only limited ground-truth data exists to validate their ability to accurately simulate MV closure and function. The validation of the underlying models will enhance modeling accuracy and confidence in the simulated results. A necessity towards this aim is to develop an integrated pipeline based on a comprehensive in-vitro flow loop setup including echocardiography techniques (Echo) and micro-computed tomography. Building on [1] we improved the acquisition protocol of the proposed experimental setup for in-vitro Echo imaging, which enables the extraction of more reproducible and accurate geometrical models, using state-of-the art image processing and geometric modeling techniques. Based on the geometrical parameters from the Echo MV models captured during diastole, a bio-mechanical model is derived to estimate MV closure geometry. We illustrate the framework on two data sets and show the improvements obtained from the novel Echo acquisition protocol and improved bio-mechanical model.

1 Introduction

Cardiovascular Disease causes approximately 30% of deaths worldwide among which heart failure is one of the most frequent causes [2,3]. One of the main contributors to heart failure is mitral valve (MV) disease, especially MV regurgitation (MR) where the MV closure is impaired causing regurgitant back-flow of blood from the left ventricle to the left atrium. Treatment of MR often requires MV replacement or repair surgery to sustain or improve heart function. In recent

© Springer International Publishing Switzerland 2015
O. Camara et al. (Eds.): STACOM 2014, LNCS 8896, pp. 239–248, 2015.
DOI: 10.1007/978-3-319-14678-2_25

years, MV repair procedures, where the valve is surgically altered in order to restore its proper hemodynamic function, are being substituted for classical valve replacements [4–6], showing improved outcomes by demonstrating lower operative mortality, improved long-term survival, and preserved left ventricular function. As the procedures are technically challenging, they require an experienced surgical team to achieve optimal results [5], since the deformation of complex valve anatomy during the intervention, where the heart is stopped, has to be predicted and associated with post-operative implications regarding valve anatomy and function. Having a framework to explore different surgical repair strategies for an individual patient and virtually compute their immediate outcomes would be a desired tool in current clinical practice. It would enable the surgeon to plan the surgical intervention with respect to the direct outcome.

Driven by the widespread prevalence of MV diseases, researchers are developing methods to assess MV anatomy from multiple imaging modalities and simulate its physiology using biomechanical models [7,8]. However, they do not enable patient-specific personalization of the geometric model, or this process requires tedious manual interactions which limits their clinical applicability.

In recent years, methods have been proposed to personalize the geometric model of the MV using semi-manual or advanced automated algorithms [9]. Using these models, biomechanical computations can be performed based on a personalized patient-specific geometry as in [10]. However, these models rely on a simplified geometrical model, mainly due to the limitations of in-vivo Echo imaging. In order to apply such methods in clinical practice, the first step is to validate the predictive capabilities of simplified models extracted from Echo against ideal models extracted from micro-computed tomography data (μCT) in a controlled in-vitro environment.

We propose a validation framework for both geometric and biomechanical models extracted from non-invasive modalities. A new controlled experimental setup was developed for MV in-vitro imaging to acquire functional Echo data and high-resolution μCT images of the MV. Building on [1], we developed a new Echo imaging protocol which significantly improved the image quality. We utilize novel image processing and geometric modeling techniques to extract reproducible geometrical models from both modalities. From the Echo geometrical model during diastole we derive a biomechanical model to estimate MV closure geometry. Compared to the biomechanical model used in [1] we are able to personalize the chordae tree by applying chordae specific rest length parameters. As the in-vitro Echo imaging is similar to routinely acquired transesophageal echocardiogram (TEE) in clinical practice, our framework could be easily transferred to the clinical setting. We illustrate the framework on two in-vitro data sets.

2   In-Vitro Setup

2.1   Mitral Valve Selection and Preparation

Ovine hearts were obtained through a local farmers market and the MVs excised preserving their annular and subvalvular structures. The valve was then mounted

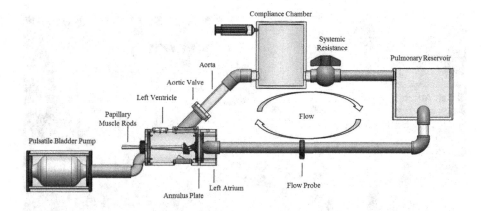

Fig. 1. Schematic of the Georgia Tech Left Heart Simulator (GTLHS) with components identified

to the annulus plate and mechanical PM positioning system (rods) of the extensively studied Georgia Tech Left Heart Simulator (GTLHS) (Fig. 1) [11,12].

While suturing the MV to the simulator's annulus, normal annular-leaflet geometric relationships were respected (anterior leaflet occupying 1/3rd of annular circumference, and commissures in the 2 and 10 oclock positions).

2.2   Establish Healthy Mitral Valve Geometry and Function In-Vitro

In establishing healthy MV geometry and function, the papillary muscles of the MV were carefully adjusted to positions apically of their respective commissures using previously published techniques [13]. The simulator was tuned to pulsatile human left heart hemodynamics (120 mmHg peak LVP, 5.0 L/min cardiac output, 70 beats/min). Fine adjustments were made to achieve ≈6-8 mm coaptation height at the A2-P2 diameter, minimal leaflet tenting (<1 mm), and the anterior leaflet consuming 2/3rd of the septal-lateral annular diameter [11]. Upon reaching a healthy control state, the hemodynamics of each valve was recorded over 15 consecutive cardiac cycles. The established healthy control geometry of each valve was held constant over each testing procedure.

2.3   In-Vitro Echocardiography

An novel acoustic window (Fig. 2) was developed for the GTLHS to be used in the new imaging protocol. The acoustic window installed in the posterior of the left ventricle allowed for higher quality acquisition of Rt3DE images compared to the atrial acquisition protocol used in [1]. The window provided a direct echocardiographic view of the chordae and chordal insertions on both the leaflet and the papillary muscles. This view was also closer to the MV leaflets

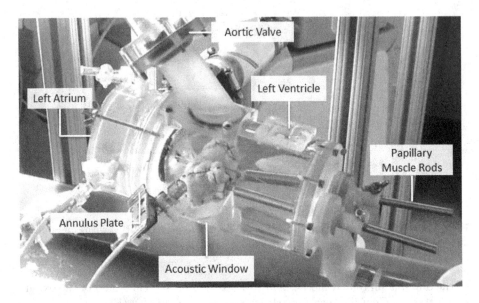

Fig. 2. New left heart chamber for the GTLHS with a smaller size and cylindrical shape for CT scanning, and acoustic window for echocardiography from the left ventricle perspective

and annulus, allowing the use of a smaller pyramid volume to maximize frame rate. Three-dimensional echocardiography imaging of MVs mounted within the GTLHS was performed using an ie33 Matrix ultrasound system and x7-2 probe (Philips Healthcare; Andover, MA). Zoomed 3D images of the entire mitral complex, including annulus, leaflets, chordae, and papillary muscles were acquired. Acquisition was repeated multiple times from different viewpoints (atrial and ventricular) for optimal image selection. DICOM images were exported for valve segmentation and model generation.

2.4   In-Vitro Micro-computed Tomography

Following echocardiography, the GTLHS was drained of saline and loaded into the new, state-of-the-art Inveon micro-computed tomography scanner (Siemens Medical Solutions USA, Inc.; Malvern, PA). The left heart chamber (LHC) was modified to a smaller size with a cylindrical shape (Fig. 2), which allowed it to fit inside the machine without LHC disassembly. This, in turn, ensured consistent valve geometry (PM positioning) between CT and Rt3DE data sets. The dataset contained the entire mitral valve and was composed of 43.29 μm isotropic voxels. The scan was conducted in air with parameters optimized for soft tissue (80 kV energy, 500 μA intensity, 500-650 ms integration time). Scans were performed under two MV configurations: open-leaflets (ambient pressure, $\approx$0 mmHg), and closed-leaflets ($\approx$120 mmHg left ventricular pressure). Acquisitions took under 7 minutes each, leading to minimal tissue dehydration as compared to

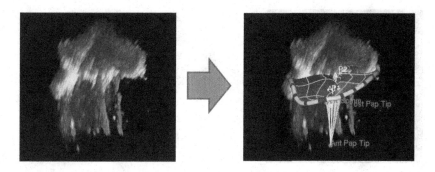

Fig. 3. Left: Echo scan of mitral valve (MV) within the in-vitro setting, right: extracted geometric model of the MV. A parachute model of the marginal chordae tendineae are shown in yellow.

previous studies. The μCT data was exported from the scanners computer and then converted to DICOMs using Siemens Inveon Research Workplace. The DICOMs were then used for computational modeling.

3   Computational Modeling

3.1   Extraction of MV Geometric Model from In-Vitro Echo

We use the anatomical point distribution model of the MV and its subvalvular components from [9,14] estimated from 3D Echo. The model is hierarchically parametrized containing nine landmarks on the coarse level and two parametric surfaces on the finer scale. The nine landmarks (two trigones, two commissures, one posterior annulus mid-point, two leaflet tips, and two papillary tips) are representing key anatomical landmarks and are capable of capturing a broad spectrum of morphological and physiological variations of the MV physiology. On the finest scale, the model is comprised of the MV annulus, the anterior and posterior leaflets represented as dense surface models.

As the Echo in the in-vitro environment deviates significantly compared to the human TEE scan we adapted our software to manually initialize the geometric model in the in-vitro Echo images. The geometric MV model is further manually refined to match the images. Fig. 3 depicts the extracted model based on the Echo image.

3.2   Biomechanical Model of the Mitral Valve from Echo

We use an extension of the model proposed in [10] to compute the MV closure based on the Echo anatomy. Hereby, the dynamics system $M\ddot{u} + C\dot{u} + Ku = f_t + f_p + f_c$ is solved, where M is the diagonal mass matrix calculated from the mass density $\rho = 1040\,g/L$, C is the Rayleigh damping matrix with coefficients $1e4\,s^{-1}$ and $0.1\,s$ for the mass and stiffness matrix respectively, K is the

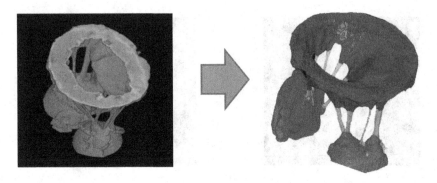

Fig. 4. Left: μCT scan of mitral valve (MV) within the in-vitro setting, right: extracted geometric model of the MV

stiffness matrix, $\boldsymbol{f}_t$ is the force created by the chords on the leaflets, $\boldsymbol{f}_p$ the pressure force, $\boldsymbol{f}_c$ the contact forces and $\boldsymbol{u}$ the displacement. We rely on transverse isotropic linear tissue elasticity, motivated by findings in [15], implemented using a co-rotational finite elements method (FEM) to cope with large deformations. Poisson ratio is set as $\nu = 0.488$ for both leaflets, fiber Young's modulus is $E_{AL} = 6.23\,MPa$ and $E_{PL} = 2.09\,MPa$ for the anterior and posterior leaflets, cross-fiber Young's modulus is $E_{AL} = 2.35\,MPa$ and $E_{PL} = 1.88\,MPa$, and shear modulus is $1.37\,MPa$. The MV annulus and PMs are fixed. Chordae are modeled as described in [10]: twenty-eight marginal chordae are evenly attached at the free-edges of the leaflets and four chordae are tethered at the base of the leaflets, following an exponential law. The model in [10] was extended to allow personalization of the chordae rest length for each chordae. Self collisions are modeled with collision stiffness of $100\,kPa$ and friction coefficient of 0.1. We used the SOFA framework[1] to implement our MV biomechanical model.

Model Personalization. Marginal chordae are personalized in a coarse-to-fine approach such that the coaptation line matches accurately. Basal chordae and tissue stiffness are adjusted such that leaflet bellowing is captured.

3.3   Extraction of Geometric Model from In-Vitro Micro-computed Tomography

We propose a semi-automated segmentation to extract geometric models of the MV from μCT images (see Fig. 4), where the final model consists of the MV papillary muscles, chordae tree and MV anterior and posterior leaflets. In the first phase the papillary muscles are segmented by placing manually positive seed points within the anterior and posterior papillary muscles. The Random Walker algorithm [16] is used to delineate the papillary muscle geometry. Next, the MV leaflets are segmented by manually carving the areas of the MV geometric model

---

[1] http://www.sofa-framework.org/

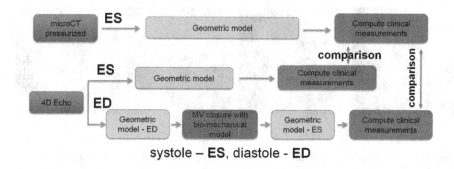

Fig. 5. Validation workflow

which does not belong to the leaflets. After 4-8 manual iterations the anterior and posterior leaflets are delineated (see red color in Fig. 4). Finally, to extract the final geometric measurements a simplified model (as described in subsection 3.1) is fitted to the extracted model. This model can also be manually refined if necessary.

4 Results

Our framework was utilized on two ovine valves to compare the geometric config-uration between the model constructed from Echo and μCT (considered ground truth) during systole (MV closed). Next, we compute the MV geometry at systole from an end-diastolic (MV open) Echo image and compare it to the ground-truth geometrical configuration obtained from the μCT image. As the geometric con-figuration of the MV in the unpressurized μCT does not correspond with the geometry in Echo during diastole, we only use the closed μCT image data in our experiments. The reason for this is without a pressure gradient, the suspension in fluid, and flow, the MV leaflets scrunch and become thicker. In addition, the chordae tendineae bunch and it is not possible to delineate the full MV chordae tendineae topology. However, with applied air pressure the leaflet fibers expand to the same geometric configuration as seen in Echo. The complete validation workflow is shown in Fig. 5.

4.1 Geometric Comparison

Based on the geometric models extracted during systole (MV closed) from Echo and μCT, we measured clinically relevant parameters for short term mitral valve repair (MR) outcome (coaptation length and coaptation area, see Fig. 7, left) in order to quantitatively compare geometric differences between the two mod-els (see Fig. 7, right). Results suggest that the simplified MV geometric model derived from Echo, similar to routinely acquired clinical data, can approximate important clinical measurements for MR within clinically relevant ranges when

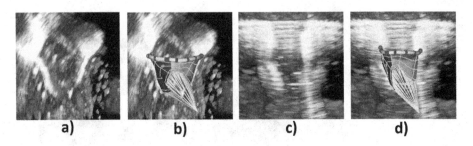

Fig. 6. Comparison of the improved Echo image quality and extracted geometric MV models from the new ventricular imaging protocol (a,b) compared to the atrial protocol used in [1] (c,d)

compared with the idealized geometric model from μCT. Due to the improved Echo imaging quality (ventricular view) in the new in-vitro setup, we can derive more accurate geometric models of the MV (see Fig. 6 and Fig. 7).

4.2   MV Closure Computation

We computed MV closure using the biomechanical model (described in Sec. 3.2) starting from the end-diastolic Echo MV model (last frame where the MV is seen open). A generic pressure profile is applied varying from 0 mmHg to 120 mmHg [10] and a time step of 10 ms.

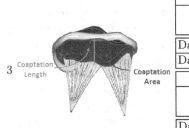

| | Coaptation Length [mm] | | | |
	Echo atrial	Echo ventricular	μCT	simEcho
Data Set 1	1.55	2.00	1.92	2.05
Data Set 2	1.46	2.25	2.12	2.32
	Coaptation Area [mm^2]			
	Echo atrial	Echo ventricular	μCT	simEcho
Data Set 1	37.93	50.07	48.23	51.47
Data Set 2	39.48	56.17	53.17	58.07

Fig. 7. Geometric comparison of clinical measurements derived from the mitral valve (MV) model at systole from μCT, old (atrial) Echo acquisition, new (ventricular) Echo acquisition and simulated closure model derived from new (ventricular) Echo acquisition protocol

The chord rest length are manually personalized in a coarse-to-fine approach such that the coaptation line matches the Echo data. Finally, to capture the fast dynamics and correctly account for collisions and inertia, pressure increase duration was scaled to last 10 s and 1000 iterations were calculated.

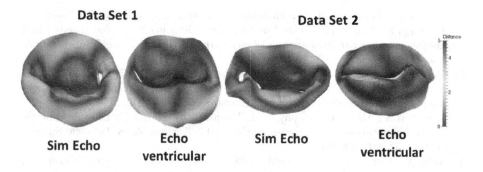

Fig. 8. Qualitative comparison of MV geometry from simulated Echo closure (Sim Echo) and ventricular Echo compared to the ground-truth μCT model

Fig. 8 illustrates the geometric distance between the simulated Echo closure (Sim Echo) model, the atrial Echo model, and the ventricular Echo model compared to the ground-truth μCT model. These results confirm that simplified models from Echo can be utilized to build biomechanical models and compute MV closure geometry in respect to relevant clinical parameters.

5   Conclusion

We extended the framework in [1] for validating geometrical and functional models of the mitral valve (MV) by utilizing a controlled in-vitro setup. We improved the Echo imaging protocol resulting in more accurate and reproducible MV models. In addition, we advanced the bio-mechanical model, allowing for a hierarchical personalization of the marginal and basal chordae rest length parameters. We evaluated our framework by using two ovine data sets. First results are promising, suggesting that the biomechanical model derived from Echo could be accurate enough to model basic clinical biomarkers of MV function. Validation on a larger cohort is under-way.

References

1. Neumann, D., et al.: Multi-modal pipeline for comprehensive validation of mitral valve geometry and functional computational models. In: Camara, O., Mansi, T., Pop, M., Rhode, K., Sermesant, M., Young, A. (eds.) STACOM 2013. LNCS, vol. 8330, pp. 188–195. Springer, Heidelberg (2014)
2. Roger, V.L., Go, A.S., Lloyd-Jones, D.M., Adams, R.J., Berry, J.D., Brown, T.M., Carnethon, M.R., Dai, S., de Simone, G., Ford, E.S., et al.: Heart disease and stroke statistics 2011 update a report from the american heart association. Circulation **123**(4), e18–e209 (2011)
3. Stewart, S., MacIntyre, K., Capewell, S., McMurray, J.: Heart failure and the aging population: an increasing burden in the 21st century? Heart **89**(1), 49–53 (2003)

4. Vassileva, C.M., Mishkel, G., McNeely, C., Boley, T., Markwell, S., Scaife, S., Hazelrigg, S.: Long-term survival of patients undergoing mitral valve repair and replacement a longitudinal analysis of medicare fee-for-service beneficiaries. Circulation 127(18), 1870–1876 (2013)

5. Kilic, A., Shah, A., Conte, J., Baumgartner, W., Yuh, D.: Operative outcomes in mitral valve surgery: Combined effect of surgeon and hospital volume in a population-based analysis. J. Thorac. Cardiovasc. Surg. (2012)

6. Borger, M.A., Alam, A., Murphy, P.M., Doenst, T., David, T.E.: Chronic ischemic mitral regurgitation: repair, replace or rethink? The Annals of Thoracic Surgery 81(3), 1153–1161 (2006)

7. Wang, Q., Sun, W.: Finite element modeling of mitral valve dynamic deformation using patient-specific multi-slices computed tomography scans. Ann. Biomed. Eng. 41(1), 142–153 (2013)

8. Stevanella, M., Maffessanti, F., Conti, C., Votta, E., Arnoldi, A., Lombardi, M., Parodi, O., Caiani, E., Redaelli, A.: Mitral valve patient-specific finite element modeling from cardiac mri: Application to an annuloplasty procedure. Cardiovascular Engineering and Technology 2(2), 66–76 (2011)

9. Ionasec, R., Voigt, I., Georgescu, B., Wang, Y., Houle, H., Vega-Higuera, F., Nassir, N., Comaniciu, D.: Patient-specific modeling and quantification of the aortic and mitral valves from 4-D cardiac CT and tee. TMI 29(9), 1636–1651 (2010)

10. Mansi, T., Voigt, I., Georgescu, B., Zheng, X., Assoumou Mengue, E., Hackl, M., Ionasec, R.T., Seeburger, J., Comaniciu, D.: An integrated framework for fnite-element modeling of mitral valve biomechanics from medical images: Application to mitralclip intervention planning. Med. Image Anal. 16(7), 1330–1346 (2012)

11. Siefert, A.W., Rabbah, J.P.M., Koomalsingh, K.J., Touchton Jr., S.A., Saikrishnan, N., McGarvey, J.R., Gorman, R.C., Gorman III, J.H., Yoganathan, A.P.: In vitro mitral valve simulator mimics systolic valvular function of chronic ischemic mitral regurgitation ovine model. Ann. Thorac. Surg. 95, 825–830 (2013)

12. Rabbah, J.P., Saikrishnan, N., Yoganathan, A.P.: A novel left heart simulator for the multi-modality characterization of native mitral valve geometry and fluid mechanics. Ann. Biomed. Eng. 31, 305–315 (2012)

13. Jimenez, J.H., Soerensen, D.D., He, Z., Ritchie, J., Yoganathan, A.P.: Effects of papillary muscle position on chordal force distribution: an in-vitro study. The Journal of Heart Valve Disease 14(3), 295–302 (2005)

14. Grbic, S., Ionasec, R., Vitanovski, D., Voigt, I., Wang, Y., Georgescu, B., Comaniciu, D.: Complete valvular heart apparatus model from 4d cardiac ct. Medical Image Analysis 16(5), 1003–1014 (2012)

15. Krishnamurthy, G., Itoh, A., Bothe, W., Swanson, J., Kuhl, E., Karlsson, M., Craig Miller, D., Ingels, N.: Stress-strain behavior of mitral valve leaflets in the beating ovine heart. J. Biomech. 42(12), 1909–1916 (2009)

16. Grady, L.: Random walks for image segmentation. IEEE Transactions on Pattern Analysis and Machine Intelligence 28(11), 1768–1783 (2006)

Robust Detection of Mitral Papillary Muscle from 4D Transesophageal Echocardiography

Mihai Scutaru[1], Ingmar Voigt[2], Tommaso Mansi[3(✉)], Anand Tatpati[4], Razvan Ionasec[5], Helene Houle[4], and Dorin Comaniciu[3]

[1] Siemens Corporate Technology, Imaging and Computer Vision, Brasov, Romania
[2] Siemens Corporate Technology, Imaging and Computer Vision, Erlangen, Germany
[3] Siemens Corporate Technology, Imaging and Computer Vision, Princeton, NJ, USA
Tommaso.mansi@siemens.com
[4] Siemens Healthcare, Clinical Products, Ultrasound, Mountain View, CA, USA
[5] Siemens Healthcare, Imaging and Therapy Systems, CR, Forchheim, Germany

Abstract. Mitral valve (MV) diseases, one of the most common valvular diseases, often require surgical repair to reduce mitral regurgitation and improve cardiac pump function. These procedures however are very complex and require careful planning. In particular, chordae replacement or sub-valvular repair demands a precise assessment of the relative position of the papillary muscles with respect to the leaflets in the beating heart. This can be achieved only before opening the chest through imaging like computerized tomography or transesophageal echocardiography (TEE). Yet, quantitative analysis of the MV structure and dynamics, in particular the papillaries, is still tedious and prone to user variability. This manuscript presents a novel approach to automatically detect and track papillary muscle tips in 4D TEE. The proposed data-driven method combines the Marginal Space Learning method with Random Sample Consensus and Belief Propagation cope with varying image quality and signal drop-offs. Experiments on 30 randomly-selected volumes show that the accuracy of our algorithm falls within inter-rater variability (5.58mm out of 6.94mm for the anterior tip and 5.75mm out of 7.06mm for the posterior tip), while being extremely fast (under 3 seconds). The proposed method could therefore provide the surgeon with quantitative MV evaluation for optimal therapy planning.

Keywords: Mitral Valve · Papillary Muscles · 4D TEE · Machine-Learning · Detection

1 Introduction

The mitral valve (MV), which ensures the unidirectional flow from the left atrium to the left ventricle, is often affected by heart failure or degenerative diseases. In particular, MV prolapse, when the leaflets billow inside the atrium during systole, is the most common source of MV regurgitation and is present in about 2% of the general population [1]. While its etiology can be diverse (e.g. chord rupture, degenerated leaflet tissues or papillary muscle displacement due to heart failure), MV prolapse is often

© Springer International Publishing Switzerland 2015
O. Camara et al. (Eds.): STACOM 2014, LNCS 8896, pp. 249–256, 2015.
DOI: 10.1007/978-3-319-14678-2_26

treated surgically through leaflet tissue resection, chord repair/replacement or papillary muscle displacement. For all these procedures, the geometry of the valve during the heartbeat must be quantified, in particular the relative position of the MV with respect to the papillary tips [2]. As this cannot be achieved during the open-heart surgery, preoperative assessment is performed using 4D trans-esophageal echocardiography (TEE). Yet, in current clinical practice this process is time consuming and prone to rater variability. More especially, automatic and robust detection of the papillary tips is challenging due to variations in image quality and the large dynamics of the organ (Fig. 1).

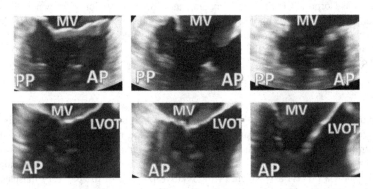

Fig. 1. Anterior (AP) and posterior (PP) papillary muscles in different cardiac phases and views. Note the variation in appearance, texture and SNR.

Methods to segment the MV and papillaries have been proposed. A first category of approaches requires user interaction to identify the landmark of interest on one frame of the cardiac sequence and then propagated automatically by using various tracking algorithms. For instance, in [6], the users identify the papillary tips on 3D TEE images according to 2D planes rotating around the mitral annulus center. In [7], the authors leverage the high spatial resolution of computed tomography (CT) to automatically segment the papillary muscles from the ventricular wall. However that method is static only and heavily relies on the details visible on the high-resolution CT to achieve correct segmentation, which is not applicable to 4D TEE. Fully automatic approaches have been pursued recently. In [3], the authors developed a method based on Marginal Space Learning to segment both aortic and mitral valves. Papillary muscles were not considered though in that work. A similar approach was introduced in [5], adding biomechanical constraints to the detection algorithm for robust leaflet tracking. Papillary tips were modeled as well, but on a frame-by-frame basis and therefore not robust to image variation and signal drop-offs.

This paper presents a novel method for robust and temporally consistent papillary tip detection and tracking from 4D TEE. Temporal boosting methods have been explored in the computer vision community [4]. Yet, because of the specificities of ultrasound imaging it is not clear how they would perform for papillary detection, in particular due to the varying image quality and the large cardiac motion, a different setup than object tracking in video. Instead, and as detailed in Section 2, we adapt the Marginal Space Learning framework presented in [3], which is particularly suited for medical images, to the papillary tips characteristics and add spatial and temporal constraints using Random Sample Consensus and Belief Propagation. Combined with the algorithm described in [3], the end result of our algorithm is a complete 4D representation of the whole MV sub-anatomy (Fig. 2). Experiments on 30 volumes show that the accuracy of the proposed method is within inter-user variability (Section 3). Section 4 concludes the manuscript.

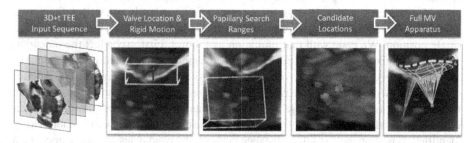

Fig. 2. Processing pipeline of the proposed algorithm: 1) MV Location & Motion estimation with MSL & RANSAC 2) Search range prediction using learned spatial coordinate mapping from MV box 3) Candidate locations estimated within search ranges 3) Final result obtained by applying spatio-temporal constraints using belief propagation

2   Method

Fig. 2 illustrates the different steps of our approach. First, an accurate and robust box is detected in the volume to identify the MV location. This is achieved using Marginal Space Learning (MSL) [8], which enables to detect the position, orientation and scale of the MV box in a 3D volume using Haar features and Probabilistic Boosting Trees [9]. In order to ensure temporal consistency throughout the sequence, in particular with large cardiac motion, the MSL is extended by using the RANSAC algorithm (RANdom SAmple Consensus) [10]. More precisely, the bounding box detection is run on a random subset of frames from the entire dynamic sequence. By running RANSAC over the resulting candidates, a best fitting box is derived for the whole subset. Specifically box candidate samples as previously estimated via MSL are incrementally clustered creating possible box hypotheses for each frame. For a finite number of 40 RANSAC iterations one box hypothesis is randomly drawn out of all frames. Subsequently distance to all remaining hypotheses is computed using a compound distance based on the valve box center and it's scaled axes. Distances that are smaller than an empirical threshold of 7mm are considered as inliers. As a result, any potential detection outliers due to signal drop-off or noise are avoided, and the overall detection method is more robust.

Once the MV box is identified, the next step consists in determining the search ranges of the papillary muscle landmarks with respect to the MV box. To achieve this, during the training phase, the expert annotations are gathered and principal component analysis (PCA) is performed on 3D landmark positions. By using all the instances of annotated muscle landmarks as input for PCA, a best fitting model is obtained, in the form of a 3D box encompassing all the positions and forming a search range. This search range is used as input to a Probabilistic Boosting Tree [9] classifier that leverages Haar features to identify the position of the landmark within the PCA-based search range.

Despite the previous spatio-temporal constraints, variations in image quality may lead to landmark candidates that are not clustered within the search range. This type of candidate distribution, spread throughout the search range makes the selection of the optimal candidates harder. In those cases, the target position is not well-defined as it would have been in the case where the majority of candidates are clustered around a single position. We cope with that limitation as follows. First, we select the 60 candidates with highest probability (number defined empirically). Then, other landmarks identified during the Mitral Valve detection process are used as reference. The anterior commissure is used for the anterior papillary muscle and the posterior commissure for the posterior papillary muscle. These landmarks are detected through similar mechanisms and thanks to more specific image features, their position is more easily identified. Based on the Euclidian distance between the candidates and these anchors, a selection is done as by excluding candidates that are not within 10mm and 30mm for the anterior tip and not within 15mm and 40mm for the posterior tip. The values were determined empirically in order to avoid detector responses on the valve leaflets or inside the ventricular wall for instance and the thresholds have been determined based on anatomical knowledge and analysis of available data (normal and pathological). For increased robustness, we further rely on temporal information from multiple frames of the TEE. The main objective is to find the most probable position of the papillary tips by gathering information from all previous frames. All the candidates that have been detected so far are organized in the form of a graphical model [11]. A small scale representation of this model is illustrated in Fig. 3. The idea is to select the appropriate candidate in each frame that minimizes the cost needed to traverse the graph.

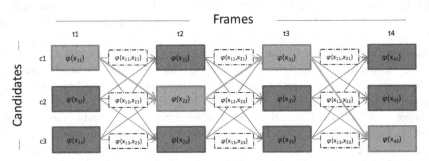

Fig. 3. Graphical model used as a basis for Belief Propagation. See text for details

Let V be the set of graph nodes and E the set of edges. We also define $x(v)$ as the random variable associated with graph node v and $\varphi(x_v)$ as the unary cost represented by the candidate's associated probability as returned by the MSL position detection. The pair-wise cost of each edge, $\varphi(x_u, x_v)$, is defined by the Euclidian distance between the candidates at either end of the edge. Therefore each graph node is characterized by two values: the unary cost used to rank between candidates on the same frame, and the pair-wise cost, used to rank the distances to candidates on the neighboring frame. The joint probability distribution of all the variables in the graph is expressed as a pair-wise Markov Random Field:

$$p(X) = \prod_{v \in V} \varphi_v(x_v) \prod_{\{u,v\} \in E} \varphi_{u,v}(x_u, x_v)$$

To find the best combination of candidates from the above described graph, max-product belief propagation is used. In this algorithm, messages are defined between neighboring nodes as a method of ranking the path taken through the graph. Let $m_{u \to v}^{(t)}(x_v)$ be the max-product message from the node u to the node v at as a function of x_v while also taking into account previous iterations.

$$m_{u \to v}^{(t)}(x_v) = \max_{x_u \in X_u} \left[\varphi_v(x_v) \varphi_{u,v}(x_u, x_v) \left(\prod_{w \in \Gamma(u) \backslash v} m_{w \to u}^{(t-1)}(x_u) \right) \right]$$

Let $\mu_v(x_v)$ be the estimated belief at node x_v and defined by the max-marginal of x_v:

$$\mu_v(x_v) = \max_{x' \mid x'_v = x_v} p(x'_1, x'_2, \dots, x'_N)$$

which can be approximated as:

$$\mu_v(x_v) \propto \varphi_v(x_v) \left(\prod_{w \in \Gamma(v)} m_{w \to v}^{(t)}(x_v) \right)$$

Given these max-marginals, the MAP (maximum a posteriori estimation) estimation is computed such that $\hat{x} \in \text{argmax}_{x'} \ p(x'_1, x'_2, \dots, x'_N)$. Based on this result, the most efficient path through the graph is obtained, as highlighted in Fig. 3, effectively providing a temporal refinement to the candidate selection process. This method is applied to all detected candidates available from the previous stages of the detection pipeline and provides the desired result, choosing the candidate in the current frame that has the closest Euclidian distance to similar candidates in neighboring frames.

3   Experiments and Results

3.1   Protocol

150 TEE volumes with variable spatial and temporal resolution were used in our experiments. Among them, 120 were randomly selected as training-set; the remaining 30 volumes were used for testing. This testing set included 5 ischemic Mitral Valve cases, 10 Mitral Valve prolapsed cases as well as 15 normal anatomies. An expert manually annotated the papillary tips in all images. For 11 volumes out of the 30 test-sets (random selection), two additional experts annotated the papillary tips for inter-rater variability assessment.

3.2   Qualitative Evaluation

Fig. 4 illustrates the detected papillary tips in one typical case. Using only a position detector yielded a large number of candidates, and for both landmarks it can be observed that further refinement is required to obtain accurate results. Due to the low level of clustering observed in the upper part of the figure concerning the anterior papillary tip, the spatial optimizations play a key role in refining the input used for the belief propagation algorithm in the final temporal optimization phase. This latter stage is crucial in obtaining accurate position estimation. As can be observed form all panels from Fig. 4 the final selected landmark is always within a small distance of the expert annotated position. The actual quantization of this accuracy can be found in section 3.3.

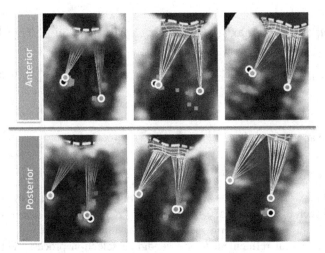

Fig. 4. Results in different examples. Landmark position candidates (green) for anterior (top row) and posterior (bottom row) papillary tip. Final estimation result obtained via temporal optimization using belief propagation are overlaid (orange / cyan for anterior and posterior papillary tip respectively) together with expert ground truth (black)

3.3   Quantitative Evaluation

Table 1 reports the results of the quantitative evaluation on the 30 test volumes. The Euclidean distance was used to assess the accuracy of the detected papillary tip position with respect to the annotated ground truth. As one can see, our proposed approach yielded significantly better results than if position detectors only were used (almost a 2-fold improvement). To further assess the obtained level of accuracy, we investigated the inter-rater variability in terms of papillary tip identification in 11 images. In these experiments, the proposed algorithm felt within rater variability (Table 1).

Table 1. Performance evaluation in mm (mean ± standard deviation). As one can see, the accuracy of the proposed algorithm was within rater variability.

	Anterior Tip Position (mm)	Posterior Tip Position (mm)
Proposed Approach	5.58 ± 3.46	5.75 ± 3.02
Detection Only	10.65 ± 4.09	11.32 ± 4.25
Inter-Rater Variability	6.94	7.06

We also evaluated the performance of the algorithm in terms of inter-papillary distance to evaluate the clinical utility of the proposed method (Fig. 5). The measurement was reported at two time points of the cardiac sequence: peak aortic (approx. mid systole) and peak mitral (approx. end diastole). Except for one case, the measurement at peak aortic was always below the 95% confidence interval defined by the raters. This was expected as papillaries are more visible during that phase of the cardiac cycle since they are normally clearly detached from the myocardial wall. At peak mitral, detection is challenged by the visual "fusion" of the papillaries with the wall, which increases uncertainty. Despite this challenge though, our algorithm was still able to recover inter-papillary distance within rater variability in about 75% of the cases.

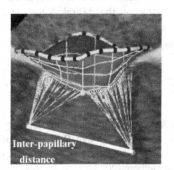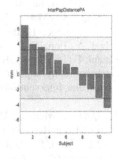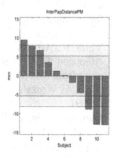

Fig. 5. Computed inter-papillary distance compared to raters at peak aortic (left panel) and peak mitral (right panel). *Blue vertical bars*: deviation of the inter-papillary distance computed from our algorithm with respect to the average expert measurements. *Light-blue and light-yellow regions*: 80 and 95% confidence intervals computed from the variation across all experts. As one can see, computed inter-papillary distance was within inter-rater variability.

4   Conclusion

This paper presented a novel algorithm for the accurate and robust detection of the left ventricular papillary muscles. In particular, clinical measurements derived from the proposed approach were within inter-user variability, while being extremely fast to compute (under 3s/frame on a test machine with a quad core processor). Such an approach could therefore constitute a surrogate tool for MV repair planning [12][13]. Future works include evaluation on more cases, extension of the method to other cardiac landmarks and application to biomechanical modeling of MV function, as for the first time robust papillary detection and tracking is available.

Acknowledgement. This paper is supported by the Sectoral Operational Programme Human Resources Development (SOP HRD), ID134378 financed from the European Social Fund and by the Romanian Government.

References

1. Lloyd-Jones, D., Adams, R., Carnethon, M., De Simone, G., Ferguson, T.B., Flegal, K., Ford, E., Furie, K., Go, A., Greenlund, K., et al.: American Heart Association Statistics Committee and Stroke Statistics Subcommittee, Heart disease and stroke statistics–2009 update: a report from the American heart association statistics committee and stroke statistics subcommittee. Circulation **119**, e21–e181 (2009)
2. Carpentier, A., Adams, D.H., Filsoufi, F.: Carpentier's Reconstructive Valve Surgery. From Valve Analysis to Valve Reconstruction. 2010 Saunders Elsevier (2010)
3. Ionasec, R., Voigt, I., Georgescu, B., Wang, Y., Houle, H., Vega, F., Navab, N., Comaniciu, D.: Patient-Specific Modeling and Quantification of the Aortic and Mitral valves from 4D Cardiac CT and TEE. IEEE Trans. Medical Imaging **29**(9), 1636–1651 (2010)
4. Kim, T., Woodley, T., Stenger, B., Cipolla, R.: Online Multiple Classifier Boosting for Object Tracking. In: IEEE Computer Vision and Pattern Recognition Workshops (2010)
5. Voigt, I., Mansi, T., Ionasec, R.I., Mengue, E.A., Houle, H., Georgescu, B., Hornegger, J., Comaniciu, D.: Robust Physically-Constrained Modeling of the Mitral Valve and Subvalvular Apparatus. In: Fichtinger, G., Martel, A., Peters, T. (eds.) MICCAI 2011, Part III. LNCS, vol. 6893, pp. 504–511. Springer, Heidelberg (2011)
6. Votta, E., Arnoldi, A., Invernizzi, A., Ponzini, R., Veronesi, F., Tamborini, G., Pepi, M., Alamanni, F., Redaelli, A., Caiani, E.G.: Mitral valve patient-specific finite element modeling from 3-D real time echocardiography: a potential new tool for surgical planning. In: MICCAI Workshop on Cardiovascular Interventional Imaging and Biophysical Modelling (2009)
7. Gao, M., Chen, C., Zhang, S., Qian, Z., Metaxas, D., Axel, L.: Segmenting the Papillary Muscles and the Trabeculae from High Resolution Cardiac CT through Restoration of Topological Handles. In: Gee, J.C., Joshi, S., Pohl, K.M., Wells, W.M., Zöllei, L. (eds.) IPMI 2013. LNCS, vol. 7917, pp. 184–195. Springer, Heidelberg (2013)
8. Zheng, Y., Georgescu, B., Lingm, H., Zhou, S.K., Scheuering, M., Comaniciu, D.: Constrained Marginal Space Learning for Efficient 3D Anatomical Structure Detection in Medical Images. In: IEEE Conf. Computer Vision and Pattern Recognition (CVPR 2009), Miami, FL (2009)
9. Tu, Z.: Probabilistic Boosting-Tree: Learning Discriminative Models for Classification, Recognition, and Clustering. In: ICCV 2005 (2005)
10. Hast, A., Nysjo, J., Marcetti, A.: Optimal RANSAC - Towards a Repeatable Algorithm for Finding the Optimal Set. Journal of WSCG (2013)
11. Kothapa, R., Pacheco, J., Sudderth, E.B.: Max-Product Particle Belief Propagation, Master Thesis, Brown (2011)
12. Kanik, J., Mansi, T., Voigt, I., Sharma, P., Ionasec, R., Comaniciu, D., Duncan, J.: Estimation of Patient-Specific Material Properties of the Mitral Valve using 4D Transesophageal Echocardiography, ISBI (2013)
13. Mansi, T., Voigt, I., Mengue, E., Ionasec, R., Georgescu, B., Noack, T., Seeburger, J., Comaniciu, D.: Towards Patient-Specific Finite-Element Simulation of MitralClip Procedure. In: Fichtinger, G., Martel, A., Peters, T. (eds.) MICCAI 2011, Part I. LNCS, vol. 6891, pp. 452–459. Springer, Heidelberg (2011)

Reusability of Statistical Shape Models for the Segmentation of Severely Abnormal Hearts

Xènia Albà[1]([✉]), Karim Lekadir[1], Corné Hoogendoorn[1], Marco Pereanez[1],
Andrew J. Swift[2], Jim M. Wild[2], and Alejandro F. Frangi[3]

[1] Center for Computational Imaging and Simulation Technologies in Biomedicine
(CISTIB), Universitat Pompeu Fabra, Barcelona, Spain
xenia.alba@upf.edu
[2] Academic Unit of Radiology, University of Sheffield, Sheffield, UK
[3] CISTIB, Department of Mechanical Engineering, University of Sheffield,
Sheffield, UK

Abstract. Statistical shape models have been widely employed in cardiac image segmentation. In practice, however, the construction of the models is faced with several challenges, in particular the need for a sufficiently large training database and a detailed delineation of the training images. Moreover, for pathologies that induce severe shape remodeling such as for pulmonary hypertension (PH), a statistical model is rarely capable of encoding the significant and complex variability of the class. This work presents a new approach for the segmentation of abnormal hearts by reusing statistical shape models built from normal population. To this end, a normalization of the pathological image data is first performed towards the space of the normal shape model, which is then used to guide the segmentation process. Subsequently, the model recovered in the space of normal anatomies is propagated back to the pathological images space. Detailed validation with PH image data shows that the method is both accurate and consistent in its segmentation of highly remodeled hearts.

1 Introduction

Automatic segmentation of severely abnormal hearts is an important yet challenging research topic in cardiac image analysis. Of the existing potential solutions, statistical models of shape have attracted significant attention due to their ability to encode the space of plausible segmentation from a training population. On the other hand, the literature on cardiac shape models in particular based on active shape models (ASMs) is mostly limited to samples of normal or mildly abnormal hearts [1–4]. Such models are known to have limited accuracy when dealing with highly remodeled ventricles. A potential solution would consist of having multiple statistical shape models for different cardiac pathologies but this is unrealistic in practice due the challenges of each model construction, which requires the collection of a sufficiently large and representative training data

O. Camara et al. (Eds.): STACOM 2014, LNCS 8896, pp. 257–264, 2015.
DOI: 10.1007/978-3-319-14678-2_27

set, as well as a detailed delineation of the ventricles with point correspondence. In this paper, we propose a method to segment severely abnormal hearts by re-using a statistical model previously constructed from a normal population.

To illustrate the potential of the proposed technique, we choose pulmonary hypertension (PH) as the exemplar application in this paper. PH describes a group of rapidly progressive conditions defined by a mean pulmonary arterial pressure greater than or equal to 25 mmHg which results in a progressive increase in pulmonary vascular resistance [5], in turn leading to complex shape remodeling of both the left and right ventricles (see Fig. 1). In a healthy heart, the RV generally has a crescent-like shape and is smaller than the more circular LV. In contrast, in a patient with PH, the RV becomes very dilated and remodeled, pushing onto the LV, which deforms and loses its roundness [6]. Such severe shape remodeling means the application of statistical shape models is challenging for PH datasets.

In this paper, we present a method for accurate segmentation of severely abnormal hearts using ASMs. More specifically, instead of segmenting directly the patient image data, we first perform a transformation of the input image data onto a reference template representing a normal heart. This allows the subsequent use of a reference point distribution model (PDM) built from a normal population for the segmentation of the abnormal case without the necessity to train and use a statistical model specifically for the pathology in question. After ASM search in the normal space, back propagation of the segmentation result onto the original image space is carried out. While conceptually simple, the proposed technique increases the re-usability of cardiac shape models and the applicability of ASMs in clinical cardiac imaging. An experimental study is also presented based on a sample of deformed hearts corresponding to 20 PH cases, with detailed comparison to the direct use of normal and pathological statistical models.

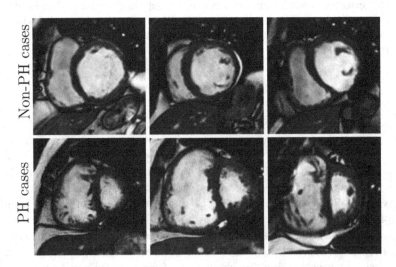

Fig. 1. Short axis MR images from non-PH (top) and PH (bottom) patients

2   Materials and Methods

The aim of this work is to automatically segment severely abnormal hearts using a statistical shape modeling approach combined with an image normalization. In this paper, we choose cases of PH as the exemplar application due to the great magnitude of the shape remodeling induced by this pathology as illustrated in Fig. 1. The proposed method is a modification of the well-known ASM technique [7], such that a standard reference PDM can be used to segment such severely abnormal shapes.

2.1   Datasets

Two sets of data are used in this study to illustrate the benefits of the proposed technique. First, we use a database that includes 20 MR datasets corresponding to 20 patients all affected with pulmonary hypertension (PH). MR imaging was performed on a 1.5T whole body scanner GE HDx (GE Healthcare, Milwaukee, USA), and comprise stacks of short axis images obtained using a bSSFP sequence (20 frames per cycle, FOV 48, matrix 256×256, bandwidth 125 KHz/pixel, TR/TE 3.7/1.6ms). Slice thickness was 8 mm, with a pixel spacing of 0.9375×0.9375 mm.

Furthermore, the aim of this work is to demonstrate that even the most severely abnormal hearts can be segmented with the proposed technique by using a unique normal PDM without the need for re-training with a group a pathological scans. To this end, we collect 20 MR datasets of healthy volunteers (with normal cardiac parameters such as ejection fraction). They were acquired using a 1.5T Philips Achieva System (Philips Healthcare, Best, The Netherlands), comprise stacks of short axis images obtained using a cine SSFP sequence (TR/TE 2.9/1.5ms, flip angle 40°, matrix 256×256). Slice thickness was 8mm, with pixel spacing of 1.42×1.42 mm.

2.2   Normal and Abnormal Shape Models

Two statistical models of shape (using the two samples) were constructed in this work to evaluate the relative strength of the proposed technique, namely one from the normal population and one from the pathological population. Both PDMs were built using the same standard approach as introduced by Cootes et al. [7].

For both PDMs, it is important to extract the training shapes with point correspondence before the building of the models. The main stages of the shape extraction include the labeling of the MRI slices (LV endocardium, RV endocardium, epicardium), thus obtaining binary masks, the derivation of volumetric meshes from the binary images using the Marching Cubes algorithm and, finally, the extraction of the surface meshes. We used the projection method in [8] to establish point correspondence across the training shapes.

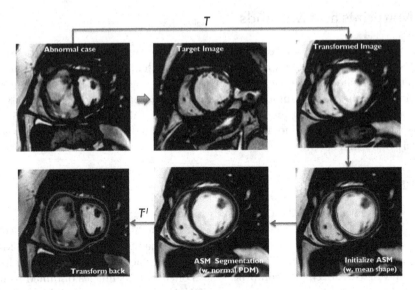

Fig. 2. Schematic workflow of the proposed method

2.3   Proposed Technique: ASMs with Image Transformation

ASMs have been widely employed in medical image segmentation. However, they rely on a (preferably large) set of training data representative of the images to be segmented. For pathological cases, both data set size and representability become increasingly difficult to achieve due to the higher and more complex variability within the class of shapes to be modeled. Furthermore, re-training of statistical models to accommodate for the new shape variability is tedious as it requires the collection and detailed delineation of a new training set.

The aim of the work is to achieve an accurate segmentation of the myocardial walls by reusing already built models and while eliminating the necessity of the cardiac model to be tailored to specific pathology and/or severity. Fig. 2 shows schematically how this is achieved. First, the image to be segmented is transformed so that the embedded shape becomes sufficiently normal (it falls within the PDM's permitted shape space). Then the transformed image is segmented and, subsequently, transformed back to match the original image.

In what follows, we describe the details of the proposed algorithm. Let us denote $\mathbf{I}_{PH}$ the new pathological scan that we want segment using ASMs and a normal PDM as previously constructed (with a mean shape $\bar{\mathbf{x}}$ and a matrix of eigenvectors $\mathbf{P}$). A standard ASM segmentation of cardiac images starts with an initialization, typically by defining key anatomical landmarks such as the apex, valve points and some landmarks on the mid-ventricular slice. Let us denote these initial points as $\mathbf{y} = (\mathbf{y}_1, ... \mathbf{y}_m)^T$. In this work, we used $m = 9$ landmarks to initialize each ventricle (four on the base, four on the mid-ventricular slice, one the apex). Subsequently, in a standard image search, these points are used to place the mean shape in the new image $\mathbf{I}_{PH}$, before the application of the ASM algorithm [7].

The problem with this approach is that the image $\mathbf{I}_{PH}$ deviates highly from the allowable shape domain as defined by the reference PDM of normality. To address this issue, the fundamental idea behind the proposed method is to apply a transformation T of $\mathbf{I}_{PH}$ onto the space of normality such that the reference PDM can then be used to guide the segmentation of the transformed image:

$$\mathbf{I}_{new} = T(\mathbf{I}_{PH}). \tag{1}$$

The estimation of T is critical in the proposed work. The simplest solution would be to perform a nonrigid image registration between $\mathbf{I}_{PH}$ and a reference image $\mathbf{I}_{ref}$ of a normal subject. Such method, however, is computationally expensive and is likely to introduce localized errors due to the significant and complex shape differences between the pathological and normal image scans. Consequently, it is not guaranteed that the deformed image will lie necessary in the space of the normal PDM.

A faster and more robust approach is used in this paper, by taking advantage of the ASM initialization, more specifically of the initial points $\mathbf{y} = (\mathbf{y}_1, ...\mathbf{y}_m)^T$, to calculate a landmark-based transformation from $\mathbf{I}_{PH}$ to the space of normality. To achieve this, the initial points are also defined on the mean normal shape $\bar{\mathbf{x}}$ and we obtain the points $\bar{\mathbf{y}} = (\bar{\mathbf{y}}_1, ...\bar{\mathbf{y}}_m)^T$. Then, we apply a thin plate spline (TPS) model [9] between the two sets of points $\mathbf{y}$ and $\bar{\bar{y}}$, and we obtain:

$$T = \mathrm{TPS}(\mathbf{y}, \bar{\mathbf{y}}). \tag{2}$$

We choose TPS in this paper as it is both smooth and invertible, which are necessary properties for the proposed technique.

As shown in Fig. 2, this approach enables to transform the image volume from a severely abnormal case to a pseudo-normal image scan. However, due to the use of only a few initial points to calculate the TPS, only a rough initial matching is obtained between the new image $\mathbf{I}_{new}$ and the mean shape. An ASM segmentation is therefore necessary to fit locally and accurately the shape model to the deformed image data. In this paper, we use a modified version of the SPASM method by van Assen et al. [10] for cardiac image segmentation as it can deal with sparse multi-slice MRI data. We obtain a segmented shape $\mathbf{x}_{new}$ in the deformed image $\mathbf{I}_{new}$.

Finally, this result is propagated back to the original pathological image space based on the transformation T, i.e., we obtain:

$$\mathbf{x}_{PH} = T^{-1}(\mathbf{x}_{new}). \tag{3}$$

3   Evaluation

In this study, we report the results of segmenting the 20 PH cases described in Sect. 2.1 using three different methods: 1) ASMs with a PDM of normal cases, 2) ASMs with a PDM of PH cases (leave-one-out basis), and 3) the proposed method

Table 1. Point-to-surface error statistics using the three segmentation approaches

	Mean	SD	Max	Min
Normal PDM	3.44	0.82	4.87	2.66
Abnormal PDM	3.01	0.50	4.04	2.38
Proposed technique	2.63	0.35	3.12	1.89

SD=Standard Deviation; Distances expressed in mm

(normal PDM combined with image normalization). For a fair comparison, the same anatomical landmarks are used in the three methods to initialize the method. To validate the resulting segmentation using the different approaches, the agreement between manual and automatic data analysis was assessed on epicardial and endocardial contours for LV and RV.

The segmentation errors for the 20 datasets are summarized in Table 1. It shows that the proposed method has greater accuracy (mean P2S error well below 3mm; max below 3.2mm) and consistency (P2S error SD below 0.5mm) than either of the other two approaches (maximal errors of 4.87 mm and 4.04 mm for the normal and PH PDMs, respectively).

The results on a per-case basis are displayed in Fig. 3, showing that the proposed technique outperforms the ASM with abnormal training data in 90% of the cases, with minimal differences in the remaining two cases (1 and 17). As expected, the normal PDM on its own generally lacks the flexibility required to segment the highly remodeled PH hearts, performing worst in 85% of the cases. It is worth noting that there are cases in which the normal PDM performs better than the PH

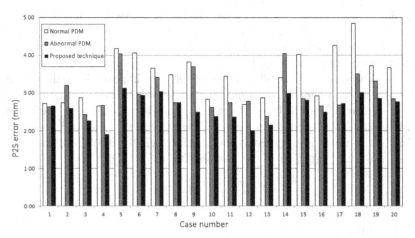

Fig. 3. Comparison of the point-to-surface (P2S) errors (in mm) between the segmentations using normal PDM (white), abnormal PDM (gray), and the proposed technique (black)

(a)   (b)   (c)

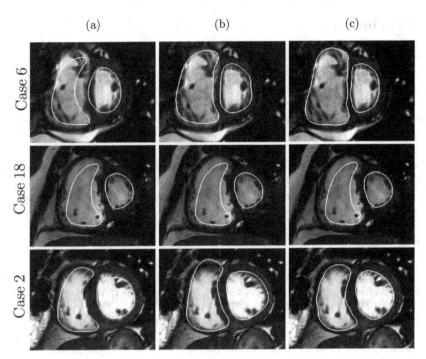

Fig. 4. Three examples showing endocardial segmentations using (a) a normal PDM, (b) an abnormal PDM, and (c) the proposed technique

PDM (cases 2, 12 and 14), illustrating the difficulty of obtaining a representative set of pathological cases for optimal model construction.

To illustrate the strength of the proposed ASM approach, visual examples are displayed in Fig. 4. The two first examples correspond to severely abnormal hearts (RV much bigger than the LV, LV very deformed), while the third example has a less pronounced abnormality. It can be seen that the proposed approach is more accurate in its segmentation of both ventricles for all the examples. For the two severe cases (6 and 18), the normal PDM naturally fails due to the change in relative ventricle size. We can also observe that the lost of roundness of the LV is not valid according to the normal PDM, resulting in an error in the LV septal wall. The abnormal PDM has a better performance but localized errors at the RV show the difficulty to correctly capture the huge RV variability in PH in a single PDM. The proposed technique, on the other hand, is accurate in all regions of the ventricles.

For the mildly abnormal case, the normal PDM performs better than the abnormal PDM due to the fact that the shape deformations are not as severe as those captured from the PH training sample. In particular, the RV is not very dilated in this case and falls instead in the acceptable range of the normal PDM. The proposed method still performs well in such example.

4   Conclusions

In this paper, we have presented a method that enables accurate and consistent LV-RV myocardial segmentation in MRI for abnormally-shaped hearts. The focal point of the study is the use of point distribution models of a normal population in the segmentation of images in the presence of pathology and related remodeling. While demonstrated on PH cases, the method can be applied to other cardiac pathologies such as hypertrophic cardiomyopathy (HCM).

Acknowledgments. The work of X. Albà was supported by an FPU grant from the Spanish Ministry of Education Culture and Sport. The work of K. Lekadir was supported by a Juan de la Cierva research fellowship from the Spanish Ministry of Science and Innovation.

References

1. Zhu, Y., Papademetris, X., Sinusas, A.J., Duncan, J.S.: Segmentation of the left ventricle from cardiac MR images using a subject-specific dynamical model. IEEE Trans. Med. Imaging **29**(3), 669–687 (2010)
2. Lekadir, K., Merrifield, R., Yang, G.Z.: Outlier detection and handling for robust 3-D active shape models search. IEEE Trans. Med. Imaging **26**(2), 212–222 (2007)
3. ElBaz, M.S., Fahmy, A.S.: Active shape model with inter-profile modeling paradigm for cardiac right ventricle segmentation. In: Ayache, N., Delingette, H., Golland, P., Mori, K. (eds.) MICCAI 2012, Part I. LNCS, vol. 7510, pp. 691–698. Springer, Heidelberg (2012)
4. Hoogendoorn, C., Duchateau, N., Snchez-Quintana, D., Whitmarsh, T., Sukno, F.M., De Craene, M., Lekadir, K., Frangi, A.: A high-resolution atlas and statistical model of the human heart from multislice CT. IEEE Trans. Med. Imaging **32**(1), 28–44 (2013)
5. Swift, A., Rajaram, S., Condliffe, R., Capener, D., Hurdman, J., Elliot, C., Wild, J., Kiely, D.: Diagnostic accuracy of cardiovascular magnetic resonance imaging of right ventricular morphology and function in the assessment of suspected pulmonary hypertension results from the ASPIRE registry. J. Cardiovasc. Magn. Reson. **14**(40) (2012)
6. Voelkel, N., Quaife, R., Leinwand, L., Barst, R., McGoon, M., Meldrum, D., Dupuis, J., Long, C., Rubin, L., Smart, F., Suzuki, Y., Gladwin, M., Denholm, E., Gail, D.: Right ventricular function and failure: report of a National Heart, Lung, and Blood institute working group on cellular and molecular mechanisms of right heart failure. Circulation **114**(17), 1883–91 (2006)
7. Cootes, T., Taylor, C.J., Cooper, D.H., Graham, J.: Active shape models - their training and application. Comput. Vis. Image Und. **61**(1), 38–59 (1995)
8. Pereanez, M., Lekadir, K., Butakoff, C., Hoogendoorn, C., Frangi, A.F.: A framework for the merging of pre-existing and correspondenceless 3D statistical shape models. Med. Image Anal. (2014). doi:10.1016/j.media.2014.05.009
9. Bookstein, F.L.: Principal warps: Thin-plate splines and the decomposition of deformations. IEEE Trans. Pattern Anal. Mach. Intell. **11**(6), 567–585 (1989)
10. van Assen, H.C., Danilouchkine, M.G., Frangi, A.F., Ordas, S., Westenberg, J.J., Reiber, J.H., Lelieveldt, B.P.: SPASM: A 3D-ASM for segmentation of sparse and arbitrarily oriented cardiac MRI data. Med. Image Anal. **10**(2), 286–303 (2006)

Registration of Real-Time and Prior Imaging Data with Applications to MR Guided Cardiac Interventions

Robert Xu[1,2,3](✉) and Graham A. Wright[1,2,3]

[1] Department of Medical Biophysics, University of Toronto, Toronto, ON, Canada
[2] Physical Sciences Platform, Sunnybrook Research Institute, Toronto, ON, Canada
[3] Schulich Heart Research Program, Sunnybrook Research Institute,
Toronto, ON, Canada
robert.xu@mail.utoronto.ca

Abstract. Recently, there has been increased interest in using magnetic resonance imaging (MRI) to guide interventional procedures due to its excellent soft tissue contrast and lack of ionizing radiation. One of the applications is the use of MRI to guide radio-frequency (RF) ablations for the treatment of cardiac arrhythmia. However, MRI is challenging as there exists significant tradeoffs between the imaging quality and acquisition time. High quality, pre-operative 3D MR images can be acquired with excellent spatial resolution at the expense of long acquisitions. Alternatively, 2D real-time MR imaging during the intervention sacrifices image quality for the ability to visualize dynamic motion of the heart. Therefore, to improve the MRI guidance capabilities for cardiac interventions, we propose a novel registration method to align the real-time and prior imaging data, which corrects for motion errors between the two datasets. The proposed method uses a hybrid metric within a multi-resolution registration framework to achieve the desired clinical accuracy for cardiac interventions. Registration experiments were performed with *in vivo* human images, and the mean alignment error between real-time and prior images after registration was 3.91 ± 1.52 mm.

Keywords: Cardiac MRI · Image guided therapy · Image registration · Motion correction

1 Introduction

Although death rates from heart disease and stroke have steadily declined in recent years, cardiovascular complications remain among the most common causes of death [8]. One of the sources of cardiac death is ventricular tachycardia (VT), which can be triggered by structural heart disease due to previous myocardial infarctions. Currently, the curative treatment of susceptibility to VT involves radio frequency (RF) ablation of anatomical substrates inside the heart. This is a challenging task due to the small size of the anatomical substrate, and the fact that the heart is

© Springer International Publishing Switzerland 2015
O. Camara et al. (Eds.): STACOM 2014, LNCS 8896, pp. 265–274, 2015.
DOI: 10.1007/978-3-319-14678-2_28

in constant motion. Therefore, an effective visual guidance protocol for this procedure has not been established and is the focus of a number of research studies [2,6,11,14].

In current clinical practice, electrophysiologists use x-ray fluoroscopy and electroanatomical mapping (EAM) to guide the interventional catheter towards the anatomical substrate. However, magnetic resonance imaging (MRI) has been proposed recently as an alternative interventional guidance tool, due to its superior soft tissue contrast and lack of ionizing radiation [6,14]. Previously, authors in [2,7,14] have shown promising feasibility results through the use of high quality pre-procedural 3D MR images to guide cardiac interventions. However, this is not ideal, as the heart is a mobile organ that moves during the procedure due to cardiac and respiratory motions. Alternatively, other studies have relied on 2D real-time (RT) intra-procedural MR images for guiding cardiac interventions [1,5,6]. Higher acquisition frame rates of RT images enable visualization of the heart motions in real-time, at the expense of reduced image quality, and restriction to imaging a single 2D plane [5]. Ideally, one should combine the advantages of RT imaging and high image resolution from pre-procedural images by registering the two datasets together. To this extent, a pre-clinical study [13] demonstrated the feasibility of intra-modality registration between real-time 2D MR images and pre-procedural 3D MR images. In their optimal setting, the capture range of the algorithm was reported for up to 10 mm of initial mis-alignment. Although promising, this could be a limitation in human studies, where the heart can potentially move by more than 10 mm due to respiratory motion [12]. Therefore, in this study, we chose to extend the work of [13] for intra-modality registration of MR images for humans. In particular, we evaluated a novel multi-resolution registration approach using a hybrid combination of distance metrics, and assessed the feasibility of registering prior 3D roadmaps to 2D real-time data for MRI-based cardiac interventions.

2   Methods

2.1   Image Acquisition

Prior roadmap image: The cardiac images for the experiments described in this study were acquired from four volunteers on a 1.5T MRI scanner (GE Healthcare, Waukesha, WI). For the pre-procedural roadmap images, multi-slice 3D volumes were acquired at end expiration breath-hold and during the end-diastolic cardiac phase. Each volume consists of a stack of short-axis (SAX) slices of the heart. The electrocardiogram (ECG) gated, GE FIESTA pulse sequence was used to obtain resolution of $1.37 \times 1.37 \times 8$ mm^3 with a field of view (FOV) = 350 mm.

Real-time images: A fast spiral balanced-stead state free precision sequence was used to acquire the real-time images. The obtained resolution was $2.3 \times 2.3 \times 8$ mm^3 with a frame rate of 8 Hz and FOV = 350 mm. The geometrical locations of the real-time slice prescriptions were equivalent to the slice locations in the pre-procedural scans, and the acquisitions were also performed at end-expiration breath-hold. This stack of 2D RT imaging slices was also cardiac gated to end-diastole and is thus optimally aligned with the multi-slice images in the 3D pre-procedural volume.

2.2   Multi-resolution Registration Framework

In general, solving a registration problem between a template image T and a reference image R amounts to finding an optimal transformation w that is applied to T, such that the difference between the transformed image $T[w]$ and the reference image R would be minimized. Mathematically, this task can be formulated as an optimization problem as follows:

$$\arg \min_{w} \left\{ \mathcal{D}(T[w], R) \right\},$$

(1)

where $\mathcal{D}$ measures the difference between the two images. In this study, R corresponds to a single 2D RT image, whereas T corresponds to an imaging slice from the 3D prior roadmap volume. Specifically, the 2D RT image intersects the 3D prior roadmap image at a known slice location given by the physical MR scanner coordinates, and the difference is measured between these two overlapping slice images. As we apply transformations w to the 3D prior image, the intersecting slice is updated correspondingly, and a difference measure is computed between the 2D RT and the updated intersecting slice image from the 3D prior. The search space of w is constrained to 3D rigid body transformations because the acquired RT and prior images are both ECG gated to the same cardiac phase. The minimization procedure in the registration framework was implemented using the simplex algorithm [10]. Furthermore, the optimization problem is solved in a multi-resolution framework. This is demonstrated in Fig. 1, where the original images are down-sampled and registered at 3 resolution levels in a coarse-to-fine manner.

2.3   Distance Measures

The choice of distance measure is critical to the success of the optimization in (1). Hence, a number of different metrics were evaluated for the purpose of this study. One of the commonly used metrics described in registration literature [9] is sum of squared differences (SSD). SSD is computationally inexpensive, and is excellent for mono-modality datasets where it assumes the registered images differ by Gaussian noise. Another prevalent registration metric, MI [15], is derived from information theory. MI is a robust metric, which only assumes that a probabilistic relationship between voxel intensities is maximized at optimal registration. More recently, normalized gradient fields (NGF) [4], has been proposed as an alternative to mutual information, and is defined as:

$$\text{NGF} = \frac{1}{2} \int_{\Omega} \langle \mathbf{n}(T, \mathbf{x}), \mathbf{n}(R, \mathbf{x}) \rangle^2,$$

$$\mathbf{n}(I, \mathbf{x}) := \frac{\nabla I(\mathbf{x})}{\|\nabla I(\mathbf{x})\|_{\varepsilon}} \cdot$$

(2)

where $\langle \cdot, \cdot \rangle$ denotes the inner product, and $\mathbf{n}$ represents the normalized gradient of the image. For $\mathbf{x} \in \mathbb{R}^d$, $\|\mathbf{x}\|_{\varepsilon} = \sqrt{\sum_{l=1}^{d} x_l^2 + \varepsilon^2}$ and $\nabla I := (\partial_1 I, \cdots, \partial_d I)$. The edge parameter ϵ distinguishes between edges from noise and is empirically set to

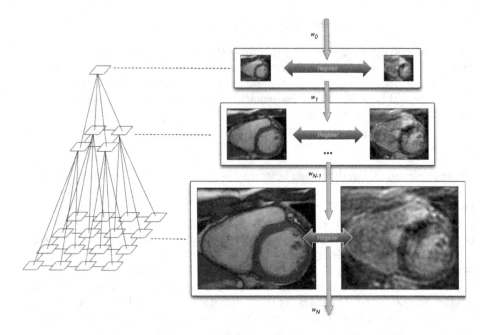

Fig. 1. Multi-resolution registration framework. Original input images are down-sampled and registered iteratively in a coarse-to-fine manner, where w_0 and w_N represent the first and final estimate respectively.

10 for our experiments. The concept behind NGF is derived from the observation that if two images are similar, then many intensity changes should occur at the same locations, leading to a large value for the inner product between the two image gradients.

Note that for image registration, the reference and template images are well aligned when the value for SSD is low, or when values for MI or NGF are high. Therefore, we wish to minimize SSD, or negative MI and negative NGF to ensure a consistent minimization framework for the image registration experiments.

2.4 Hybrid Registration

Typically, intensity based multi-resolution registrations are performed with the same distance measure at every resolution level [9,13]. However, in this study, we propose a hybrid metric approach, which uses a combination of metrics and takes advantage of their individual properties as assessed by the cost function profiles in Fig. 2. These profiles were obtained by translating or rotating a pair of aligned real-time and prior images with respect to each other along the (x, y, z) axes respectively. It is observed that the overall SSD cost function is generally smooth, which allows the optimizer to converge to a global optimum. However, for the translational cost function profiles, the global optima did not correspond to the correct image alignment, which should occur at the zero crossings. In contrast, for the MI and NGF distance metrics, sharp optimal peaks are detected near the expected zero crossings of the cost function (Fig. 2 b-c), which is a desirable property. However, the disadvantage of these metrics is that the overall landscape of the cost function consists of many local optimums. Therefore, when the initial misalignment is large, the optimizer can converge to a non-optimal local solution. Hence, in the hybrid registration approach, we propose to use SSD as the distance metric at coarse resolutions, and use MI or NGF at the finest resolution level to achieve the optimal registration results. The proposed method was evaluated against registrations using a single distance measure across all resolutions.

2.5   Experimental Setting

To quantitatively evaluate the performance of the registration algorithm, a controlled experiment was carried out in this study. For each subject, a 3D pre-procedural volume and 2D RT slices were acquired within the same scan session using the image acquisition protocols described in Sect. 2.1. In this experiment, the RT and prior imaging slices were gated to the same cardiac and respiratory phase cycles. Therefore, the two imaging datasets are optimally aligned, and provides us with the ground truth for registration. To test the registration algorithm, landmarks within the heart (e.g. LV apex, papillary muscles, and aortic valve annulus) were manually selected in the 3D pre-procedural dataset by an expert, and their corresponding (x, y, z) coordinates were recorded. Next, a known distance transformation ω consisting of rotations and translations $\omega := (\theta_x, \theta_y, \theta_z, t_x, t_y, t_z)$ along the 3 axes was applied to move the 3D prior volume out of alignment with the 2D RT slices. For each distance transformation ω, the rotation and translation parameters were randomly generated with independent and identically distributed distributions. Moreover, each transformation would cause a mean displacement d of the selected landmarks. We generated 100 transformations for each displacement $d = 5, 10, 15$, and 20 mm for every volunteer dataset. Thus, a total of 400 registration trials were performed for each dataset. After the transformation is applied, the proposed registration framework is used to register mis-aligned datasets, and the objective is to recover the original optimal alignment. The target registration error (TRE) was assessed by measuring the final displacement, in units of mm, from the original landmarks after registration recovery.

3   Results

For each of the volunteer studies, a number of distance measures were evaluated in the registration framework described in Sect. 2.2. In three approaches, registration was performed with a single metric across all resolution levels. The three metrics were SSD, MI, and NGF. Alternatively, a hybrid metric approach is employed, which uses SSD as the registration similarity metric at coarse resolution levels, and MI (SSD-MI) or NGF (SSD-NGF) at the finest resolution level.

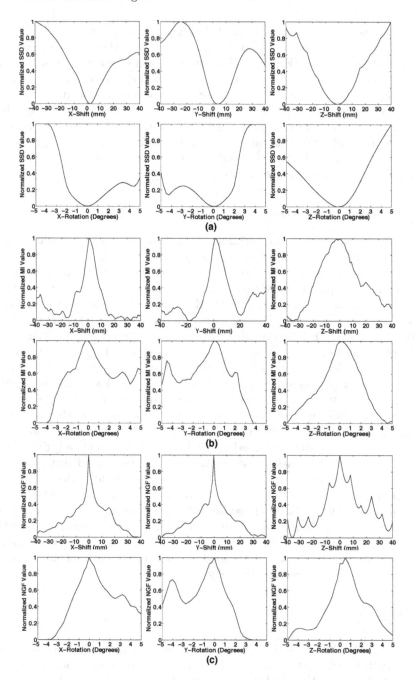

Fig. 2. Cost function analysis was performed for real-time and prior images that were aligned in the same cardiac and respiratory phase. Known translations and rotations along the x, y, and z axes were applied to the prior image and the resulting cost functions were mapped for different metrics: (a) SSD, (b) MI, and (c) NGF.

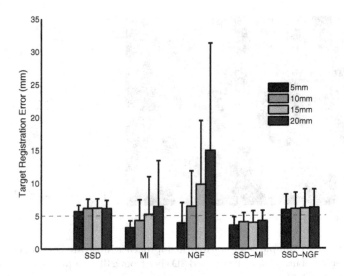

Fig. 3. Mean target registration errors and standard deviations are shown for all 4 initial displacement distances after registration. The mean values are grouped together based on the similarity metric used and are visualized within the group from left to right in ascending order, representing 5, 10, 15, 20 mm initial displacements respectively.

From Fig. 3, we observe that for the single metric approaches, registration using MI or NGF both outperformed registration with SSD when the initial misalignment is low ($d = 5$ mm). However, as the initial misalignment increased, the target registration errors for SSD stayed consistent, whereas the TREs for MI and NGF were markedly increased. Alternatively, the hybrid metric approach with SSD-MI achieved comparable results to registration with MI at $d = 5$ mm, and lower TREs than all the other metrics for $d > 5$ mm. A paired t-test was used to assess the statistical significance between the mean TREs in a pairwise manner between each metric and SSD-MI at the 1% significance level. It was determined that registration with SSD-MI achieved the lowest overall TRE (3.91 ± 1.52 mm) compared to registrations with SSD, MI, NGF, and SSD-NGF ($p < 0.01$). A typical registration example using SSD-MI in a controlled experiment is shown in Fig. 4.

4 Discussions and Conclusions

In this study, we evaluated a number of metrics in the context of registration for real-time and prior MR images and showed that each metric has its own advantages and disadvantages. Evaluation of the distance measures in the controlled experiment demonstrated that registration using the SSD distance metric achieved robust target registration errors of approximately 6 mm (Fig. 3), regardless of the initial magnitude of misalignment. Although this is a desirable property, the optimal target registration error was not achieved. This correlates well to the fact that

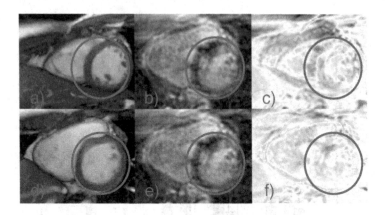

Fig. 4. Registration example using the hybrid approach is illustrated, where the contours indicate the region of interest. a) Extracted 2D slice from a 3D pre-procedural volume. b) Real-time image. c) Difference image between a) and b) before registration. d) Extracted 2D slice from the same 3D pre-procedural volume after registration. e) Real-time image. f) Difference image between d) and e) after registration.

the SSD cost function is relatively smooth, but did not have an accurate global optimum as seen in Fig. 2. A number of factors could have contributed to this phenomenon. The assumption that the voxel intensities in the RT and prior images are only different by Gaussian noise, implicit to registrations using the SSD metric, is not true for the acquired MR images. It is known that the noise characteristics of the MR magnitude images obey a Rician distribution[3]. Moreover, due to the use of different acquisition schemes for the RT and prior images, the imaging artifacts and signal-to-noise ratios also differ for the respective datasets. Nevertheless, registration using the SSD metric demonstrated good robustness, and showed it can converge to the near vicinity of the desired optimum. On the other hand, the use of MI and NGF metrics demonstrates good registration accuracy when the initial misalignment is low (i.e. $d = 5$ mm), but appears to converge to wrong local optimums as the magnitude of initial misalignment increases (Fig. 3). This is also reflected in the cost function profiles (Fig. 2), where the global optima are closer to the expected zero-crossings, but contains many local optima in the respective cost functions. In particular, the NGF cost function appears to have many local optima in the through-plane direction (i.e. Z-Shift) as illustrated in Fig. 2(c), which may explain the higher observed TREs for registrations with NGF compared to MI (Fig. 3). The undesirable local optima shown in the thorough-plane translation may be due to interpolation artifacts and poor resolution along that direction. Specifically, through-plane displacements that result in non-integer slice thickness shifts require interpolation in the corresponding direction before calculation of the associated distance measure. The image blurring introduced by interpolation inherently reduces the value of the NGF measure, which negatively impacts the smoothness of the cost function profile.

In conclusion, after considering the different characteristics of the various registration metrics, we presented a hybrid registration approach in a multi-resolution framework for aligning real-time and pre-procedural MR images for the purpose of guiding cardiac interventions. In the proposed approach, we used SSD as the registration metric at coarse resolution levels and subsequently switched to MI at the original image resolution to achieve the best overall registration results (SSD-MI in Fig. 3). The motivation behind this strategy was to take advantage of distinct characteristics belonging to different registration metrics. Notably, the robustness of the SSD metric and the accuracy of the MI metric. Experiments using *in vivo* volunteer data demonstrated that the hybrid approach (SSD-MI) was able to achieve a mean target registration error of 3.91 ±1.52 mm for initial mis-alignments in the range of 5-20 mm. Therefore, the feasibility of fusion of motion corrected pre-procedural datasets and real-time interventional images has been evaluated. This could potentially lead to better ablation targeting outcomes in future clinical practice.

Acknowledgments. The authors would like to thank GE Healthcare and Federal Development Agency of Canada for their funding support.

References

1. Dick, A.J., Guttman, M.A., Raman, V.K., Peters, D.C., Pessanha, B.S., Hill, J.M., Smith, S., Scott, G., McVeigh, E.R., Lederman, R.J.: Magnetic resonance fluoroscopy allows targeted delivery of mesenchymal stem cells to infarct borders in swine. Circulation **108**, 2899–2904 (2003)
2. Dukkipati, S.R., Mallozzi, R., Schmidt, E.J., Holmvang, G., d'Avila, A., et al.: Electroanatomic mapping of the left ventricle in a porcine model of chronic myocardial infarction with magnetic resonance based catheter tracking. Circulation **118**, 853–862 (2008)
3. Gudbjartsson, H., Patz, S.: The rician distribution of noisy MRI data. Magn. Reson. Med. **34**(6), 910–914 (2005)
4. Haber, E., Modersitzki, J.: Intensity gradient based registration and fusion of multimodal images. In: Larsen, R., Nielsen, M., Sporring, J. (eds.) MICCAI 2006. LNCS, vol. 4191, pp. 726–733. Springer, Heidelberg (2006)
5. Hoffmann, B.A., Koops, A., Rostock, T., Mullerleile, K., Steven, D., et al.: Interactive real-time mapping and catheter ablation of the cavotricuspid isthmus guided by magnetic resonance imaging in a porcine model. European Heart Journal **31**, 450–456 (2010)
6. Lardo, A.C.: Real-time magnetic resonance imaging: Diagnostic and interventional applications. Pediatr. Cardiol. **21**, 80–98 (2000)
7. Malchano, Z.J., Neuzil, P., Cury, R.C., Holmvang, G., Weichet, J., Schmidt, E.J., Ruskin, J.N., Reddy, V.: Integration of cardiac CT/MR imaging with three-dimensional electroanatomical mapping to guide catheter manipulation in the left atrium: implications for catheter ablation of atrial fibrillation. J. Cardiovasc. Electrophysiol. **17**, 1221–1229 (2006)

8. Mendis, S., Puska, P., Norrving, B.: Global atlas on cardiovascular disease prevention and control. World Health Organization (2011)
9. Modersitzki, J.: Numerical Methods for Image Registration. Oxford University Press, New York (2004)
10. Nelder, J.A., Mead, R.: A simplex method for function minimization. The Computer Journal **7**, 308–313 (1965)
11. Rhode, K.S., Hill, D.L.G., Edwards, P.J., Hipwell, J., Rueckert, D., et al.: Registration and tracking to integrate X-ray and MR images in an XMR facility. IEEE Trans. Med. Imaging **22**(11), 1369–1378 (2003)
12. Scott, A.D., Keegan, J., Firmin, D.N.: Motion in cardiovascular MR imaging. Radiology **250**(2), 331–351 (2009)
13. Smolíková-Wachowiak, R., Wachowiak, M.P., Fenster, A., Drangova, M.: Registration of two-dimensional cardiac images to preprocedural three-dimensional images for interventional applications. J. Magn. Reson. Imaging **22**, 219–228 (2005)
14. Tao, Q., Milles, J., Van Huls Van Taxis, C., Lamb, H.J., et al.: Toward magnetic resonance-guided electroanatomical voltage mapping for catheter ablation of scar-related ventricular tachycardia: A comparison of registration methods. J. Cardiovasc. Electr. **23**(1), 74–80 (2012)
15. Viola, P., Wells, W.M.: Alignment by maximization of mutual information. Int. J. Comput. Vision **24**(2), 137–154 (1997)

Restoration of Phase-Contrast Cardiovascular MRI for the Construction of Cardiac Contractility Atlases

Christina Koutsoumpa[1(✉)], Robin Simpson[2], Jennifer Keegan[3],
David Firmin[3], and Guang-Zhong Yang[1]

[1] The Hamlyn Centre for Robotic Surgery, Imperial College London, London, UK
{c.koutsoumpa13,g.z.yang}@imperial.ac.uk
[2] Radiological Physics, University of Freiburg, Freiburg, Germany
[3] Cardiovascular Biomedical Research Unit, Royal Brompton Hospital, London, UK

Abstract. Cardiac Atlases are promising tools for the interpretation of functional and anatomical structures of the heart. Myocardial viability is reflected by both global and regional contractile abnormalities. Atlases incorporating contractility information of a population can assist the diagnosis of myocardial disease and myocardial infarction. For the analysis of myocardial contractility phase-contrast MRI (PC-MRI) is emerging as a valuable clinical tool. The myocardial velocity distribution depicted by PC-MRI provides important insights into the intrinsic mechanics of the heart. As with many imaging techniques, there is an inherent trade-off between imaging resolution and noise. The main purpose of this study is to reduce the noise exhibited in phase-contrast MRI by applying a total variation restoration algorithm. The restoration algorithm has been evaluated on a spiral phase-contrast MRI sequence from a group of normal subjects. The results have shown that the proposed method is able to restore the myocardial velocity distribution whilst preserving the fidelity of the underlying contractile behavior.

Keywords: Restoration · Total Variation · Contractor Atlas · Cardiac Atlas · Phase Contrast MRI · Myocardial Contractility

1   Introduction

Quantitative analysis of the deformation of the left ventricle (LV) enables the assessment of cardiac contractility, which is associated with symptoms such as cardiomyopathies, myocardial ischemia and myocardial infarction [1]. The introduction of statistical cardiac atlases as population reference templates opens new doors to the automatic and reliable diagnosis of myocardial disease [2]. In this context statistical atlases of heart anatomy [3-5] and myocardial motion were introduced [6-8]. However the work on cardiac atlases for the assessment of myocardial contractility has been limited.

Among the established Cardiovascular MRI techniques [9] PC-MRI has shown significant promise for myocardial contractility assessment. The high spatial and temporal resolution velocity images acquired with this technique can be used directly or

© Springer International Publishing Switzerland 2015
O. Camara et al. (Eds.): STACOM 2014, LNCS 8896, pp. 275–283, 2015.
DOI: 10.1007/978-3-319-14678-2_29

constitute the basis for a number of contractility assessment and visualization approaches including myocardial virtual tagging [10] and strain rate mapping [11]. The majority of such studies involve spatial differentiation or integration of PC-MRI velocities for the generation of regional myocardial strain rates or displacement and strain tensors respectively. The integration and differentiation processes are particularly sensitive to noise and, in addition, the PC-MRI technique is itself prone to motion artifacts and other distortions. Therefore, effective restoration of the underlying noise-free velocity data is necessary.

The key requirement for PC-MRI restoration is the preservation of detailed contractile patterns of myocardial motion [12], which are formed by the complex structure of the myocardium and the mechanism of cardiac conduction. The anisotropic discontinuities of myocardial contraction can be interpreted by the "myocardial band model" [13] and the organization of cardiac muscle fibers [14], as well as the discontinuous propagation of action potentials across the cardiac muscle [15]. Due to structure and electric conduction properties of the heart, neighboring myocardial regions which belong to different fiber bundles are likely to contract in different directions and time phases, forming velocity field boundaries in between them. Unlike linear filtering, which blurs edges, non-linear filtering methods and particularly Total Variation (TV) restoration seem promising for the maintenance of fidelity of this complex underlying myocardial motion.

The basis for TV restoration is Laplace's L1 estimation algorithms. The TV restoration algorithm for scalar images was first introduced by Rudin et al. [16] and was extended for vector-valued images by Blomgren and Chan [17] who then developed a version of this multidimensional restoration algorithm for non-flat images [18], as well as CB and HSV images [19], and proposed a digital TV filter [20]. The directional TV version was developed and first applied to CMR data by Ng and Yang for the restoration of blood flow [21]. In [22] Huntbach presents a maximum a posteriori restoration technique that relies on Bayes theory.

The present work is for the construction of a statistical cardiac contractility atlas of the LV based on PC-MR velocity images and addresses the pre-processing stage of this procedure, which is the restoration of training data. To this end, it presents a robust restoration method based on the Digital TV filter with reduced complexities. The method is evaluated on both simulated and in vivo data with detailed analysis of its robustness and fidelity.

2   Methods

Myocardial Contractility Analysis: In the process of constructing a cardiac contractility atlas, the following main stages are involved, which include restoration of PC-MR images of the LV, registration, and statistical analysis. Because of their size, position, shape and time variations, all multi-subject and intra-subject images require spatiotemporal alignment to a common reference template. The restored data undergo statistical analysis for the construction of the atlas. Efficient restoration of the initial PC-MRI data can facilitate and improve the registration process, as well as increase the fidelity of the constructed statistical cardiac atlas. In this paper, we focus on the restoration process.

PC-MRI Restoration: The objective of a TV restoration algorithm is to minimize the total variation of velocity fields based on prior information on noise level, which is expressed by its variance. Let $u_0(a)$ denote the noisy version of a clean underlying image $u(a)$ corrupted by white Gaussian noise $n(a)$, i.e.,

$$u_0(a) = u(a) + n(a) \tag{1}$$

where $a = (x, y) \in \Omega$ is the set of pixels. The TV Restoration approach indicates the minimization of the L1 norm of the total variation

$$TV\left(u(a)\right) = \iint_\Omega |\nabla u(a)| dx dy \tag{2}$$

over the image, under the constraint

$$\sigma^2 = \frac{1}{|\Omega|} \iint_\Omega (u - u_0)^2 dx dy \tag{3}$$

where σ^2 is the variance of noise n and $|\Omega|$ the number of pixels on the image. The discrete solution to the above minimization problem given in [20] is

$$\hat{u}_t(a) = \sum_{b \sim a} h_{ab}\left(a; b\right) u(b) + h_{aa}(a; a) u_o(a) \tag{4}$$

where $\hat{u}_t(a)$ denotes the calculated value of the restored image on t iteration on pixel a. In the above equation, b denotes the neighboring pixels of pixel a, excluding the pixel a. The coefficients h_{ab} and h_{aa} are calculated by the formulae:

$$h_{ab}(a; b) = \frac{w_{ab}(a;b)}{\lambda + \sum_{\gamma \sim a} w_{a\gamma}(a;\gamma)} \quad \text{and} \quad h_{aa}(a; a) = \frac{\lambda}{\lambda + \sum_{\gamma \sim a} w_{a\gamma}(a;\gamma)} \tag{5}$$

where $w_{a\gamma}$ is the weight indicating the level of likeness of the pixels a and γ compared to their neighbors [20].

Regularization Parameter λ: For consistent results, the choice of regularization parameter λ is critical. The amount of smoothing and preservation of the initial value of a pixel are controlled by the coefficients h_{ab} and h_{aa} respectively and, hence, by the "fitting" parameter λ. This parameter incorporates the prior noise information into the restoration algorithm, and therefore its value is essential for convergence to the real underlying image. In this study, a constant value of $1/\sqrt{(\sigma^2)}$, the optimum value of λ, is used. The noise variance σ^2 is estimated from a uniform small area whose velocity is regarded constant. In this study a 25 x 25 pixel region located on the chest wall was chosen for this purpose.

Evaluation: For the assessment of the suggested restoration algorithm, the following estimation criteria are introduced: Mode of Removed Noise (MRN), Modified-MRN (MMRN) and Percentage Variance Reduction (PVR).

The MRN criterion is denoted as the mode of the distribution of the PRN measure, which expresses the Percentage Removed Noise (PRN) on each pixel **a**.

$$PRN(\boldsymbol{a}) = 100 * \frac{u_0(a) - \hat{u}_t(a)}{u_0(a) - u(a)} (\%) \qquad (6)$$

The MRN criterion requires knowledge of the underlying image and, therefore, it can be applied only to synthetic images of known noise. For the evaluation of the algorithm on real data, PRN is replaced by its estimation, the MMRN criterion, which is denoted as the mode of the distribution of the Modified-PRN measure (MPRN).

$$MPRN(\boldsymbol{a}) = 100 * \frac{u_0(a) - \hat{u}_t(a)}{u_0(a) - \hat{\bar{u}}_t(a)} (\%) \qquad (7)$$

The MMRN criterion is applied to a uniform area of an image, where it can be assumed that $\bar{u}_0(\boldsymbol{a}) \approx u(\boldsymbol{a}) \approx \hat{\bar{u}}_t(\boldsymbol{a})$, and therefore, the values of the underlying area can be replaced by the mean value of the restored area without significant loss of accuracy.

The PVR criterion expresses the percentage reduction of variance and it is defined as

$$PVR = 100 * \frac{\sigma^2 - \widehat{\sigma^2}}{\sigma^2} (\%) \qquad (8)$$

where σ^2 and $\widehat{\sigma^2}$ denote the noise variances of the noisy and restored images respectively, as they are estimated from the selected uniform area. PVR applies both to trial and real images.

The optimum value for all criteria is 100. For MRN and MMRN, a value over 100 indicates under-denoising whereas a value under 100 over-denoising. PVR ranges from 0 to 100.

Data: To evaluate the proposed restoration algorithm, the method was first applied to a synthetic RGB image corrupted with white Gaussian noise of known variance. For *in vivo* validation, images from 10 healthy volunteers were analyzed for this study. Each subject was scanned with the spiral PC-MRI sequence described in [23]. For each subject, 11 short axis slices were acquired with 1.7 x 1.7mm spatial resolution (reconstructed to 0.85 x 0.85 mm) on a Siemens 3 Tesla scanner (MAGNETOM Skyra, Siemens AG Healthcare Sector, Germany). For one subject, the proposed restoration approach was applied to an entire ventricular stack. For each of the 10 subjects, a single mid-ventricular slice consisting of 50 image frames over a full cardiac cycle was restored.

3   Results

Figure 1 shows the proposed restoration technique applied to a synthetic RGB image. The original image was augmented with Gaussian white noise with a variance of 0.01. The suggested TV restoration technique was then used to restore the original image.

All the three images are presented in (a). The λ parameters were calculated based on the variance of the marked uniform area. For each color component, the PVR, MRN and MMRN criteria as well as the corresponding PRN and MPRN distributions are shown in graph (c). The values of variance σ^2, parameter λ and the aforementioned estimation criteria for each color component are presented in table (b) of the same figure.

It can be seen that the RGB image was successfully restored. The noise was removed while maintaining the visual image features and intensity of the colors. The efficacy of the algorithm was also quantified by the MRN and MMRN criteria. With a total value of $(98.4\pm1.1)\%$ and $(101.82\pm1.6)\%$ respectively, MRN and MMRN lie very close to the desired value of 100%. The error in the estimation of noise variance is no more than 7% for all color components, indicating a good approximation of the real noise variance and, consequently, a good estimation of the optimum λ parameter.

(a) Original, noisy and restored 3-component image

Parameter	Red	Green	Blue
Estimated Variance	0.0107	0.0103	0.0101
λ Parameter	9.68	9.90	10.36
MRN(%)	98.32	97.15	99.86
MMRN(%)	9.73	103.52	102.21
PVR(%)	99.86	99.97	99.17

Red   PRN
Green PRN
Blue PRN
Red   MPRN
Green MPRN
Blue MPRN

0   50   100   150   200
         Mode   Criteria Value

(b) Parameters and Criteria

(c) Distributions of PRN and MPRN

Fig. 1. (a) Original RGB image, its noisy version, restored image and uniform area for the calculation of λ marked in blue. (b) Estimated variance, parameter λ, MRN, MMRN and PVR criteria for each color component. (c) Corresponding distributions of PRN and MPRN.

Figure 2 presents the first group of restoration results from in-vivo data. Our method was applied to a left ventricular short axis stack from an asymptomatic subject at peak expansion, for each of the 3 velocity components, over 1 cardiac cycle.

The MMRN and PVR criteria, which are presented in Table 1, have a total value of $(95.7\pm15.5)\%$ and $(83.8\pm11.9)\%$, respectively, approaching the optimum value of 100%. It can be claimed, therefore, that the in-vivo myocardial velocities were successfully restored.

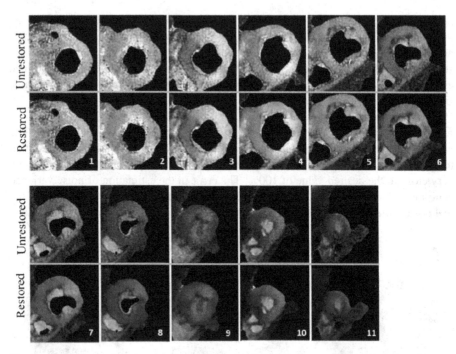

Fig. 2. Unrestored and restored velocity field of a full stack from an asymptomatic subject at peak expansion. The RGB colors represent 3D velocity components.

Table 1. MMRN and PVR criteria for each velocity component on the 11 slices of the stack

Slice	MMRN			PVR		
	1	2	3	1	2	3
1	89.79	97.47	70.38	82.64	84.83	72.97
2	104.89	100.44	105.85	71.79	95.64	97.06
3	118.36	67.58	106.64	80.99	57.14	85.00
4	102.02	57.67	120.80	90.61	69.08	81.24
5	103.86	109.97	125.05	90.58	82.83	85.45
6	117.00	102.57	78.15	71.22	78.37	56.20
7	89.82	95.73	94.77	84.79	80.60	97.32
8	85.02	107.29	76.82	98.38	90.83	85.19
9	105.15	99.39	89.15	99.49	99.45	74.83
10	84.62	91.89	106.98	71.68	91.29	56.72
11	98.77	72.35	87.72	96.38	87.62	83.21

The proposed TV Restoration technique was also applied to a mid-ventricular slice from 10 asymptomatic subjects, on the 3 velocity components, over 1 cardiac cycle. A sample of this second group of results from in-vivo data is demonstrated in Figure 3. The figure illustrates the unrestored (b) and restored (c) velocity fields in yellow and removed noise (c) in red at peak anticlockwise rotation, peak contraction, peak clockwise rotation and peak expansion respectively. The yellow frame in (a) encloses the corresponding illustrated region of the myocardium.

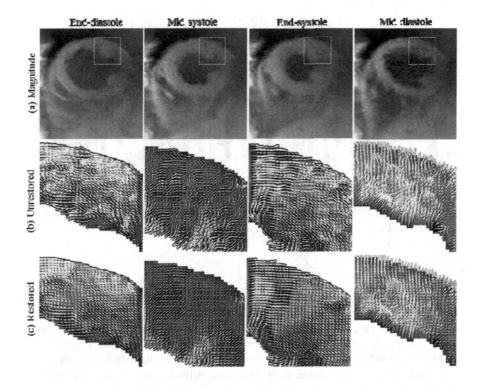

Fig. 3. (a) Mid-ventricular slice at peak anticlockwise rotation, peak contraction, peak clockwise rotation and peak expansion respectively and selected region for illustration. (b) Unrestored velocity field (c) Restored velocity field in yellow and removed noise vectors in red.

Significant improvement in the myocardial velocity field is visually observed. Discrete myocardial regions comprising smooth velocities are revealed by the proposed restoration process. This myocardial velocity pattern is in accordance with studies in the myocardium structure and function mentioned in the introduction.

Figure 4 presents the MMRN and PVR criteria calculated for the above application for the 3 velocity components at peak contraction. Their values, which lie in (84.1±12.2)% and (88.3±8.5)% respectively, confirm the successful restoration observed in the visual representation of myocardial velocities above.

The proposed restoration method assumes a constant value of the regularization parameter λ rather than calculating it with iterative formulae, as seen in other TV problems in the literature. In this way, the computation complexity of restoration process is reduced while the efficacy of the method remains high. Cautious selection of a uniform area, as performed in this study, allows for a good estimation of noise variance and, therefore, the calculation of an appropriate value for λ.

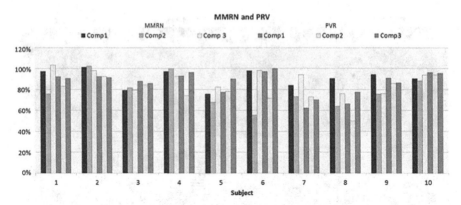

Fig. 4. MMRN and PRN criteria for the proposed restoration technique applied to a left ventricular short axis mid-slice for 10 asymptomatic subjects at peak contraction.

4   Conclusions

In this study, we have demonstrated a robust restoration method for PC-MR velocity images from the left ventricle based on the Digital TV Filter. The restoration technique was tested on a trial image and was applied to mid-ventricular slices from 10 healthy volunteers and one full stack from 1 healthy volunteer over one cardiac cycle. The MRN, MMRN and PVR criteria are introduced to evaluate the effectiveness of the method. The main advantage of the proposed method is its efficacy to restore PC-MR data, while being simple and computationally inexpensive. The restoration of myocardial velocity images will contribute to the fidelity of a future cardiac contractility atlas from PC-MRI data.

Acknowledgements. This project was supported by the NIHR Royal Brompton Cardiovascular Biomedical Research Unit. This report is independent research by the National Institute for Health Research Biomedical Research Unit Funding Scheme. The views expressed in this publication are those of the authors and not necessarily those of the NHS, the National Institute for Health Research or the Department of Health. The authors wish to thank Dr. Robert Merrifield from the Hamlyn Centre for Robotic Surgery for useful discussions.

References

1. Gault, J.H., Ross, J., Braunwald, E.: Contractile state of the left ventricle in man: instantaneous tension-velocity-length relations in patients with and without disease of the left ventricular myocardium. Circ. Res. **22**(4), 451–463 (1968)
2. Young, A.A., Frangi, A.F.: Computational cardiac atlases: from patient to population and back. Exp. Physiol. **94**(5), 578–596 (2009)
3. Ordas, S., Oubel, S., Sebastian, R., Frangi, A.F.: Computational anatomy atlas of the heart. In: Proceedings of the 5th ISPA 2007, vol. 8, pp. 338–342 (2007)
4. Fonseca, C.G., Backhaus, M., Bluemke, D.A., Britten, R.D., Do Chung, J., Cowan, B.R., et al.: The Cardiac Atlas Project–an imaging database for computational modeling and statistical atlases of the heart. Bioinformatics **27**(16), 2288–2295 (2011)

5. Hoogendoorn, C., Duchateau, N., Sánchez-Quintana, D., Whitmarsh, T., Sukno, F.M., De Craene, M., Lekadir, K., Frangi, A.F.: A high-resolution atlas and statistical model of the human heart from multislice CT. IEEE Trans. Med. Imaging **32**(1), 28–44 (2013)
6. Chandrashekara, R., Rao, A., Sanchez-Ortiz, G.I., Mohiaddin, R.H., Rueckert, D.: Construction of a statistical model for cardiac motion analysis using nonrigid image registration. Inf. Process. Med. Imaging **18**, 599–610 (2003)
7. Duchateau, N., De Craene, M., Piella, G., Silva, E., Doltra, A., Sitges, M., et al.: A spatio-temporal statistical atlas of motion for the quantification of abnormal myocardial tissue velocities. Med. Image Anal. **15**(3), 316–328 (2011)
8. Rougon, N.F., Petitjean, C., Prêteux, F.J.: Building a 4D atlas of the cardiac anatomy and motion using MR imaging. SPIE Medical Imaging **2**, 253–264 (2004)
9. Simpson, R.M., Keegan, J., Firmin, D.N.: MR assessment of regional myocardial mechanics. J. Magn. Reson. Imaging **37**(3), 576–599 (2013)
10. Masood, S., Gao, J., Yang, G.-Z.: Virtual tagging: numerical considerations and phantom validation. IEEE Trans. Med. Imaging **21**(9), 1123–1131 (2002)
11. Wünsche, B., Young, A.A.: The visualization and measurement of left ventricular deformation using finite element models. J. Vis. Lang. Comput. **14**(4), 299–326 (2003)
12. Codreanu, I., Robson, M.D., Golding, S.J., Jung, B.A., Clarke, K., Holloway, C.J.: Longitudinally and circumferentially directed movements of the left ventricle studied by cardiovascular magnetic resonance phase contrast velocity mapping. J. Cardiovasc. Magn. Reson. **12**, 48 (2010)
13. Torrent-Guasp, F., Ballester, M., Buckberg, G.D., Carreras, F., Flotats, A., Carrió, I., et al.: Spatial orientation of the ventricular muscle band: physiologic contribution and surgical implications. J. Thorac. Cardiovasc. Surg. **122**(2), 389–392 (2001)
14. Sengupta, P.P., Korinek, J., Belohlavek, M., Narula, J., Vannan, M.A., Jahangir, A., Khandheria, B.K.: Left ventricular structure and function: basic science for cardiac imaging. J. Am. Coll. Cardiol. **48**(10), 1988–2001 (2006)
15. Veeraraghavan, R., Gourdie, R.G., Poelzing, S.: Mechanisms of cardiac conduction: a history of revisions. Am. J. Physiol. Heart Circ. Physiol. **306**(5), H619–H627 (2014)
16. Rudin, L., Osher, S., Fatemi, E.: Nonlinear total variation based noise removal algorithms. Phys. D Nonlinear Phenom. **60**, 259–268 (1992)
17. Blomgren, P., Chan, T.F.: Color TV: total variation methods for restoration of vector-valued images. IEEE Trans. Image Process. **7**(3), 304–309 (1998)
18. Shen, J., Chan, T.: Variational restoration of nonflat image features: Models and algorithms. SIAM J. Appl. Math. **61**(4), 1338–1361 (2001)
19. Chan, T.F., Kang, S.H., Shen, J.: Total Variation Denoising and Enhancement of Color Images Based on the CB and HSV Color Models. J. Vis. Commun. Image Represent. **12**(4), 422–435 (2001)
20. Chan, T.F., Osher, S., Shen, J.: The digital TV filter and nonlinear denoising. IEEE Trans. Image Process. **10**(2), 231–241 (2001)
21. Ng, Y., Yang, G.: Vector-valued image restoration with applications to magnetic resonance velocity imaging. In: WSCG, vol. 37(2), pp. 58–61 (February 2003)
22. Huntbatch, A., Lee, S.-L., Firmin, D., Yang, G.-Z.: Bayesian motion recovery framework for myocardial phase-contrast velocity MRI. Med. Image Comput. Comput. Assist. Interv. **11**(Pt 2), 79–86 (2008)
23. Simpson, R., Keegan, J., Gatehouse, P., Hansen, M., Firmin, D.: Spiral tissue phase velocity mapping in a breath-hold with non-cartesian SENSE. Magn. Reson. Med. (2013)

Manifold Learning for Cardiac Modeling and Estimation Framework

Radomir Chabiniok[1][✉], Kanwal K. Bhatia[2], Andrew P. King[1],
Daniel Rueckert[2], and Nic Smith[1]

[1] Division of Imaging Sciences and Biomedical Engineering,
King's College London, London, UK
Radomir.Chabiniok@kcl.ac.uk
[2] Department of Computing, Imperial College London, London, UK

Abstract. In this work we apply manifold learning to biophysical modeling of cardiac contraction with the aim of estimating material parameters characterizing myocardial stiffness and contractility. The set of cardiac cycle simulations spanning the parameter space of myocardial stiffness and contractility is used to create a manifold structure based on the motion pattern of the left ventricle endocardial surfaces. First, we assess the proposed method by using synthetic data generated by the model specifically to test our approach with the known ground truth parameter values. Then, we apply the method on cardiac magnetic resonance imaging (MRI) data of two healthy volunteers. The post-processed cine MRI for each volunteer were embedded into the manifold together with the simulated samples and the global parameters of contractility and stiffness for the whole myocardium were estimated. Then, we used these parameters as an initialization into an estimator of regional contractilities based on a reduced order unscented Kalman filter. The global values of stiffness and contractility obtained by manifold learning corrected the model in comparison to a standard model calibration by generic parameters, and a significantly more accurate estimation of regional contractilities was reached when using the initialization given by manifold learning.

1 Introduction

Biophysical modeling is becoming a valuable approach in clinical applications such as in computer assisted therapy planning [18] and diagnosis. Within this methodology, parameter estimation provides a way of coupling between a model and measured data to increase the model predictivity [7,11,21–23]. However, patient-specific modeling is also associated with a significant computational cost. In addition to the time required for heavy computations, there is a substantial effort necessary for setting up the model, pre-calibrating and performing the parameter estimation to obtain a quantity of clinical interest. Depending on the type of model and data used, this process can currently take many days to weeks.

Manifold learning (ML) – a type of machine learning methods allowing nonlinear reduction of dimensionality of a high-dimensional problem (see for example

© Springer International Publishing Switzerland 2015
O. Camara et al. (Eds.): STACOM 2014, LNCS 8896, pp. 284–294, 2015.
DOI: 10.1007/978-3-319-14678-2_30

[1] and references therein) – may be of help addressing this issue. First, ML can directly provide diagnostically relevant information usable for instance in stratifying of patients in therapy. Secondly, ML can be applied prior performing a very detailed modeling and has the potential to suggest the most appropriate type of biophysical model that should be employed to enrich our knowledge about the state of a given patient. Finally, ML can be used to initialize a complex data assimilation technique (in a way as also some reduced-order biophysical models can be applied [5]) in order to achieve a faster convergence and successful parameter estimation. This will be explored in the presented work.

In this study we are estimating material parameters reflecting myocardial stiffness and contractility in a biophysical model of cardiac cycle. In [7], the tissue contractility was successfully estimated by using a biophysical model and cine MRI of a real subject. Our goal is now to extend this approach. Prior estimation of the local contractility values in LV myocardium subdivided into several regions, we perform ML to obtain an initial guess of the tissue parameters. While cine MRI is used for the model creation and parameterization, the accuracy of the resulting model is assessed both by using cine and 3D tagged MRI.

In Section 2 we describe the type of image data, simulation setup and the creation of the manifold on a set of cardiac cycle simulations. In Section 3 we assess the proposed ML method using synthetic data generated by the model. Then, we embed the post-processed *real* cine MRI for each volunteer into the manifold together with the *simulated (synthetic)* samples and estimate the global parameters of contractility and stiffness. These values are finally used as an initialization to a sequential data assimilation to capture the local variations of contractility, which we compare with the estimation initialized by generic values. We discuss the obtained results in Section 4 prior to our concluding comments.

2   Methods

2.1   Image Data

The acquisition of cardiac MRI datasets of 2 healthy volunteers is performed on 1.5 T Philips Achieva system and the following data were used in this work:

- Short axis cine MRI stack covering the heart ventricles in retrospective ECG gating capturing the whole cardiac cycle with the following parameters: bSSFP, parallel imaging factor SENSE 2, FOV 350x350 mm, acquired spatial resolution ∼2x2x8mm and temporal resolution ∼20 ms (40 time frames). A severe inter-slice misregistration due to non-reproducible breath-holds was avoided by using a diaphragm navigator prior the cine sequence was launched.
- 3D tagged MRI of LV using the sequence described in [15] acquired during 3 breath-holds – each for the whole 3D volume and one orientation of the tag lines – in prospective ECG triggering, FOV 100x100x100 mm, acquired spatial resolution 3.4x7.7x7.7 mm which were merged into one resulting 3D tagged image interpolated to 1x1x1 mm voxel size, temporal resolution ∼30 ms.

The image processing is based on the image registration toolkit IRTK[1] [14, 17]. First, the inter-slice misregistration of the short axis cine stack is performed by allowing a 2D rigid registration for each cine slice and using the 3D tagged MRI as a template. Secondly, the cine series is tracked using the non-rigid image registration described in [19]. The resulting motion field obtained from the analysis of cine data is applied on the LV endo- and epicardial surface meshes, which were extracted from the myocardial volume mesh. Finally, the full tissue displacements are extracted from the 3D tagged MRI and interpolated into the internal nodes of the LV mesh by using the IRTK library (B-splines).

2.2   Model

The model used in this work is described in [8,16]. It consists of a chemically-controlled constitutive law of cardiac myofiber mechanics based on Huxley's model (Bestel-Clément-Sorine) with a key parameter of active *contractility* σ_0 representing an asymptotic active stress along the myocardial fibers developed by sarcomere. The passive part is formed by Hill-Maxwell rheological model in large strains, with passive visco-hyperelasticity. The hyperelastic potential is given by $W_e^{ref} = \kappa_1(J_1-3)+\kappa_2(J_2-3)+\kappa(J-1-\ln J)$ (Ciarlet-Geymonat), with J_1, J_2 and J being reduced invariants of the strain tensor. The parameters κ_1, κ_2 and κ represent the reference stiffness parameters with the values $\kappa_1 = 5,000$ Pa, $\kappa_2 = 33$ Pa and $\kappa = 300,000$ Pa which were used in previous physiologically and clinically oriented cardiac modeling works [6,18]. The hyperelastic potential applied in the presented work is the reference potential W_e^{ref} multiplied by a factor K, $W_e = K \cdot W_e^{ref}$, $K \in [0.8, 3.0]$. This allows a variation of passive tissue properties from soft to rather stiff, with keeping a nearly incompressibility. In the following, we will associate the multiplication factor K with the *tissue stiffness*.

We use a simplified analytically prescribed but physiologically justified electrical activation. The propagation is initiated on the endocardial side of apex from which it propagates quickly on the endocardial surfaces (along the geodesics curves) and slowly through the working myocardium. The velocities are set to 4000 m/s and 500 m/s, for the fast and slow propagation, respectively, in accordance with the physiological velocities along the Purkinje fibers and through the working myocardium. Such an activation gives a physiological propagation pattern with the QRS duration of 60–70 ms, as is presented in Figure 1.

Visco-elastic boundary conditions [12] are applied on the base of the heart – replacing atria and large vessels – and on the anterior wall and apex – to represent the contact between epicardium and thoracic cage, diaphragm, respectively. A 2-element Windkessel models replace the pulmonary and systemic circulations.

The geometrical model is created from the end-diastolic time frame of the short axis cine MRI, which was selected as a reference configuration. The manual segmentation in the Cardioviz3D software [20] is followed by regularization of

---

[1] http://www.doc.ic.ac.uk/~dr/software

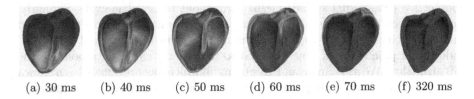

(a) 30 ms   (b) 40 ms   (c) 50 ms   (d) 60 ms   (e) 70 ms   (f) 320 ms

Fig. 1. Simulation of cardiac contraction of physiological heart of Volunteer 1

surface meshes and creating the tetrahedral mesh using the Yams and Ghs3D[2] meshing tools [9]. The final bi-ventricular meshes consist of $\sim 50,000$ tetrahedra.

2.3 Simulations

The model described in Section 2.2 is pre-calibrated manually using the cine MR images. This includes adjusting of the action potential duration to achieve the observed duration of contraction, tuning of Windkessel parameters to obtain the measured maximum systolic pressure under a physiological contractility. We vary the elevation angle of the synthetic myocardial fibers between -45 and $60°$ from LV epicardium to endocardium, -30 and $50°$ for RV, respectively. Such a fiber orientation allows a level of twist as observed in the tagged MRI, for the geometry and mesh size used. The stiffnesses of vico-elastic boundary conditions are adjusted to prevent the epicardial surface from extensive non-physiological movements. A physiological atrial pressure during diastole is prescribed.

We run the model for the stiffness and contractility values spanning the feasible range obtaining normokinetic as well as hypo- and hyperkinetic heart contractions (stiffness multiplication factor K varying between 0.8 and 3.0 with a step 0.1, contractility σ_0 between 100 kPa and 600 kPa with a step 50 kPa). Prior running the simulations, the inverse problem as described in [12] is solved to find an unloaded reference configuration of the myocardium for each myocardial stiffness used.

2.4 Manifold Learning Method

Manifold learning (ML) is a method of nonlinear dimensionality reduction which transforms high-dimensional data into a low-dimensional space, within which Euclidean (linear) distances are meaningful, thus simplifying tasks such as regression and classification [4,24,26]. From the set of simulations with varying tissue stiffness and contractility as described in Section 2.3, we aim to determine these parameters for real subjects. For each of the simulated cycles, signed LV endocardial distances from the initial surface location are evaluated point-wise (for each

---

[2] http://www.ann.jussieu.fr/frey/software.html; Ghs3D is available in Cubit meshing toolkit (https://cubit.sandia.gov)

node of LV endocardial surface mesh) throughout the cardiac cycle. Similarly, the LV endocardial distances are measured for each real subject from the tracked surfaces in cine MRI. For each simulation, these signed distances of ∼1000 LV endocardial points across time are used to represent a single data point in the ML algorithm. We use Laplacian Eigenmaps [3] which has previously been shown to be useful in cardiac image analysis [4,13]. On the resulting set of manifold co-ordinates – obtained by applying the nonlinear ML transformation – we subsequently apply linear regression on the parameter space to estimate the stiffness and contractility of the volunteers based on their clinical MRI data.

2.5   Sequential Estimation of Tissue Contractility

After obtaining the optimal values of tissue stiffness and contractility using our ML technique, we input these values as an initialization for the nonlinear model-based sequential parameter estimation technique [7] (using reduced order unscented Kalman filter) to estimate the contractility in 6 radial regions of LV. We compare the performance of the filter by using a nominal stiffness value 1 and contractility 200 kPa – the values providing sufficient pre-calibration of the model – and with the initialization suggested by the result of ML.

3   Results

3.1   Embedding of Synthetic Data

To test if the manifold can accurately represent a population with varying stiffness and contractility parameters, we first construct the manifold using the synthetic data generated by all the simulations (of which the combinations of contractility and stiffness parameters – ground truth – are known). A leave-one-out regression analysis is then performed on all these synthetic data points. The manifold will characterize the most dominant feature in the data. In order to estimate the contractility we found that the first half of the cycle is most accurate, giving a mean absolute error of 18 kPa (±16 kPa). In contrast, for estimating the stiffness we found that the second half of the cycle contains the most useful information, with a mean absolute error of 0.05 (±0.12). From our cross-validation tests on these synthetic data it was found that a manifold dimension of 10 gives good results without overfitting for both cases.

3.2   Embedding of Real Data

Using the parts of cardiac cycles and the manifold parameters determined from the synthetic data tests (Section 3.1), for each subject we construct two manifolds (for stiffness and contractility). These manifolds contain all the simulated cycles and also the subject dataset. The parameters of stiffness and contractility are then estimated using linear regression on the manifolds obtained by mapping each 3D+t simulation to a single point, see table in Figure 2(a). Figures 2(b-c)

	Contractility	Stiffness multiplication factor
Volunteer 1	190 kPa	2.2
Volunteer 2	204 kPa	2.26

(a) Estimated values by using manifold learning

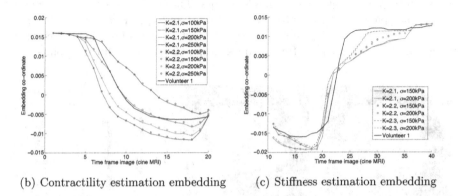

(b) Contractility estimation embedding   (c) Stiffness estimation embedding

Fig. 2. Embedding of real data. Note that (b) and (c) are separate embeddings and therefore the plots cannot overlap.

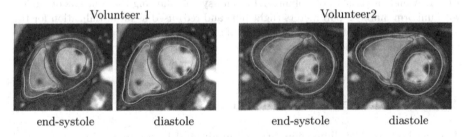

Fig. 3. Mid-cavity slices showing the segmented contours (observations, in green) and contours of model given by a generic pre-calibration (light blue) and with the material parameters obtained by ML (red). Note a slower relaxation for the generic case in the beginning of diastole while the ML initialized model follows the data more accurately.

show for illustration the motion state embeddings for Volunteer 1, where the manifolds are constructed using the LV endocardial distances (as described in Section 2.4) at each data sampling time frame as a separate data point. These 1D plots demonstrate how the embedding of the real data clusters with data with similar parameters. Figure 3 shows a visible improvement of the contours if the model is parameterized by ML.

Figure 4 shows that the locally estimated parameters bring the model closer to the image contours both with and without the ML initialization. However, we can see that by using the generic initialization the lateral wall undergoes some unphysiological thinning at end-systole. In the values of estimated parameters we can see that the compensation is achieved by a massive decrease of contractility in the antero-lateral region. If ML is used for the initialization, the final correction is given by an increase of contractility in the septal regions and the contractility of the lateral wall drops less. Finally, the bar plots in Fig. 4(c) demonstrate the relative improvement of the data-model errors. Those are assessed by summing up the discrepancies of simulated vs. real endo- and epicardial surfaces ("cine error") or discrepancies of the nodal displacement magnitudes ("3D tag error") over all the LV endocardium (inner nodes, respectively) and all time points.

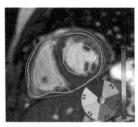 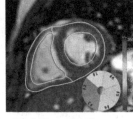 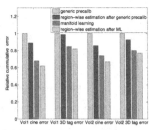

(a)   Generic   material   (b) ML pre-calibration   (c) Relative errors (sum over
parameters initialization   all nodes and time points)

Fig. 4. A mid-cavity slice of Volunteer 1 at end-systole showing the contours of models with uniform material parameters (light blue and red) used as an initialization for the regional contractility estimation. The results of these estimations are displayed in the bull's eye plots and the corresponding corrected models are in purple and yellow.

4   Discussion and Conclusion

The methodology of dimensionality reduction and linear regression of material parameters used in the presented paper has similarities with the methodologies proposed in [10,25]. In comparison to [10], in addition to the technical differences (e.g. type of estimated parameters, metrics used for- and type of dimensionality reduction), the main difference in our approach is that after performing an initial synthetic data study we applied the method on *real* clinical datasets. Succeeding in such a step strongly supports the idea of compatibility between the methods based on machine learning and biophysical modeling.

In [25], machine learning was linked to an electrophysiological model and the whole method was then finally preliminarily tested using patient ECG data. The achieved result was compared using the same metrics as the one used in the machine learning step (QRS duration and electrical axis of the heart). Although a ground truth is often inaccessible in such *in vivo* works, a drop in error measured on independently acquired and processed 3D tagged MRI data (Figure 4(c)) is a promising sign of a correction towards the true solution, and provides additional support for our framework in comparison to assessing the error by using only the LV contours of cine MRI, on which the parameter estimation was based.

Separating the manifolds for estimating the contractility and stiffness improves the predictive accuracy as it eliminates confounding motions. The manifold produced characterizes the data in terms of the most dominant underlying features of the data. Using different parts of the cycle therefore produces different manifolds depending on the dominant cause of motion captured during that time period. During our synthetic data tests (Section 3.1) we found that the stiffness is estimated using only the second half of the cycle to reduce the confounding effects of the contraction present during the early cycle. Similarly, the contractility is only estimated using the first half of the cycle in order to exclude excess data where contractility has no role. However, we emphasize that for both our parameters the manifolds jointly contain the contractility and stiffness information, and the statistical method then provides the best possible estimates within the ML method. Those are subsequently used to initialize the nonlinear biophysical model-based estimation, in which the two material properties are completely coupled in a physical sense.

From a qualitative assessment, the synthetic data curves may seem not to accurately embed the clinical data (Fig. 2(c)) and the initial LV contours of model seem to be quite far from the segmented contours of cine MRI (Fig. 3). It is certain that a manual pre-calibration – of which the level of necessary accuracy is a non-trivial question within the modeling and data assimilation framework – will always be involved. However, we proved that even with such a level of discrepancy we are able to estimate the meaningful values. The additional ML pre-initialization leads to physiologically more plausible results and possibly reduces the ill-posedness of the inverse problem. Both these components are topics of our further research. In addition, we need to emphasize that the image observations obtained automatically by tracking of LV endo- and epicardial surfaces from cine MRI using the IRTK library – although introducing some image processing error – allow parameter estimation combining ML and a complex biophysical model.

The real data within our manifold learning step could have been implemented as an out-of-sample extension. However, it is often more accurate to embed all data simultaneously and since there is significantly more training data than test data, this does not affect the shape of the manifold. Furthermore, since training is fast, there is little computational gain from using an out-of-sample extension.

In the regional estimations, only the contractility was estimated. This is given by our intention to follow [7] – where the contractility estimation (and not the stiffness) was performed on real cine MRI. For the same reason, we did not use the "richer" information from the 3D tagged MRI. Adding a level of complexity and estimating both the regionalized contractility and stiffness using real cine and in addition tagged MRI will be addressed in our future works.

There are various perspectives of ML within the modeling framework. If considering a new estimated parameter, we would similarly first identify from synthetic data the part of the cardiac cycle within which the new parameter is the most observable. Secondly, a valuable step will be to create a single "population-wide" manifold, which would require running the hundreds of cardiac cycles only for a limited number of subjects and the method would then provide a fast clustering for new subjects. In such an extension we would practically consider subjects of a similar pathology and the spatial alignment could be performed using some techniques from [2]. We should mention that in this case, the pressure indicator (at least peak aortic pressure) will need to be incorporated within the ML to give an absolute sense to the estimated material parameters.

The other possibility is to span the parameter space by "cheap" simulations (for a given subject) for instance on a very reduced mesh size. This could suggest some parameter initializations – though of a limited accuracy – useful in a detailed regional estimation. The confidence intervals for manifold sampling might even suggest parameter covariances for the sequential parameter estimation.

To conclude, we managed to put the manifold learning into a framework of biophysical modeling. The preliminary results obtained on estimating the tissue stiffness and contractility, as well as connecting the approach with the established parameter estimation techniques in cardiac modeling are promising and will trigger our further efforts.

Acknowledgments. The authors acknowledge the support of Engineering and Physical Sciences Research Council EP/H046410/1 and of the British Heart Foundation grant NH/11/5/29058. In addition, the authors thank P. Moireau and D. Chapelle (Inria, France) for providing the HeartLab software library, used in this work for all modeling and regional estimation computations, and for valuable discussions. This research was supported by the National Institute for Health Research (NIHR) Biomedical Research Centre at Guy's and St Thomas' NHS Foundation Trust and King's College London. The views expressed are those of the author(s) and not necessarily those of the NHS, the NIHR or the Department of Health.

References

1. Aljabar, P., Wolz, R., Rueckert, D.: Manifold learning for medical image registration, segmentation, and classification. In: Machine Learning in Computer-Aided Diagnosis: Medical Imaging Intelligence and Analysis. IGI Global (2012)
2. Bai, W., Shi, W., O'Regan, D.P., Tong, T., Wang, H., Jamil-Copley, S., Peters, N.S., Rueckert, D.: A probabilistic patch-based label fusion model for multi-atlas segmentation with registration refinement: Application to cardiac MR images. IEEE Trans. Med. Imaging **32**(7), 1302–1315 (2013)
3. Belkin, M., Niyogi, P.: Laplacian Eigenmaps for dimensionality reduction and data representation. Neural Computat. **15**(6), 1373–1396 (2003)
4. Bhatia, K.K., Rao, A., Price, A.N., Wolz, R., Hajnal, J.V., Rueckert, D.: Hierarchical manifold learning for regional image analysis. IEEE TMI **33**(2), 444–461 (2014)
5. Caruel, M., Chabiniok, R., Moireau, P., Lecarpentier, Y., Chapelle, D.: Dimensional reductions of a cardiac model for effective validation and calibration. Biomech Model Mechanobiol **13**(4), 897–914 (2014)
6. Chabiniok, R., Chapelle, D., Lesault, P.-F., Rahmouni, A., Deux, J.-F.: Validation of a biomechanical heart model using animal data with acute myocardial infarction. In: CI2BM09 - MICCAI Workshop, London, UK (2009)

7. Chabiniok, R., Moireau, P., Lesault, P.-F., Rahmouni, A., Deux, J.-F., Chapelle, D.: Estimation of tissue contractility from cardiac cine-MRI using a biomechanical heart model. Biomech Model Mechanobiol **11**(5), 609–30 (2012)
8. Chapelle, D., Le Tallec, P., Moireau, P., Sorine, M.: An energy-preserving muscle tissue model: formulation and compatible discretizations. International Journal for Multiscale Computational Engineering **10**(2), 189–211 (2012)
9. Frey, P.J., George, P.-L.: Mesh generation application to finite elements. Wiley, London (2008)
10. Le Folgoc, L., Delingette, H., Criminisi, A., Ayache, N.: Current-based 4D shape analysis for the mechanical personalization of heart models. In: Menze, B.H., Langs, G., Lu, L., Montillo, A., Tu, Z., Criminisi, A. (eds.) MCV 2012. LNCS, vol. 7766, pp. 283–292. Springer, Heidelberg (2013)
11. Marchesseau, S., Delingette, H., Sermesant, M., Ayache, N.: Fast parameter calibration of a cardiac electromechanical model from medical images based on the unscented transform. Biomech. Model Mechanobiol. **12**(5), 815–831 (2013)
12. Moireau, P., Xiao, N., Astorino, M., Figueroa, C.A., Chapelle, D., Taylor, A.C., Gerbeau, J.-F.: External tissue support and fluid-structure simulation in blood flows. Biomech. Model Mechanobiol. **11**(1–2), 1–18 (2012)
13. Perry, T.E., Zha, H., Zhou, K., Frias, P., Zeng, D., Braunstein, M.: Supervised embedding of textual predictors with applications in clinical diagnostics for paediatric cardiology. J. Am. Med. Inform. Assoc. **21**, e136–e142 (2013)
14. Rueckert, D., Sonoda, L.I., Hayes, C., Hill, D.L., Leach, M.O., Hawkes, D.J.: Non-rigid registration using free-form deformations: Application to breast MR images. IEEE Trans. Med. Imaging **18**(8), 712–721 (1999)
15. Rutz, A.K., Ryf, S., Plein, S., Boesiger, P., Kozerke, S.: Accelerated whole-heart 3D CSPAMM for myocardial motion quantification. Magn. Reson. Med. **59**, 755–763 (2008)
16. Sainte-Marie, J., Chapelle, D., Cimrman, R., Sorine, M.: Modeling and estimation of the cardiac electromechanical activity. Comput. Struct. **84**, 1743–1759 (2006)
17. Schnabel, J.A., et al.: A generic framework for non-rigid registration based on non-uniform multi-level free-form deformations. In: Niessen, W.J., Viergever, M.A. (eds.) MICCAI 2001. LNCS, vol. 2208, p. 573. Springer, Heidelberg (2001)
18. Sermesant, M., Chabiniok, R., Chinchapatnam, P., Mansi, T., Billet, F., Moireau, P., Peyrat, J.M., Wong, K., Relan, J., Rhode, K., Ginks, M., Lambiase, P., Delingette, H., Sorine, M., Rinaldi, C.A., Chapelle, D., Razavi, R., Ayache, N.: Patient-specific electromechanical models of the heart for the prediction of pacing acute effects in CRT: A preliminary clinical validation. Med. Image Anal. **16**(1), 201–215 (2012)
19. Shi, W., Zhuang, X., Wang, H., Duckett, S., Luong, D.V.N., Tobon-Gomez, C., Tung, K., Edwards, P., Rhode, K., Razavi, R., Ourselin, S., Rueckert, D.: A comprehensive cardiac motion estimation framework using both untagged and 3D tagged MR images based on non-rigid registration. IEEE Trans. Med. Imaging **31**(6), 1263–1275 (2012)
20. Toussaint, N., Mansi, T., Delingette, H., Ayache, N., Sermesant, M.: An integrated platform for dynamic cardiac simulation and image processing: application to personalised tetralogy of Fallot simulation. In: Proc.of VCBM. Delft, NL (2008)
21. Wang, V.Y., Lam, H.I., Ennis, D.B., Cowan, B.R., Young, A.A., Nash, M.P.: Modelling passive diastolic mechanics with quantitative MRI of cardiac structure and function. Med. Image Anal. **13**(5), 773–784 (2009)

22. Xi, J., Lamata, P., Lee, J., Moireau, P., Chapelle, D., Smith, N.: Myocardial transversely isotropic material parameter estimation from in-silico measurements based on reduced-order unscented Kalman filter. Journal of the Mechanical Behavior of Biomedical Materials 4(7), 1090–1102 (2011)

23. Xi, J., Lamata, P., Niederer, S., Land, S., Shi, W., Zhuang, X., Ourselin, S., Duckett, S., Shetty, A., Rinaldi, C., Rueckert, D., Razavi, R., Smith, N.: The estimation of patient-specific cardiac diastolic functions from clinical measurements. Med. Image Anal. 17(2), 133–146 (2013)

24. Ye, D.H., Desjardins, B., Hamm, J., Litt, H., Pohl, K.M.: Regional manifold learning for disease classification. IEEE TMI 33(6), 1236–1247 (2014)

25. Zettinig, O., Mansi, T., Georgescu, B., Kayvanpour, E., Sedaghat-Hamedani, F., Amr, A., Haas, J., Steen, H., Meder, B., Katus, H., Navab, N., Kamen, A., Comaniciu, D.: Fast data-driven calibration of a cardiac electrophysiology model from images and ECG. In: Mori, K., Sakuma, I., Sato, Y., Barillot, C., Navab, N. (eds.) MICCAI 2013, Part I. LNCS, vol. 8149, pp. 1–8. Springer, Heidelberg (2013)

26. Zhang, Q., Souvenir, R., Pless, R.: On manifold structure of cardiac MRI data: application to segmentation. In: CVPR, pp. 1092–1098. IEEE Comp. Soc. (2006)

Author Index

Printed in the United States
By Bookmasters